THE HERBALIST'S GUIDE TO PREGNANCY, CHILDBIRTH AND BEYOND

THE HERBALIST'S GUIDE TO PREGNANCY, CHILDBIRTH AND BEYOND
Herbal Therapeutics for the Childbearing Year

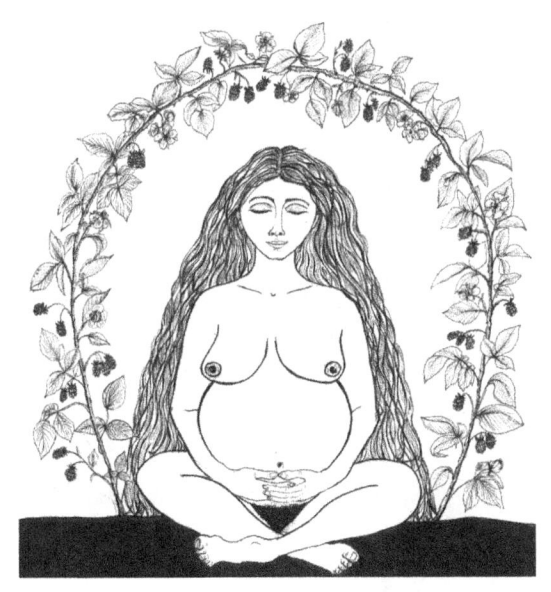

Carole Guyett

AEON

First published in 2022 by
Aeon Books

Copyright © 2022 by Carole Guyett

The right of contributors to be identified as the authors of this work has been asserted in accordance with §§ 77 and 78 of the Copyright Design and Patents Act 1988.

All rights reserved. No part of this publication may be reproduced, stored in a retrieval system, or transmitted, in any form or by any means, electronic, mechanical, photocopying, recording, or otherwise, without the prior written permission of the publisher.

British Library Cataloguing in Publication Data

A C.I.P. for this book is available from the British Library

ISBN-13: 978-1-91280-765-9

Cover illustrations by India Elyn
Cover design by Jessica Coomber
Illustrations by India Elyn and Judith Evans
Typeset by Medlar Publishing Solutions Pvt Ltd, India

www.aeonbooks.co.uk

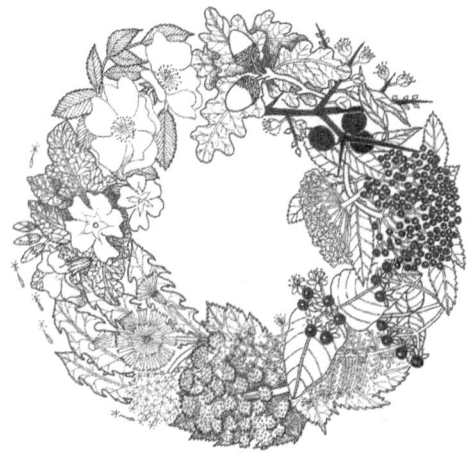

Dedicated to herbalists, past, present, and future, that our work may continue to thrive for the benefit of childbearing women and the children yet to come.

In love and honour of the plants who bring so much medicine into the lives of humans.

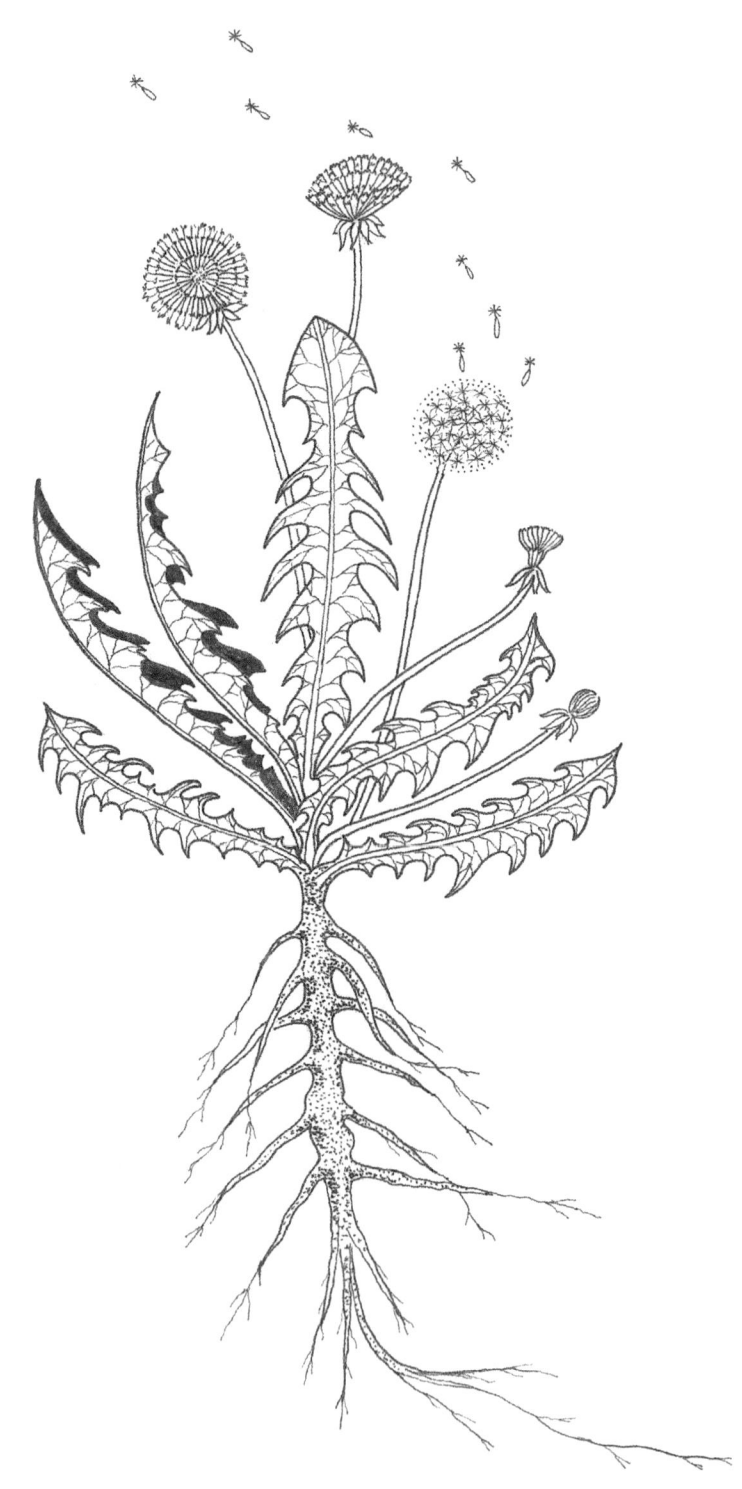

TABLE OF CONTENTS

GUIDELINES FOR USING THIS BOOK	ix
INTRODUCTION	xiii
1. Herbal prescribing and safety	1
2. Herbal care of the pregnant woman	19
3. Nutrition	29
4. Exercise and lifestyle	41
5. Stages of pregnancy	51
6. Herbal pharmacy	59
7. Materia medica	73
8. Conditions of pregnancy	103
9. Healing after loss	175
10. Preparation for labour and birth: week 36 onwards	189
11. The process of labour	207
12. Herbs for labour and delivery	225
13. Postpartum care	237
14. Lactation	267
15. Care of the newborn	283
16. Vibrational essences	301

GLOSSARY OF HERBAL ACTIONS	*309*
RESOURCES	*313*
BIBLIOGRAPHY	*315*
ACKNOWLEDGEMENTS	*319*
AUTHOR BIOGRAPHY	*321*
INDEX OF GODDESS ILLUSTRATIONS	*323*
INDEX	*325*

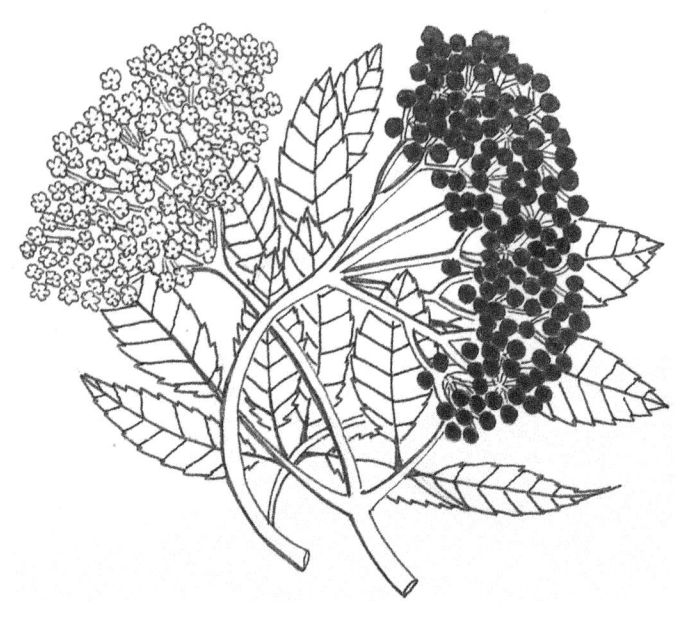

GUIDELINES FOR USING THIS BOOK

Chapter 1 'Herbal Prescribing and Safety' contains important information on prescribing, safety, and contraindicated herbs. **This is required reading for herbal practitioners and anyone intending to prescribe or use the herbs or essential oils recommended in this book.**

Chapter 6 'Herbal Pharmacy' contains instructions and quantities for the standard preparation of herbs, essential oils, and herbal applications for pregnancy, breastfeeding, and the newborn as outlined herein. These may differ from preparations made by herbalists for other purposes and should be checked before preparing any of the herbs recommended in this book.

Chapter 7 'Materia Medica' describes the plants referred to in the text with particular emphasis on their use for pregnancy, lactation, and the newborn. Dosages given are the typical adult dosage range considered safe for childbearing women. Tincture dosages are for 1:4 dried herb tincture or 1:2 specific tincture unless stated otherwise. **Check this chapter to find maximum dosages, cautions, and further information about each herb. Essential oils are listed in Chapter 1.**

NOTE: Certain treatments described in this book should only be undertaken by a trained medical herbalist. Teas are generally safe for non-herbalist use when taken at the doses recommended here. For other herbal treatments, non-herbalist practitioners should consult a trained herbalist. If you are new to working with herbs, be cautious and stick to the gentlest of remedies until you gain experience. If in any doubt, consult a herbal practitioner.

Throughout the text ♣ indicates a **Schedule 20 herb**.

Schedule 20 herbs are toxic at high dosages and are restricted to herbal practitioner use only in the UK with a maximum permitted dosage. These herbs are not available for prescribing in the Republic of Ireland.

Practitioners should check their own country's legislation for all herbal prescribing. Herbs are predominately prescribed in combination.

Herbal medicine is not prescribed in the first trimester of pregnancy unless specifically indicated.

The remaining chapters can be read sequentially or dipped into depending on requirements. Chapter 2 starts by describing herbal care of the pregnant woman, followed in Chapters 3 and 4 by advice on nutrition, exercise, and lifestyle for pregnancy. Chapter 5 describes what happens at the various stages of pregnancy. This is followed by Herbal Pharmacy and Materia Medica as described above. Next is an A–Z of conditions that may be encountered during pregnancy. This is the place to go for a quick reference to particular conditions of pregnancy, appropriate herbal medicines, and other treatments. Healing after loss has its own chapter, as does the preparation for birth, including preparatory herbs, herbal induction, and a suggested birthing kit. Chapter 11 describes the process and stages of labour, followed by a chapter on herbs for labour and delivery. Chapters 13 and 14 outline herbal therapeutics for postpartum care and lactation, while Chapter 15 describes the herbal treatment of common conditions of the newborn. The final chapter gives information on vibrational essences. The glossary contains an explanatory list of plant actions used throughout the book.

Pregnancy does not fit neatly into boxes and many issues may occur at several stages of pregnancy or postpartum. Inevitably there may be some cross-referencing needed. Please refer to the index.

I am using the terms "woman/women" throughout this book. Some mothers may identify differently. The text includes all mothers, regardless of their chosen terminology.

I have taken the decision to capitalise all plant names in honour of their status.

Standard abbreviations used in the text

aa	of each
bd	twice daily
mane	in the morning
nocte	at night
qds	to be taken four times daily
tds	to be taken three times daily
ac	before food
pc	after food
sig	let it be labeled
aq cal	warm water
gtt	drops

Cort	Cortex, bark
EO	Essential oil
Fl	Flos, Flowers
Fol	Folia, Leaves
Fr	Fruct, Fruit
Rad	Radix, Root
Rx	Prescription
Tr	Tincture

Notice to health professionals and disclaimer

Health professionals should use clinical knowledge and judgement in applying the principles and recommendations contained in this book. These recommendations may not be appropriate in all circumstances. Practitioners without appropriate herbal training should consult an experienced medical herbalist for professional advice. New research and clinical experience of herbal medicine may reveal new safety precautions necessitating changes in prescribing practice. It is the responsibility of individual health practitioners, relying on experience and knowledge of the patient, to determine the best treatment and dosages for each individual patient. Neither the publisher nor the author assumes any liability for any injury and/or damage to persons or property arising from this publication.

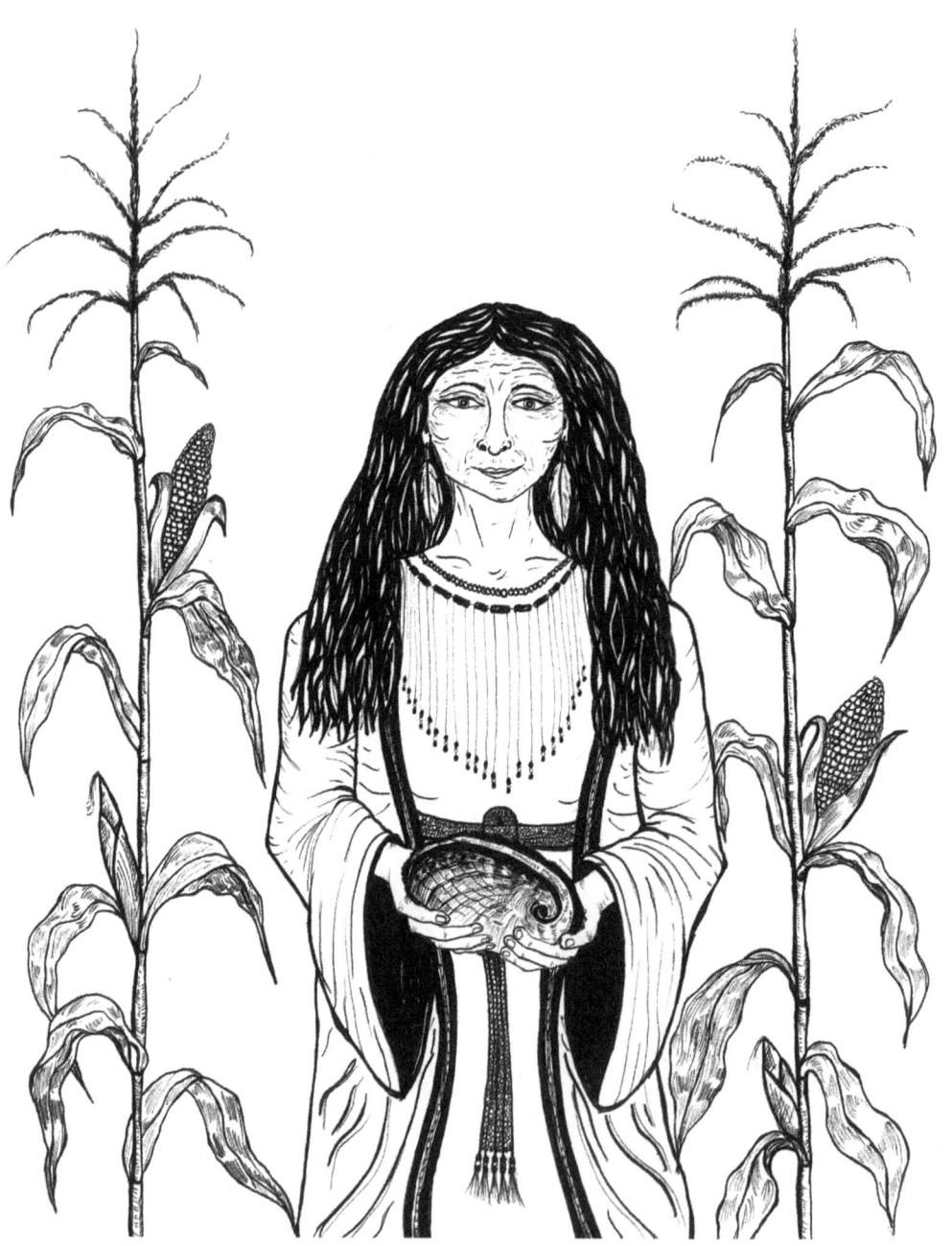

White Shell Woman. Creator and sustainer of life, enabler of beauty.
Corn (*Zea mays*). The abundant one who nourishes all and promotes alignment with the Earth.

INTRODUCTION

Throughout history, medicinal plants have played a significant role during pregnancy, birth, and postpartum. This is still true today in many rural areas of the world. Since ancient times, midwives have attended women in childbirth and very often these midwives were also herbalists, relying on the food and medicine of the plants around them to assist the women in their care. Midwifery and herbalism have traditionally been woven together, with herbs bringing their abundant gifts to support women and their babies throughout all stages of childbearing, promoting optimum health while treating any problems that might arise. This precious herbal wisdom is a legacy for the herbalists of today to preserve for the well-being of women and future generations.

In modern times, more and more women are looking for natural ways to care for their health during pregnancy, seeking to reclaim this ancient knowledge for themselves and their families. Pregnancy is a unique moment of time for a woman, an opportunity for joy and celebration as she prepares for the arrival of a new being, as well as the transformation of her own life. Herbal medicine is a natural choice for many women at this time, offering valuable support for both mother and child.

While public interest in herbs increases, there is also a considerable amount of misinformation and fear surrounding the use of herbs in pregnancy. The media and the internet are full of unsubstantiated scare stories about herbs, as well as some recklessly dangerous advice. In the medical model, pregnancy is sometimes seen as an illness that needs managing rather than a natural state, and herbal medicine may be considered 'too risky' by health care professionals and members of the public alike. Certain herbs are contraindicated in pregnancy for very good reasons, others are safe but discredited due to ignorance or theory rather than evidence. Still, others have reasonable but unproven question marks hanging over them, indicating the need for caution and appropriate targeted research. The entire area can feel like a minefield, with some herbalists fearing to prescribe any herbs in pregnancy as a consequence. The knock-on effect can be that student herbalists receive less experience of treating pregnant women during their training and may enter herbal practice without sufficient confidence or skill to undertake this work. In turn, this means that our knowledge and expertise may dwindle and disappear.

Such a decline in our herbalist repertoire would be a tragic loss. What we do have is a safety record based on the time-tested foundation of empirical evidence from centuries of traditional use. This book is written as a way of recording and sharing a tiny piece of that massive body of knowledge, born from the generous teachings of so many plants, herbalists, and midwives before me, and of course, not forgetting the pregnant women and their babies. It offers an account of herbs and therapeutic methods found to be helpful from experience in clinical practice, both mine and some of my colleagues. This is an undoubtedly personal account, backed up by whatever meaningful studies, literature, and surveys I have found. This book comes in response to requests by students and other herbalists, as well as my desire to preserve and promote the continued safe practice of herbal medicine for pregnancy and childbirth.

Herbs have a wealth of virtues to offer throughout the time of childbearing and it is important that women and their babies are not denied these benefits. My hope is that the material in this book may in some way contribute to ensuring that practitioners of the future are equipped with the information, skill, and confidence to continue this respected tradition.

I am a medical herbalist (not a midwife), with a passion for herbal medicine and women's health, particularly the areas of fertility, pregnancy, and birthing. These have been particular interests of mine over my thirty-five years of herbal practice and I have been privileged to work with many women at this unique stage of their lives, witnessing the profound gifts that herbal medicine has to offer.

I undertook my herbal training with the School of Phytotherapy in England in the 1980s. With a keen interest in women's health, I was fortunate to do much of my clinical training with Janet Hicks, an inspirational herbal practitioner who herself had been taught by a herbalist/gynaecologist. Janet ran a busy practice from her home in Winchester, which she generously opened to students and shared her expertise with enthusiasm. Working at her clinic provided an opportunity to see a large number of women with gynaecological and obstetric conditions, while receiving expert tuition in clinical care and examination. I was deeply impressed by Janet's integrity and respect for patients and plants, combined with her skilful, thorough, and gentle care. The healing virtues of the plants themselves have never ceased to amaze and impress me!

At the end of my herbalist training, I became pregnant with my first child who was born during my initial year of practice. This immersed me in a world of pregnancy, birth, and babies, attracting many pregnant women to my clinic and offering me the opportunity to attend births as a birth assistant. Attending births is something

I love and have continued to do. In 1995, I moved to rural Ireland and have been in practice here ever since. For more than thirty years, my work has included teaching students and herbalists on the subject of herbal therapeutics for fertility, pregnancy, and childbirth.

This book describes my personal therapeutic approach and reflects what I have learned and found useful from experience in practice over the years. It is primarily a practical, hands-on manual of tried and tested herbal therapeutics and does not set out to provide a fully referenced compendium of possible herbs for pregnancy. Herbal medicine treats the whole person. Therefore, as well as prescribing herbs, a herbalist's remit includes providing information and guiding patients in areas of diet and lifestyle, stress management, and simple self-help strategies. In holistic herbal medicine, the physical, emotional, mental, and spiritual aspects of an individual are recognised as being intimately entwined. Plants work on all these levels and my therapeutic approach may include advocating a number of different ways to access plant medicine, whether it is drinking an infusion, spending time in nature, working with living plants, taking a flower essence, or performing a simple ceremony.

This book is primarily aimed at students and practitioners of herbal medicine or other medical disciplines that use medicinal herbs. It may also be of interest to midwives, doulas, and other health practitioners who work with women during childbearing. In fact, anyone with an interest in pregnancy, childbirth and postnatal care, can dip into the relevant sections, and find information that I hope may be useful. Some of the conditions described are not suitable for herbal treatment by those without adequate training in herbal medicine. If in any doubt, consult a herbal practitioner. Other therapeutic methods described are completely safe for non-herbalists.

I am repeatedly struck by the sheer miracle of pregnancy and birth. Witnessing a baby being born into the world or feeling a child kicking inside her mother's belly, I am constantly reminded of the wonder of life and creation. As such common occurrences, it is easy to take pregnancy and birth for granted but these everyday miracles continue to fill me with awe. Pregnancy itself is a mystery and birth is a sacred act that I am always honoured to be part of.

Likewise, the plant world offers magnificent and sometimes miraculous medicines with which to assist pregnancy and childbirth. We should never underestimate the capacity of herbal medicine to support, heal, and regenerate the human being at all stages of life. As practitioners we are in a position to facilitate this exceptional process. We can also empower women, encouraging them to take responsibility for their lives and make their own choices. We can help build a woman's confidence and self-esteem, assisting her to view childbirth with excitement and helping to make her experience as healthy, rewarding, and pleasurable as possible.

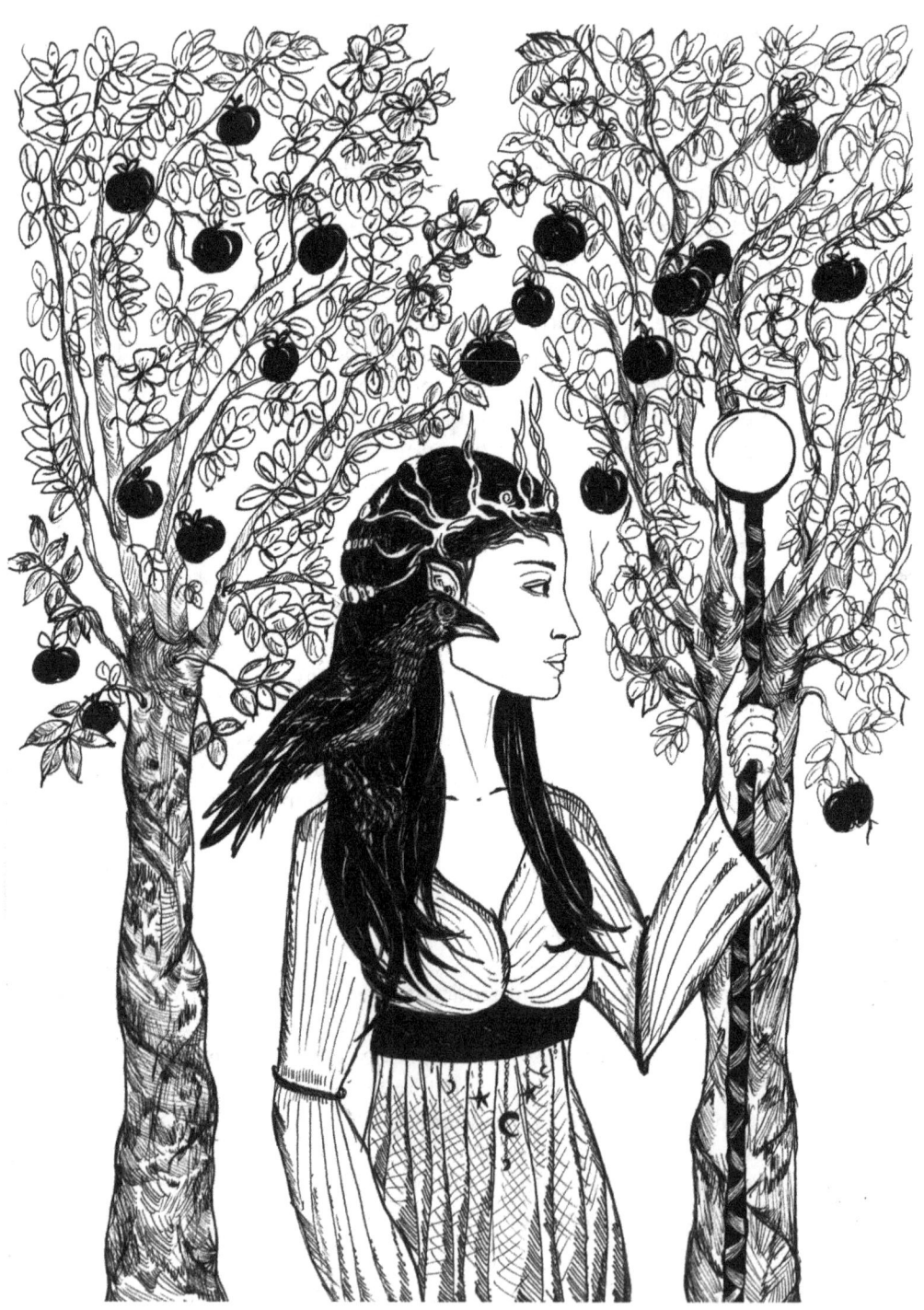

Morgan Le Fay. Lady of healing, herbs and magic, midwife.
Apple (*Malus spp.*) Purveyor of beauty, abundance, love, and magic.

CHAPTER 1

Herbal prescribing and safety

First some background...

Physiomedicalism and non-native herbs

Contemporary Western herbal medicine is frequently a blend of many traditions, both modern and historical. My own formal training is rooted in Physiomedicalism, which works with the concept of enhancing the 'vital force' and combines European herbalism with the herbal wisdom of the native Americans.

While my personal therapeutic approach has evolved considerably over time, the herbs I prescribe in pregnancy have remained primarily a combination of European and North American native plants and this is what is represented here. For me, this is a harmonious mix of cultural origins, aligned with my lifelong interest in native American culture that eventually led me to undertake a ten-year apprenticeship with a métis Medicine Woman from Arizona. However, with current global concerns, I now seek to avoid imported plants as far as possible and it is not my intention to promote the importation of herbs from other lands. I urge all herbalists to consider air miles, fair trade, and sustainable practice (see 'Endangered plants', below) when buying herbs and extracts. Now, more and more herbalists are seeking to use exclusively the plants that grow around them, and this must surely be commended.

This text offers a historical account of herbs and methods that I have found effective and dependable over my years of practice. I can only authentically describe what I know. It goes without saying that a large number of alternative and effective herbs exist that are outside the scope of my experience and therefore this book. My hope is that readers can draw useful information from these pages and that this may inform their own ways of practising. By referencing herbs from two continents, I hope the text may at least have the advantage of having relevance for international readers.

Endangered plants

In the past forty years, an increasing number of plants have become at risk or endangered. This is due to a variety of reasons including habitat loss, climate change, unsustainable wildcrafting, and heavy use of over-the-counter herbal medicines. The situation is constantly changing with some plants being rescued while others become newly at risk. As practitioners, we have a responsibility to keep informed of changes, seeking out sustainable sources and harvesting with care. Information on threatened wild medicinal plants can be found through resources such as United Plant Savers,[1] the Earth's Endangered list,[2] the European Red List,[3] and CITES (the Convention on International Trade in Endangered Species of Wild Fauna and Flora).[4] United Plant Savers aims not to prohibit the use of threatened plants but to initiate programs that will preserve them. At the time of writing, several plants described in this book are currently under threat. These herbs are included, not to promote the use of endangered species, but both as a historical record and in order to acknowledge and give thanks for their remarkable gifts. This information is also offered in the hope that the value of these plants be recognised and they may thrive and become available to herbalists in the future. ALWAYS USE PLANTS FROM A SUSTAINABLE SOURCE.

Principles of herbal practice

This book is in no way a treatise on herbal medicine but it feels important to start by offering a little background information, both to clarify my approach and to provide information for non-herbalists.

Western herbal medicine is a holistic system focused on returning a person to a healthy state of homeostasis or balance. My personal therapeutic approach is a synthesis of various traditions and systems, with Physiomedicalism sitting firmly at its foundation. Treatment seeks to enhance the natural functions of the body, supporting vital function, harmonising the endocrine and nervous systems, and paying particular attention to both circulation and elimination. My aim is to resolve underlying causes and relieve symptoms without suppressing the efforts of the vital force or impeding the soul's journey. Herbs are prescribed on an individual basis to treat the person rather than the disease. In this way, a prescription is tailored to an individual and herbs are chosen to match the patient. This 'matching' of herbs works on many levels and needs to be mentioned here even though a full discussion is far outside the scope of this book.

Interpretation of principles in obstetric care

Real clinical practice is not as simple as theory, and in obstetric care practitioners find themselves in a unique situation. We are often faced with acute or superficial conditions that need fast remedial action, and it may be neither safe nor appropriate to attempt changes to background physiology. While our aim is always to treat the whole person (or rather, two or more together in the case of a pregnant woman and her unborn child), in obstetrics, if there is an underlying chronic condition (sometimes more than one), our best strategy is usually to give gentle, supportive care and reserve more intensive treatment until after lactation. We avoid heroic measures and radical treatments, not wanting to stir up a chronic condition. In general, this is not a time for strong alterative herbs, which may throw out more toxicity before improving the situation. We do not want to precipitate a healing crisis during pregnancy or lactation. Instead, we aim to support and strengthen vital reserves, giving low dosages of gentle herbs.

General approach to herbal prescribing

From the previous comments, you can see that in obstetric care we may need to treat more symptomatically than usual. We gently treat underlying imbalances as best we can, while acknowledging that certain aspects just cannot be addressed until later. It also becomes appropriate to take a more standardised approach than we usually might, typically selecting from a smaller range of trusted herbs, and often requiring them to be fast-acting.

The gentlest approach is to support the body's self-healing mechanisms through diet, lifestyle, use of vibrational essences, and topical applications. Nutrient and tonic herb teas, such as Nettle (*Urtica dioica*), Chamomile (*Chamomilla recutita*), Chickweed (*Stellaria media*), Dandelion leaf and root (*Taraxacum officinalis*), Elderberries (*Sambucus nigra*), Ground Ivy (*Glechoma hederacea*), Hawthorn tops (*Crataegus monogyna/oxacanthoides*), Oatstraw (*Avena sativa*), Raspberry leaf (*Rubus idaeus*), Dog Rosehips (*Rosa canina*), Lemon Balm (*Melissa officinalis*), and Plantain (*Plantago lanceolata/major*) can be considered as a beneficial part of the diet.

If stronger internal herbs are needed, choose the most gentle medicine that will be effective. Teas are generally milder than tinctures at the dosages given. Avoid giving any internal treatment unless it is really necessary, particularly in the first trimester. Exceptions are partus-preparators and postpartum tonics, which are invaluable.

Key considerations in prescribing herbs

- Avoid giving herbs in the first trimester unless absolutely necessary.
- Be rigorous and thorough in your history taking and documentation.
- Know your herbs and how to use them safely.

Given the high safety record of herbs properly prescribed in clinical practice, risks are usually minimal and potential benefits great. Herbs are prescribed on a risk versus benefit basis, and a practitioner must assess the severity of a patient's condition and weigh up the possible risks and benefits of herbal treatment compared to a pharmaceutical approach or to no treatment at all. Clinical decisions will depend on the practitioner's individual perspective of the potential risks involved (see 'Herbal Safety' below). Where appropriate and necessary, herbs may sometimes be prescribed alongside pharmaceuticals, for instance to protect against side effects (such as taking Slippery Elm (*Ulmus rubra*) to protect the gut lining from damage), or to enable a reduction in dosage of prescription drugs. Particular care must be taken with concurrent prescribing during pregnancy and this should only be undertaken by experienced herbal practitioners.

Heightened sensitivity of pregnancy

It is usually the case that women are more sensitive on all levels (physically, emotionally, psychologically, and spiritually) during pregnancy. Consequently, lower doses of herbs than usual are effective. Unless faced with a medical emergency, it is wise to start with a low dose and work upwards if necessary. In sensitive patients it may be necessary to give simples (a single herb at a time) and carefully monitor the response. Idiosyncratic reactions can occur with anyone and any substance. If an adverse reaction is suspected, stop treatment immediately. Trust your inner guidance and if something does not feel right, don't do it.

Alcohol in tinctures

Alcohol is best avoided in the first three months and where possible, it is preferable to prescribe water-based extracts rather than tinctures in the first twelve weeks. However, sometimes tinctures are needed and if tolerated, can be prescribed in small amounts, even in the first trimester. This is especially true for threatened miscarriage. Teas, glycerites, syrups, vinegars, and capsules provide an alternative option to alcohol if needed. I mainly use tinctures and teas in my practice and therefore these are what I have described here. See Chapter 6 for further information on tinctures.

Tinctures compared to powders

Tincture strength cannot be directly compared to the equivalent amount of a powder or capsule, since the bioavailability of an alcohol extract is far higher than a powder. Liquids, such as tinctures, are absorbed very quickly and efficiently by the body. Capsules and tablets, on the other hand, need to be broken down in the stomach and assimilated in the intestines. This can lead to a wide variation in absorption rates in different individuals. If you are prescribing capsules or powders in pregnancy and lactation, the safest option is to use an exact equivalent of dried plant material as in a tincture, being aware that absorption may not be as efficient. Where necessary, digestive function and the health of the gut microbiome can be enhanced by herbs and diet.

Tincture strength and quality

Where herbal tinctures are listed in this text, dosages are for 1:4 dried herb tincture or up to 1:2 fresh herb tincture (specific tincture), unless otherwise specified. If you are using different strength tinctures in your practice, you should adjust the dosage accordingly. See Chapter 6 Herbal Pharmacy for more information on tinctures.

Tinctures must always be of the highest quality possible. Bear in mind that "the medicine a herbalist gives a patient will embody for the patient the standards of the practitioner—the care, the sincerity and the conviction in what he or she does" (Unknown).

Use of the whole plant

For readers who are new to herbal medicine, it is important to note that a single isolated compound from a herb (sometimes sold in tablet or capsule form as the 'active ingredient') will not have the same effect as the whole plant, which contains a mix of compounds. Plants are complex beings containing many compounds that interact. For treatments described in this book, it is imperative to use whole plant extracts. Avoid standardised extracts, since they may behave differently.

The role of synergy in a herbal prescription

When herbs are combined in a blend they act synergistically, meaning that they potentiate, enhance, or balance each other. I tend to experience this like a new plant coming together in the patient's bottle. Last century, more than a few UK practitioners prescribed using the concepts of polypharmacy, where a single prescription might include small amounts of forty or fifty herbs (sometimes more). Working as a dispenser in this kind of clinic was a time-consuming activity! I did not incorporate polypharmacy into my own practice but nevertheless I was imbued with the understanding that, whether using five herbs or fifty in a mix, the synergistic blend creates the equivalent of a 'new' herb with a combined effect greater than the sum of their separate parts. It was also understood that a combination of small amounts of herbs generally confers greater safety than the comparative total amount of a single herb.

Sometimes in herbal practice, 'less is more' and this is especially valuable to bear in mind when treating pregnant women.

The therapeutic relationship or the 'golden triangle'

Herbal prescribing involves a three-way relationship between patient, practitioner, and plants. All sorts of hidden dynamics take place, incorporating the powers of intention, belief, and trust to name but a few. At times, an unexpected herb will work superbly for the most unlikely condition. You might call this the placebo effect or something else, it doesn't really matter as long as we prescribe safely and the patient benefits. There is much we do not understand.

Trust the process

It is clear from all of the above that herbal medicine is not an exact science. Many factors are involved, some of them mysterious. This is true of all of life, including human healthcare. Prescribing involves much more than simply choosing herbs with the required physical actions. As well as understanding the pharmacology and physiological actions of herbs, we can develop a deeper relationship with the plants, truly listen to them, and get to know their personalities and more subtle virtues. This enables us to fine-tune our prescribing to find the best herbs to match our patients, as well as being a way to honour our beloved herbs and their gifts. Plants are manifestations of consciousness, and this can be naturally transferred to us when we are regularly in their presence (whether out in nature or in the dispensary). It is my belief that most experienced herbal practitioners learn to integrate this kind of awareness with scientific knowledge and this integration is crucial for best practice. Trust the plants, trust your intuition, and trust the therapeutic process!

Summary of prescribing guidelines

Safety and efficacy of treatment rely not only on choice of herbs but also on proper dosage and preparation. For any medicine, first ensure that you have the correct plant and of the highest quality possible. Be sure you know the appropriate dosage (check in Chapter 7 'Materia Medica') and familiarise yourself with Chapter 6 'Herbal Pharmacy', for methods of use. Be aware that most of the infusions I am recommending for pregnancy and lactation are a much weaker dilution than those often prescribed in general herbal practice or described by other authors. Work with caution, bearing in mind that every woman and child is different. Respect the plants and their virtues. Build a relationship of reciprocity with your herbs. Silently talk to the plants as you harvest, prepare, or dispense, praising their virtues, describing the patient/s and requesting help from the herbs. Give thanks to the plants. Commit to doing no harm. Enjoy your work and your life!

Flower essences and other vibrational essences

My herbal practice often incorporates the use of vibrational essences. These are safe and effective to use alongside conventional herbal treatment and are particularly beneficial for issues stemming from psychological, emotional, and spiritual causes. Throughout this text, I have suggested optional essences that can be added as part of a synergistic blend of herbs or given as a separate preparation. My examples refer to the Derrynagittah essences, and these may be substituted by any other essences of choice. See Chapter 16 for further details.

Use of nutritional supplements

Various supplements are suggested throughout this text. Unless stated otherwise, these can be taken in addition to the herbal medicine indicated. This is not always necessary, but in specific conditions, and particularly where a woman has a low nutritional status, extra supplementation is extremely valuable. See Chapter 3 'Nutrition'.

Herbal legislation

Legislation affecting herbs and herbalists varies around the world. This book primarily describes herbs currently available to practitioners in the UK and Ireland, although a few of the herbs mentioned in prescriptions are no longer permitted in the Republic of Ireland. Schedule 20 herbs (☙) (previously 'Schedule 3') are restricted to herbal practitioner use only in the UK with a maximum permitted dosage. These include Lobelia (*Lobelia inflata*), Gelsemium (*Gelsemium sempervirens*), and Ephedra (*Ephedra sinica*), which are not available for prescribing in the Republic of Ireland.

These matters are constantly changing and readers ought to check the legislation in their own countries. Similarly, medical procedures and practice vary from place to place and you should inform yourself of current practices in your country.

Herbal safety

There is a notable lack of consensus regarding the safety of herbal medicine in pregnancy.

Accurate data about herbs known to adversely affect pregnancy is scarce, often contradictory, and of dubious origin. Many regulatory authorities recommend that a herb should not be used unless controlled clinical trials exist to prove its safety. Other recommendations are based on speculation of harmful effects rather than any real evidence. Most often, this guidance comes from people who have little or no experience of prescribing herbs in pregnancy. Sometimes, the view is expressed that if any possible risk of harm exists, however unlikely, then a herb is unsafe and should not be used—a view which takes no account of the enormous benefits herbs can offer. In fact, most herbs have a high record of safety. Aside from cases of intentional overdose, very few adverse effects in pregnancy have been reported, with most of these resulting from the consumption of adulterants or toxic plants.

Limited clinical studies exist and most of what is currently known about the use of herbs in pregnancy is based on empirical, historical, and observational evidence. Herbal medicine can claim generations of safe usage in this field and we need to use careful discernment about the relevance and reliability of some published research studies. However, we cannot be complacent and it is essential that readers remain open to new research findings as well as always being vigilant to seek out the highest quality, non-adulterated herbal products for our patients. In listing contraindicated herbs, I have erred on the side of caution, including some herbs that I have used without problems in earlier times but I have now stopped prescribing due to recent scientific concerns, even if unproven.

Readers may be surprised to realise that very little safety data exists for conventional pharmaceuticals and most drug companies avoid studying pregnant women preferring to publish results of animal studies. This is discussed in detail by Simon Mills and Kerry Bone in *The Essential Guide to Herbal Safety*.[5]

The area of herbal safety in pregnancy can be a minefield of myths, inconsistencies, and misinformation. In my opinion, *The Essential Guide to Herbal Safety* offers a reliable reference text and contains data aligned with my own experience. Readers are encouraged to consult this text for more detailed information. Naturally, new research and clinical experience are constantly emerging and all practitioners need to keep abreast of current findings.

There is a widely held view that large amounts of emmenagogue herbs are likely to cause uterine contractions and potential miscarriage. I am certainly not advocating such reckless practice but it is interesting to note, that according to Mills and Bone "many of the commonly used emmenagogue herbs may be excluded from use during pregnancy because of potential toxicity, undesirable hormonal effects, or other possible detrimental effects. However, abortifacient activity is probably the least likely reason for any safety concerns regarding their use during pregnancy".

Correct dosage is key to safety. I suspect that in many cases where a herb is denigrated as unsafe, it is a result of an excessive dose being used and many herbs that may prove dangerous in large amounts can be perfectly safe in low doses. In general prescribing, aside from in acute conditions, I usually give herbs at relatively low doses and this is particularly true in obstetric care. I believe this approach to be typical of most medical herbalists. It seems that many pharmaceutical trials test herbs at dosage levels that would be unthinkable in clinical practice and do not accurately reflect the complexities of practitioner use.

It should be remembered that herbs and spices are safely consumed on a daily basis by pregnant women around the world. Certain culinary herbs may be contraindicated in large doses. These include Cinnamon, Fennel, Fenugreek, Oregano, Parsley, Rosemary, Saffron, and Sage. However, these are perfectly safe in normal use, as is the non-excessive drinking of most regular herb teas.

Below, I have listed herbs contraindicated in pregnancy and lactation.

Refer to Chapter 7 'Materia Medica' for information on herbs including maximum dosages for pregnancy and lactation. Typically, when prescribing herbs in my practice, I am using therapeutic doses that are considerably lower than the maximum limits given.

Herbs contraindicated in pregnancy and lactation

In herbal training, I was taught to avoid prescribing all contraindicated herbs to any woman who *could* become pregnant. This is the safest way to proceed since we cannot predict when an unexpected pregnancy might occur. In exceptional circumstances, if a contraindicated herb is crucial to a prescription for a woman in this category, the importance of not becoming pregnant during treatment needs to be made crystal clear to the patient. For instance, this might occur if I want to prescribe *Artemisia absinthe* or *Tanacetum vulgaris* in a short-term mix for parasites in a non-pregnant, non-lactating woman. Similarly, *Thuja occidentalis* can be valuable in many conditions but possible pregnancy must always be considered. If conception is even a possibility, treatment with a contraindicated herb needs to be as short-term as possible and if pregnancy should arise unexpectedly, the herb must be stopped immediately. In clinical practice, there is only a handful of contraindicated herbs that I give to fertile women, and most of these are rarely prescribed apart from in the very short term.

See relevant sections in Chapter 7 'Materia Medica' for further information on Caulophyllum as well as Symphytum and pyrrolizidine alkaloids. Some of these herbs e.g. *Angelica sinensis*, are included as a caution due to adverse reporting that needs further research.

Unless medically indicated, **avoid giving any herbs in the first trimester of pregnancy**.

Where herbal treatment is medically indicated in the first trimester, proceed with caution and be sure to avoid all herbs that are contra-indicated (check Chapter 7 for individual herbs).

Herbs not to be taken in pregnancy or lactation

Aconitum spp. ☘	Aconite
Acorus calamus	Sweet Flag
Anemone pulsatilla	Pulsatilla, Pasque Flower *safe for childbirth*
Angelica sinensis	Chinese Angelica *safe in lactation*
Arnica spp.	Arnica *external use only*
Artemisia absinthe	Wormwood
Arctostaphylos uva-ursi	Bearberry *risk is theoretical*
Atropa belladonna ☘	Deadly Nightshade
Berberis spp.	Barberry, Oregon Grape
Borago officinalis	Borage *pyrollizidine alkaloids*
Byronia alba	Byrony
Caulophyllum thalictroides	Blue Cohosh *labour only (see pages 79 and 234)*
Chelidonium majus ☘	Greater Celandine
Convallaria majalis ☘	Lily of the Valley
Datura spp. ☘	Datura
Gelsemium sempervirens ☘	Gelsemium *safe for childbirth*

Hydrastis Canadensis	Golden Seal *safe for childbirth*
Hyoscyamus niger ❦	Henbane
Juniperus communis	Juniper
Lobelia inflata ❦	Lobelia *safe for threatened miscarriage and childbirth*
Lycopus spp	Bugleweed, Gypsywort
Mentha pulegium	Pennyroyal
Peganum harmala	Wild Rue, Syrian Rue
Petasites spp.	Butterbur
Peumus boldus	Boldo
Phytolacca decandra	Poke Root
Piscidia erythrina	Jamaican Dogwood
Ruta graveolens	Rue
Salvia officinalis	Sage *safe for weaning*
Sanguinaria canadensis	Bloodroot
Sarothamnus scoparius	Broom
Senecio spp.	Senecio
Symphytum officinale	Comfrey *pyrollizidine alkaloids*
Tanacetum parthenium	Feverfew *safe for childbirth*
Tanacetum vulgaris	Tansy
Thuja occidentalis	Thuja
Tussilago farfara	Coltsfoot *pyrollizidine alkaloids*

Caution in pregnancy and lactation

Laxative herbs containing anthraquinones

Aloe barbadensis	Aloe resin no more than 200mg/day powdered resin, 4ml/day 1:10 tincture
Rhamnus purshiana	Cascara no more than 1g/day dried bark, 4ml/day tincture
Rheum spp.	Rhubarb no more than 3g/day dried root/rhizome, 4ml/day tincture

Additional cautions in lactation

Avoid Ma huang (*Ephedra sinica*) during lactation. Elecampane (*Inula helenium*) should not be given in lactation at doses above 3g daily.

Avoid Willow bark (*Salix alba*) during lactation due to risk of salicylate hypersensitivity reaction.

Sage (*Salvia off.*) is contraindicated in lactation except to stop milk flow.

Essential oils

Essential oils should not be administered orally, vaginally, or rectally throughout pregnancy or lactation. They can cross the placenta and may affect foetal growth and development during pregnancy. Most are best avoided altogether in the first trimester. Small quantities are safe when used as flavourings, such as Peppermint, Orange, or Aniseed. Note that Peppermint and strong menthol essential oils can cause respiratory distress in the newborn if used externally during labour or delivery.

Avoid essential oils with epilepsy, high-risk pregnancies, major cardiac, liver or renal disease, pre-eclampsia, eclampsia, pyrexia, anticoagulant therapy, polyhydramnios, placenta previa, reduced foetal movements, higher multiple pregnancies. Room spray only with preterm labour.

Certain oils can be used in pregnancy with good effect at low dilution (1%) in carrier oils for massage, ointments, creams, lotions, inhalations, room sprays, burners, and other purposes.

Particular caution is needed for lactation and the newborn since essential oils can be overpowering for a newborn infant's delicate developing systems, both physically and energetically. Some practitioners recommend delaying infant exposure to essential oils in any form until 3–6 months of age. This text includes a limited selection of essential oils considered safe to use in the postpartum period and with the newborn. Whatever is used by the mother will generally affect the infant, even in a non-breastfeeding woman. Professional opinion varies significantly in this area and practitioners must exercise common sense and keep up to date with current understanding. When using any essential oil during lactation or with the newborn, even at the lowest dilution, be aware of any changes in the baby, even if there is no obvious visible skin reaction.

The information offered here is to the best of my knowledge and experience to date. Essential oils are strong medicine and must always be prescribed on an individual basis. In labour and postpartum, essential oils can be diluted up to 2% although it is advisable to start at a weaker dilution. For babies, dilute up to 1%. Use patch testing before using any essential oil directly on the skin.

Do not give essential oils internally to pregnant or lactating women or newborn infants.

Avoid essential oils in the first trimester (see exceptions below).

Never apply essential oils undiluted on the skin.

Dilute essential oils in a suitable carrier oil/cream prior to applying to the skin or carrying out a patch test.

Use patch testing before using any diluted essential oil directly on the skin.

Any essential oil may irritate sensitive skin.

Essential oils generally accepted as safe in pregnancy

1st trimester:

Ginger	*Zingiber officinalis*—as inhalations for nausea and vomiting
Lemon	*Citrus limonum*—as inhalations for nausea and vomiting

2nd and 3rd trimesters, including labour:

Bergamot	*Citrus bergamia*—Relaxing, uplifting. Used for anxiety, depression, stress, pain relief.
Black Pepper	*Piper nigrum*—Circulatory stimulant, digestive tonic.
Chamomile (Roman)	*Chamaemelum nobile/Anthemis nobilis*—Calming, anti-spasmodic, nerve tonic, analgesic. For allergic skin response (may cause allergy, patch test before use).
Chamomile (German)	*Chamomilla recutita/Matricaria chamomilla/Matricaria recutita*—Strongly anti-inflammatory, actions overlap with Roman Chamomile.
Clary Sage*	*Salvia sclarea*—**Labour and delivery only**. Oestrogen-like action, anti-spasmodic, circulatory tonic tonic. Caution in hypotension. Do not give with oxytocin/pitocin, avoid with epidural until blood pressure normalises.
Eucalyptus	*Eucalyptus smithii* or *radiate*—Anti-infectious, anti-bacterial. Avoid in labour with diabetes.
Frankincense	*Boswellia carterii*—Soothes the mind, promotes clear thought, calms anxiety, uterine tonic, enhances spiritual practice.
Geranium	*Pelargonium graveolens (Pelargonum x asperum)*—Balances mood/hormones, soothes anxiety and agitation, calms atmosphere.
Ginger	*Zingiber officinalis*—Analgesic, carminative, stomachic, warming stimulant.
Grapefruit	*Citrus racemosa*—Actions similar to Lemon.
Jasmine*	*Jasminum grandiflorum* **Labour and delivery only**. Antidepressive, eases anxiety, provides inner strength.
Lavender	*Lavandula officinalis, vera, angustifolia*—Calming, soothing, anti-spasmodic, active against MRSI and Staph. Inhalation best for spasmolytic effect. For liniment, use whole plant rather than essential oil. Caution in hypotension. In labour: Avoid with epidural until blood pressure normalises.
Lemon	*Citrus limonum*—Emotionally uplifting, antibacterial, circulatory tonic, nerve restorative.

Lime	*Citrus medica* var. *acida/ aurantifolia/ latifolia*—Similar to lemon.
Mandarin	*Citrus reticulata*—Uplifting and relaxing.
Neroli	*Citrus aurantium bigarade* (flos)—Calming for panic and anxiety, antidepressant, sedative.
Orange (sweet)	*Citrus sinensis per.*—Sedative, antidepressant.
Petitgrain	*Citrus aurantium* (leaves and twigs)—Similar to Neroli but more delicate
Rose otto*	*Rosa damascena/centifolia/gallica flos.*—Calming, uplifting, restores self-love and self-worth, antidepressant, reproductive tonic. Avoid with haemorrhage.
Rosewood	*Aniba roseodora*—Anti-microbial, slightly antidepressant.
Sandalwood	*Santalum album*—Anti-infectious, sedative, anti-spasmodic, tension and anxiety associated with depression, antidepressant.
Tangerine	*Citrus reticulata*—Uplifting and relaxing.
Tea tree (Ti-Tree)	*Melaleuca alternifolia*—Anti-microbial. Avoid in labour.
Ylang-ylang	*Cananga odorata*—Relaxing and uplifting. Anxiety, stress, panic attacks, lowered libido. Caution in hypotension.

*do not use in labour with previous uterine scar, VBAC.

Essential oils generally considered safe for external use with lactating women

Use at 1–2% dilution. Patch test with diluted essential oil before using on skin.

Bergamot	*Citrus bergamia*—Relaxing, uplifting. Used for anxiety, depression, stress, pain relief.
Black Pepper	*Piper nigrum*—Circulatory stimulant, digestive tonic.
Chamomile (Roman)	*Chamaemelum nobile/Anthemis nobilis*—Calming, anti-spasmodic, nerve tonic, analgesic. For allergic skin response (may cause allergy, patch test before use).
Chamomile (German)	*Chamomilla recutita/Matricaria chamomilla/Matricaria recutita*—Strongly anti-inflammatory, actions overlap with Roman Chamomile.
Lavender	*Lavandula officinalis, vera, angustifolia*—Calming, soothing, anti-spasmodic, active against MRSI and Staph. Inhalation best for spasmolytic effect. For liniment, use whole plant rather than essential oil.

Lime — *Citrus medica* var. *acida/ aurantifolia/ latifolia*—Uplifting.
Mandarin — *Citrus reticulata*—Uplifting and relaxing.
Petitgrain — *Citrus aurantium* (leaves and twigs)—Similar to Neroli but more delicate.
Tangerine — *Citrus reticulata*—Uplifting and relaxing.

Essential oils to be used with caution for external use with lactating women

Eucalyptus — *Eucalyptus smithii* or *radiata*—Anti-infectious, antibacterial.
Frankincense — *Boswellia carterii*—Soothes the mind, promotes clear thought, calms anxiety, uterine tonic, enhances spiritual practice.
Geranium — *Pelargonium graveolens (Pelargonum x asperum)*—Balances mood/hormones, soothes anxiety and agitation, calms atmosphere.
Ginger — *Zingiber officinalis*—Analgesic, carminative, stomachic, warming stimulant.
Grapefruit — *Citrus racemosa*—Similar to Lemon.
Lemon — *Citrus limonum*—Emotionally uplifting, antibacterial, circulatory tonic, nerve restorative.
Neroli — *Citrus aurantium bigarade* (flos)—Calming for panic and anxiety, antidepressant, sedative.
Orange (sweet) — *Citrus sinensis per.*—Sedative, antidepressant.
Rose otto — *Rosa damascena/centifolia/gallica flos.*—Calming, uplifting, restores self-love and self-worth, antidepressant, reproductive tonic.
Rosewood — *Aniba roseodora*—Anti-microbial, slightly antidepressant.
Sandalwood — *Santalum album*—Anti-infectious, sedative, anti-spasmodic. Tension and anxiety associated with depression, antidepressant.
Tea tree — *Melaleuca alternifolia*—Anti-microbial.
Ylang-ylang — *Cananga odorata*—Relaxing and uplifting. Anxiety, stress, panic attacks, lowered libido. Caution in hypotension.

Essential oils generally considered safe for external use for newborn infants (weeks 1–12)

Use at up to 1% dilution. Patch test with diluted essential oil before use on skin. Be aware of any changes in the baby.

Suitable oils: Chamomile Roman (*Chamaemelum nobile/Anthemis nobilis*), Chamomile German (*Chamomilla recutita/Matricaria chamomilla/Matricaria recutita*), Lavender (*Lavandula officinalis, vera, angustifolia*)

Use with caution: Eucalyptus (*Eucalyptus smithii* or *radiata*)

Essential oils contraindicated in pregnancy, lactation, and the newborn (*not an exhaustive list*)

Aniseed	*Pimpinella anisum*
Arnica	*Arnica spp.*
Basil	*Ocimum basilicum*
Birch	*Betula spp.*
Cedarwood	*Cedrus atlantica, Cedrus deodara, Juniperus mexicana, Juniperus virginiana*
Chamomile, Moroccan	*Tanacetum anuum*
Cinnamon	*Cinnamomum zeylanicum*
Clary sage	*safe for delivery Salvia sclarea*
Clove	*Syzygium aromaticum*
Cypress	*Cupressus sempervirens*
Fennel	*Foeniculum vulgare*
Hyssop	*Hyssopus officinalis*
Jasmine	*safe for delivery Jasminum grandiflorum*
Juniper	*Juniperis communis*
Marjoram	*Oreganum majorana, Thymus mastichina*
Mugwort	*Artemisia vulgaris, Artemisia arborescens, Artemisia herba-alba, and other species*
Myrrh	*Commiphora molmol*
Nutmeg	*Myristica fragrans*
Oregano	*Oreganum vulgare*
Pennyroyal	*Mentha pulegium*
Peppermint	*Mentha x piperita*
Rosemary	*Rosemarinus officinalis*
Rue	*Ruta graveolens*
Sage	*Salvia officinalis*
Sassafras	*Sassafras albidum*
Savory	*Satureja hortensis*
Thuja	*Thuja occidentalis*
Thyme	*Thymus vulgaris*
Wintergreen	*Gaultheria fragrantissima*
Wormwood	*Artemisia absinthe*

Notes

1. United Plant Savers. https://unitedplantsavers.org/species-at-risk/ [last accessed 10/7/21].
2. Earth's Endangered Creatures. www.earthsendangered.com/plantlist.asp [last accessed 18/7/21].
3. European Union. https://ec.europa.eu/environment/nature/conservation/species/redlist/downloads/European_med_plants.pdf [last accessed 10/7/21].
4. CITES is an international agreement between governments. Its aim is to ensure that international trade in specimens of wild animals and plants does not threaten the survival of the species. https://cites.org/eng/prog/medplants [last accessed 10/7/21].
5. Simon Mills and Kerry Bone, *The Essential Guide to Herbal Safety*, (Missouri: Churchill Livingstone, 2005), 90.

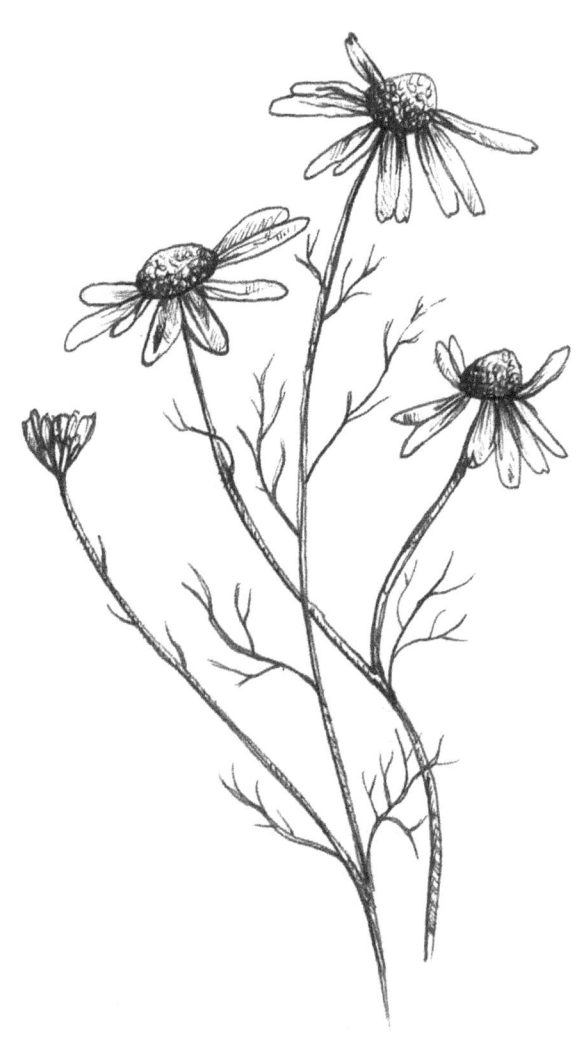

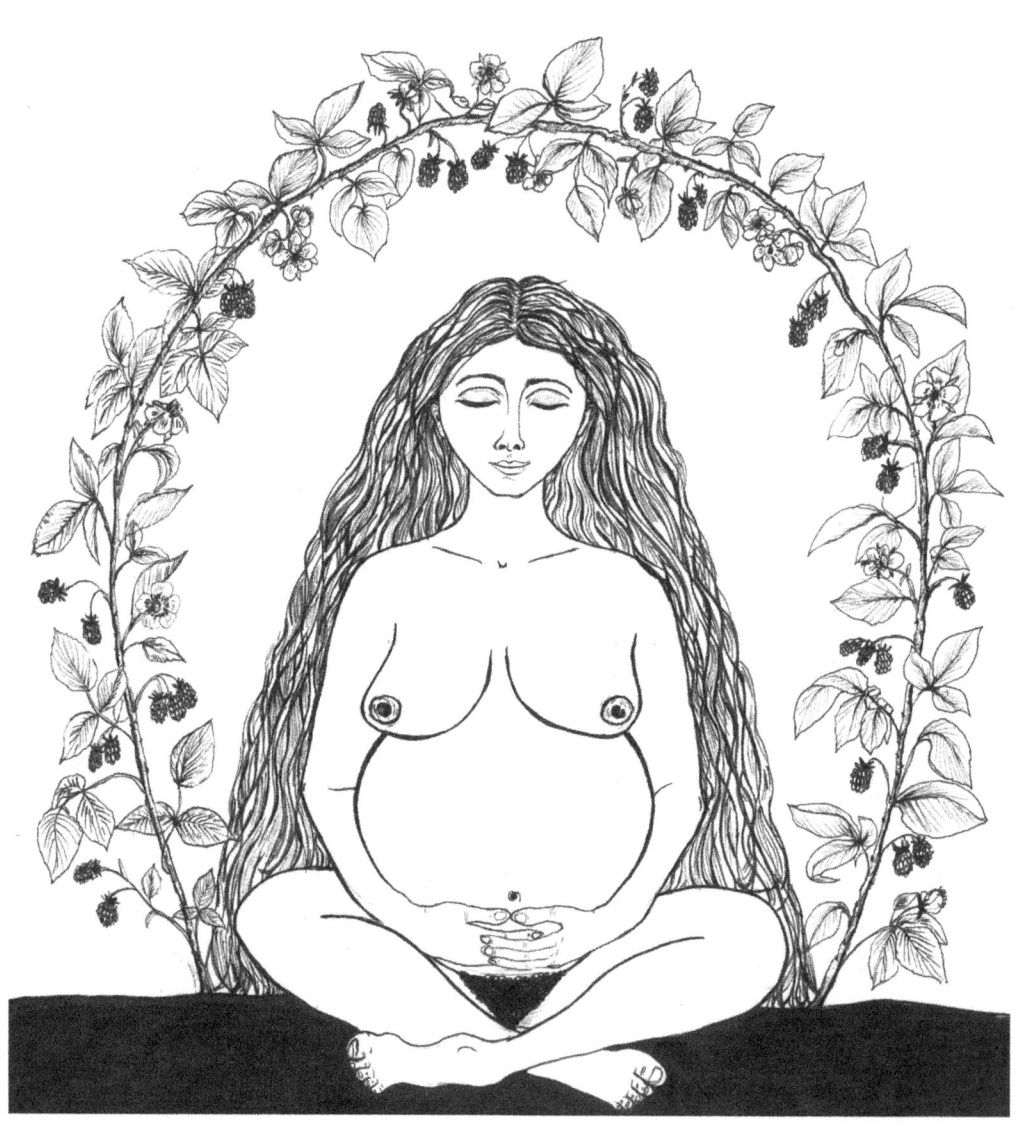

Gaia, Mother Earth. Fertility incarnate, mysterious, moist, strong.
Raspberry (*Rubus idaeus*). The receptive, fertile, intuitive mother.

CHAPTER 2

Herbal care of the pregnant woman

Reasons why a pregnant woman comes to a herbalist

There are endless scenarios and reasons why women come for herbal treatment in pregnancy. All women want their babies to be healthy, and this is often the time when a woman most seeks to take care of her health, prevent illness, and where possible, avoid pharmaceutical medication.

Ideally, antenatal care should begin before pregnancy, providing the opportunity to cleanse, nourish, and balance in preparation for healthy childbearing. Of course, this does not always happen in clinical practice. Many women attend my clinic as soon as they discover they are pregnant. Of these, some are already in good health, wanting the support of a herbalist to maintain optimum health for themselves and their baby throughout their pregnancy and birthing. Some women may have been receiving treatment to aid fertility (if you treat women for fertility problems in your practice, you will almost certainly end up with pregnant patients). Others may have a history of previous miscarriage or various problems of pregnancy, while some may have a deep-rooted fear of giving birth or have different psychological issues they would like to address. Other women may have been diagnosed with a complication in their current pregnancy and be seeking to treat this with herbs. This could occur at any stage during the pregnancy. There will also be new or existing patients who present with chronic health conditions that need to be managed throughout their pregnancy, for instance allergies, multiple sclerosis, or chronic asthma. Others may simply attend during their final weeks, seeking to avoid a hospital induction or to receive advice and support.

Treatment of chronic conditions

When a pregnant woman presents with a pre-existing health concern, unless their condition is interfering with the progress of the pregnancy, best practice is not to treat the chronic condition unless absolutely essential, particularly in the first trimester. However, in some cases, an untreated chronic condition could undermine the health of the mother and/or the course of the pregnancy. Also, pregnancy puts numerous additional demands on a woman's health, which may adversely affect an existing condition. Clinical judgement must be exercised, weighing up risk versus benefit. Most commonly, the best course of action if herbs are indeed needed is to give gentle restorative and supportive tonics, postponing deeper treatment until after lactation. Bearing in mind that it is common for pre-existing symptoms to change when a women is pregnant, sometimes a 'wait and see' approach is preferable. Either way, any prescription should be tailored for pregnancy and the dosage kept as low as possible.

As well as conditions specific to pregnancy, a woman may also require treatment for any of the usual complaints faced by a non-pregnant woman. At this time, herbalists tend to be treating acute and superficial problems that need to be addressed quickly, ensuring that an acute problem does not become chronic. We must proceed gently, emphasising dietary and lifestyle changes along with appropriate herbs as needed.

The herbal consultation

For any new patient, my initial consultation usually lasts two hours, allowing me plenty of time to undertake a detailed medical, family, social, and personal history. For a pregnant woman, this involves carefully listening to her concerns and includes looking at all the body systems, absorption, elimination, relaxation, level of toxicity, growth, repair, and nourishment. I pay particular attention to kidneys, liver, circulatory, and adrenal function, since these can be especially vulnerable under the considerable demands of pregnancy. I also assess her general vitality and energy reserves, nutrition, exercise, attitudes, social circumstances, home and work environment, and the quality of her relationships. Allergic or atopic tendencies should be noted, being aware that idiosyncratic reactions to herbs are always possible and this likelihood is increased in patients with pre-existing sensitivities. By careful and thorough case taking and prescribing, idiosyncratic reactions are minimised or avoided altogether. After making a clear assessment of a woman's needs, I can formulate a treatment plan. Part of the value of the consultation is also about building a good relationship between the patient and myself, encouraging a positive psychological approach and fostering trust, hope, and motivation.

Pregnancy is, of course, a healthy state and not an illness. That said, many women appreciate monthly appointments throughout their pregnancy, regardless of whether or not they have a particular health issue to treat. Even though most women in developed society will be receiving regular medical check-ups, many welcome the opportunity to visit a herbalist to discuss their concerns and receive support, information, and guidance. Relieving fear and anxiety are often high on the list of priorities. As well as medical treatment and advice, pregnancy is a time when women need strong social supports and herbal practitioners can play a vital role in empowering women on their journey to motherhood.

Herbal care in an uncomplicated pregnancy

For some women, if their health is good and there is no requirement for them to see me regularly, I give advice at the first consultation and arrange to see them at around twenty-eight weeks (always with the proviso that they contact me sooner if needed), usually seeing them once per month in the third trimester. For a healthy woman with an uncomplicated pregnancy and no significant history, from a herbal perspective the best practice is to do nothing, especially in the first twelve weeks. It may be that nothing is required until the third trimester when we begin preparing for labour and delivery. Alternatively, if there is a complaint that needs treating or an area requiring support, appropriate herbs can be prescribed at any stage (see Chapter 8). Flower essences (vibrational essences) can also be given throughout as needed (see Chapter 16).

Typically, a midwife will be carrying out regular physical examinations (such as checking the height of the fundus after twenty-four weeks and routine urinalysis) and recording findings in the woman's notes, which you can ask her to bring to each visit. You can make your own examinations and refer back to midwifery care if needed.

See Table 1.1 for a typical herbalist antenatal care schedule in an uncomplicated pregnancy.

Table 1.1 Herbalist antenatal care schedule in an uncomplicated pregnancy

As early as possible	Full case history including wishes for pregnancy and full medical history, including previous pregnancies/problems and blood group.
	Discuss pregnancy care and choices for place of birth.
	Discuss nutrition including supplementation, healthy lifestyle, exercise including pelvic floor.
	Discuss screening, risks and benefits.
	Discuss breastfeeding.
	Assess for any additional needs, both physical and psychosocial.
	Arrange timing of future appointments.
	Exam: Height, weight, blood pressure, urinalysis.
Monthly *if desired*	General check-up.
	Exam: weight, blood pressure, urinalysis
Week 28	General check-up.
	Give Raspberry leaf (*Rubus idaeus*) tea 1 cup daily,
	Or appropriate partus preparator(s).
	Exam: weight, blood pressure, urinalysis, ankle oedema.

(*Continued*)

Table 1.1 Herbalist antenatal care schedule in an uncomplicated pregnancy (continued)

Week 32	General check-up. Discuss preparation for labour and birth outline herbal options. Exam: weight, blood pressure, urinalysis, ankle oedema. Continue with Raspberry leaf tea 1 cup daily (or appropriate herbs).
Week 36 onwards	General check-up. Discuss labour and delivery. Birth plan Explain Birthing Pack and discuss individual requirements. Discuss breastfeeding and care of new baby. Exam: weight, blood pressure, urinalysis, ankle oedema. Increase Raspberry leaf tea to 3 cups daily (or appropriate herbs). Give Birthing Pack and postnatal tonic according to individual requirements (to be used at appropriate times).
Week 39/40	General check-up. Discuss options for prolonged pregnancy. Exam: weight, blood pressure, urinalysis, ankle oedema. Continue with Raspberry leaf tea, 3 cups daily (or appropriate herbs).
Week 40/41+	Give induction mix if required (see page 202).

Birth attendants

If it appeals to you, it is well worth considering offering your services as a herbalist birth attendant. A birth attendant (often called a *doula* or a labour coach) is someone (typically non-medical) who accompanies a woman during labour and delivery, providing comfort, guidance, encouragement, and support. As a herbalist, you can provide appropriate herbal care at the same time. This may be at home or in hospital and can be as well as or instead of the baby's father or another family member or friend. Unless you are a trained midwife yourself, there will almost certainly be a midwife present for the baby's delivery.

I attend both home and hospital births, sometimes with the baby's father present, sometimes with the woman's mother or other relative, sometimes with no-one except the midwife. Usually, the pregnant woman calls me at the start of labour and I may spend a short or long time with her before the midwife needs to come (in the case of a home birth) or before we leave for the hospital (in the case of a hospital delivery). It depends on the woman's circumstances and personal requirements, as well as practical considerations. As a herbalist caring for pregnant women, you can of course provide excellent care without ever attending a birth. Being a birth attendant can be a demanding role and is not for everyone. You need to be available on call, you may need to stay awake for hours, and occasionally it can be very stressful, especially in a hospital environment. However, being present for the birth of a baby can be a beautiful and awe-inspiring experience. It is a lovely way to support a woman and an amazing privilege to be present as a new soul enters the world. From the perspective of the woman giving birth, having an experienced support person who has no prior social bond with the mother can be enormously helpful and has been shown to have a very positive effect in terms of outcome and duration of labour. This is the case in any circumstance and is particularly important if the woman is on her own with no other trusted support. It is only in recent times that it has become acceptable for men, as husbands and partners, to be present at labour and birth. Research suggests that women report higher levels of support from their partners when there is an additional trained support person present who can give encouragement and advice.

There is no requirement for formal training to be a birth assistant. However, if you have not given birth yourself or would simply like more experience or training as an assistant, you can undertake training as a doula.[1]

To support a woman in this way is richly rewarding work and, in my experience, most midwives welcome the presence of a herbalist birth attendant.

Some hospitals have policies limiting a woman to one partner only, but this can be negotiated. Therefore, if your patient is planning a hospital birth, make sure she makes prior arrangements to have the people of her choice accompany her.

Antenatal screening and medical prophylaxis options

In developed countries, women are generally offered routine screening in pregnancy. Deciding whether or not to have screening tests can be a difficult decision for a woman and is a subject she may want to discuss with her herbalist.

Pregnancy screening includes blood tests and ultrasound scans. It is standard practice to check if a woman's blood type is rhesus positive or rhesus negative. Fifteen percent of the population in the UK and Ireland have rhesus negative blood. If a woman is rhesus negative and her baby's father is rhesus positive, the risk of rhesus incompatibility problems rises with each successive pregnancy. If a rhesus negative mother carries a rhesus positive baby, their blood does not usually mix during pregnancy. However, during the process of pregnancy, labour and birth, a small amount of the baby's blood may enter the mother's bloodstream where it will be recognised as foreign and the mother's body will usually make anti-D antibodies against the foreign cells. The mother's blood is then described as 'sensitised'.

Sensitisation is rarely seen with a first baby, although it may occur if there has been a previous miscarriage, a termination, or a mis-matched transfusion. Once a woman has anti-D antibodies in her bloodstream, any subsequent rhesus positive baby will be at risk of an immune attack from these antibodies since they can cross the placental membrane and may cause haemolytic disease of the foetus and newborn. This can result in problems for the baby varying from mild jaundice to death.

A woman with rhesus negative blood who gives birth to a rhesus positive baby is generally given an injection of anti-D (a manufactured blood product) within 72 hours of giving birth or after any traumatising event during pregnancy (such as bleeding episode, pelvic injury, or amniocentesis), where the two bloodstreams may have mixed. This neutralises any rhesus positive antigens that have entered the mother's blood during pregnancy.

Rhesus negative women in the UK are currently offered routine antenatal anti-D prophylaxis (RAADP), either in one dose between 28–30 weeks of pregnancy or in a 2-dose treatment received during week 28 and week 34. The offering of one or two doses depends on the policy of the local hospital trust. Some midwives do not advise women to accept anti-D prenatally, unless there has been a traumatising event.[2]

Ultrasound uses high frequency sound waves rather than ionizing radiation like X-rays. However, research into its safety has been limited and while in the short-term, no problems have been detected for children exposed during pregnancy and labour, we actually have no idea of its long term effects. Many women are happy to have ultrasound scans, especially when offered the excitement or reassurance of seeing a picture of their baby. However, it would be wise to avoid excessive exposure to ultrasound and it is best reserved for use when there are medical indications. It can be useful to diagnose if the foetus is alive, accurate dating if this is uncertain, how many babies there are, the location of the placenta, the position of the baby and to assess how the baby is growing. In the UK, a first scan for gestational age is usually done between weeks 10–14 with a follow-up scan at 18–20 weeks for structural anomalies.

Additional screening tests may be offered. The following are the most common:

Chorionic villus sampling (CVS)	Carried out between weeks 10–13. Used to detect chromosomal abnormalities such as Down syndrome. A sample of chorionic villus (placental) tissue is extracted by inserting a needle either through the abdominal wall or the cervix. There is around 4% chance of miscarriage being caused and rarely damage to arms, legs, fingers, and toes of the embryo. CVS can provide a quick and early diagnosis but there are risks to the embryo and the test cannot detect all the problems that can be picked up by amniocentesis.
Amniocentesis	Carried out after week 15. Used to detect chromosomal abnormalities and neural tube defects such as Down syndrome, spina bifida, cystic fibrosis, sickle cell anaemia, and anencephaly. It can be used to determine lung maturity if a woman goes into premature labour. A needle is used to extract a sample of amniotic fluid from the amniotic sac. There is around 1.5% chance of foetal damage or miscarriage.
Alpha-fetoprotein (AFP)	Carried out at week 16. A blood test used to indicate the *possibility* of a foetus being affected by spina bifida or anencephaly. If AFP screening indicates a possible abnormality then usually the woman will be offered follow-up amniocentesis or ultrasound. Sometimes the foetus is completely healthy. This is not a harmful test, but there is a high rate of false positives. In diabetic women, this test is more likely to give an inaccurate result than in non-diabetic women, so, it is helpful if a woman knows this in advance.

Each woman will have her own feelings about screening. It can help to weigh up risk versus benefit, bearing in mind that screening tests may not be of value unless the woman is willing to have a termination if a test indicates anomalies. Otherwise, receiving a worrying result will not necessarily help but will very likely make for a stressful pregnancy.

In-vitro fertilisation (IVF) and other assisted pregnancies

The field of IVF and assisted pregnancy is a vast area of which a full discussion is beyond the scope of this book. Reproductive technologies have been linked with a range of problems in children, from birth defects to childhood leukaemia, as well as health issues for the mother ranging from ectopic pregnancy to increased risk of ovarian cancer. With a lack of long-term studies it is impossible to have a clear view of the risks.

In my experience, an assisted pregnancy raises potential areas of concern for both mother and child. Every woman needs to be assessed individually but key areas for a herbalist to consider in the mother are possible liver dysfunction, thought to be due to elevated oestrogen concentrations as well as circulatory dysfunction, both of which may impact upon a pregnancy. In most cases, full restorative treatment will need to be postponed until after lactation.

Pregnancy as a rite of passage—the journey to motherhood

Pregnancy and birth, however common, are awesome and wondrous events. A woman's body has the capacity to receive another being and birth it into the world. Together with menarche and menopause, childbearing is considered one of the traditional women's blood mysteries, a biological turning point and a major initiation for a woman. The womb is considered a sacred temple and giving birth an important rite of passage, the significance of which is rarely recognised in today's society. Pregnancy is a liminal phase when a woman can more easily encounter and identify with the Sacred Feminine within herself, sometimes spontaneously and perhaps for the first time in her life. Doing so can bring enormous strength, healing, and personal growth. Many women find that connecting with the archetype of the Goddess or the Divine Feminine helps them to experience the sacredness of pregnancy and birth, assisting them to see their body as a temple and ultimately in seeing their entire life as sacred.

Whether a woman has one child or several, each experience of birth is a new initiation, a new way of being in the world. Life will never be the same again. Acknowledging this transformative rite of passage helps link a mother to her new status, her community, her spiritual life. When this is overlooked, not only can it undermine the woman, it can lead on to conditions, such as postpartum depression (see Chapter 13 'Postpartum Care'). As herbal practitioners, we have the opportunity to hold a space for a woman to explore her journey to motherhood and welcome this new aspect of herself. This journey will mean different things to different women, but simply by acknowledging pregnancy as a rite of passage, mothers are facilitated in making the most of their personal process, not just as a means to an end (the birth of their baby) but as an opportunity for growth, learning, and self-development. By receiving appropriate support at this transitional time, women gain strength and empowerment from their experience, learning to trust their bodies and enhancing their spiritual awareness.

One way of acknowledging this rite of passage is by holding a blessing ceremony for the pregnant woman. This can be carried out with the intention of honouring and welcoming the woman's inner mother, nurturing her, and celebrating motherhood. It can be a private ceremony carried out alone, or a group event with a circle of trusted friends or family (usually women).

Another option is for the pregnant woman to connect with her inner Sacred Mother through a guided visualisation, such as the one below. This can be repeated as often as the woman chooses, helping her to get to know her inner mother and step fully into her new role.

Guided visualisation to connect with your inner Sacred Mother/ Mother Goddess

Dedicate a pink candle to your inner Sacred Mother. Place this in a candle holder.

Find a time and place where you will not be disturbed.

Light your candle, asking to meet your inner Sacred Mother. Place the candle in a safe place near to you.

Sit or lie comfortably with your spine straight.

Close your eyes and take a deep breath in through your nose, releasing the breath through your mouth.

Take another deep breath, and as you release it, feel all the tension leaving your body.

Take another breath and as you exhale, allow yourself to relax deeply.

Now find the place inside yourself where your Sacred Mother lives. Does she live at the bottom of a lake or beneath the sea? In a cave? Or a tree? Or a special place in nature? Does she live in your womb? Your heart? Or your head?

Once you have an image, sense, or feeling of where she is, go there and familiarise yourself with the surroundings. Use all your senses to experience this place. What are the colours? The smells? The sounds? Textures?

Once you are familiar with the surroundings you are ready to meet your inner Sacred Mother and she appears before you.

Look into her eyes and feel her loving gaze.

Ask her whatever question/s you need to ask.

She responds and you thank her.

She tells you to come back at any time. She is always here within you and you are always welcome.

> She holds you in a warm embrace and you feel the nourishment flowing from her body to yours. Breathe in this nourishing vibration and let it anchor in your body.
> Open your eyes, coming back to your ordinary reality strengthened and restored.
>
> Give thanks for the Sacred Mother/Mother Goddess within you.
> Blow out the candle, knowing that the flame of your inner Sacred Mother's heart continues to burn on the inner planes and she is always within you.
> Light the candle daily or whenever you want to consciously connect.[3]

Notes

1. Doula UK, https://doula.org.uk/ [last accessed 12/2/20]. Doula Association of Ireland, https://doula.ie/ [last accessed 12/2/20].
2. Ina May Gaskin, *Ina May's Guide to Childbirth*. (London: Vermilion, 2019), 200.
3. Meditation inspired by 'Connecting with your Inner Sophia'. Amy Sophia Marashinsky, *The Goddess Oracle*, (Stamford, CT USA, U.S. Games Systems, inc., 2006) 159.

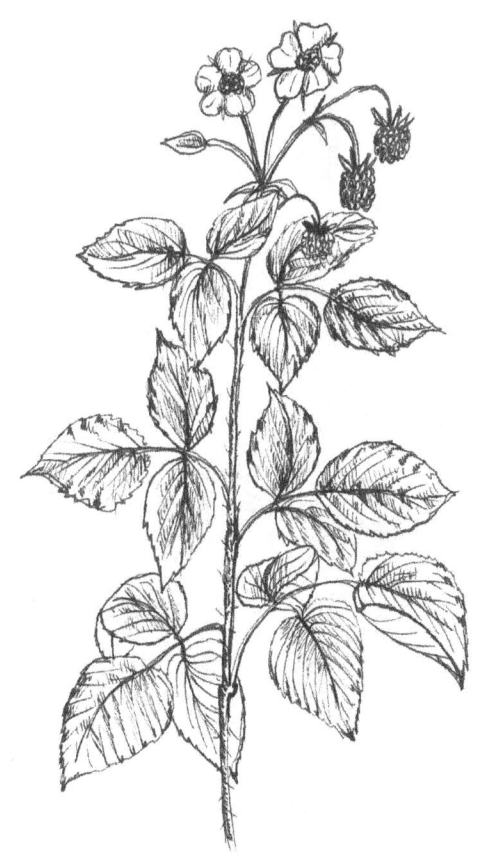

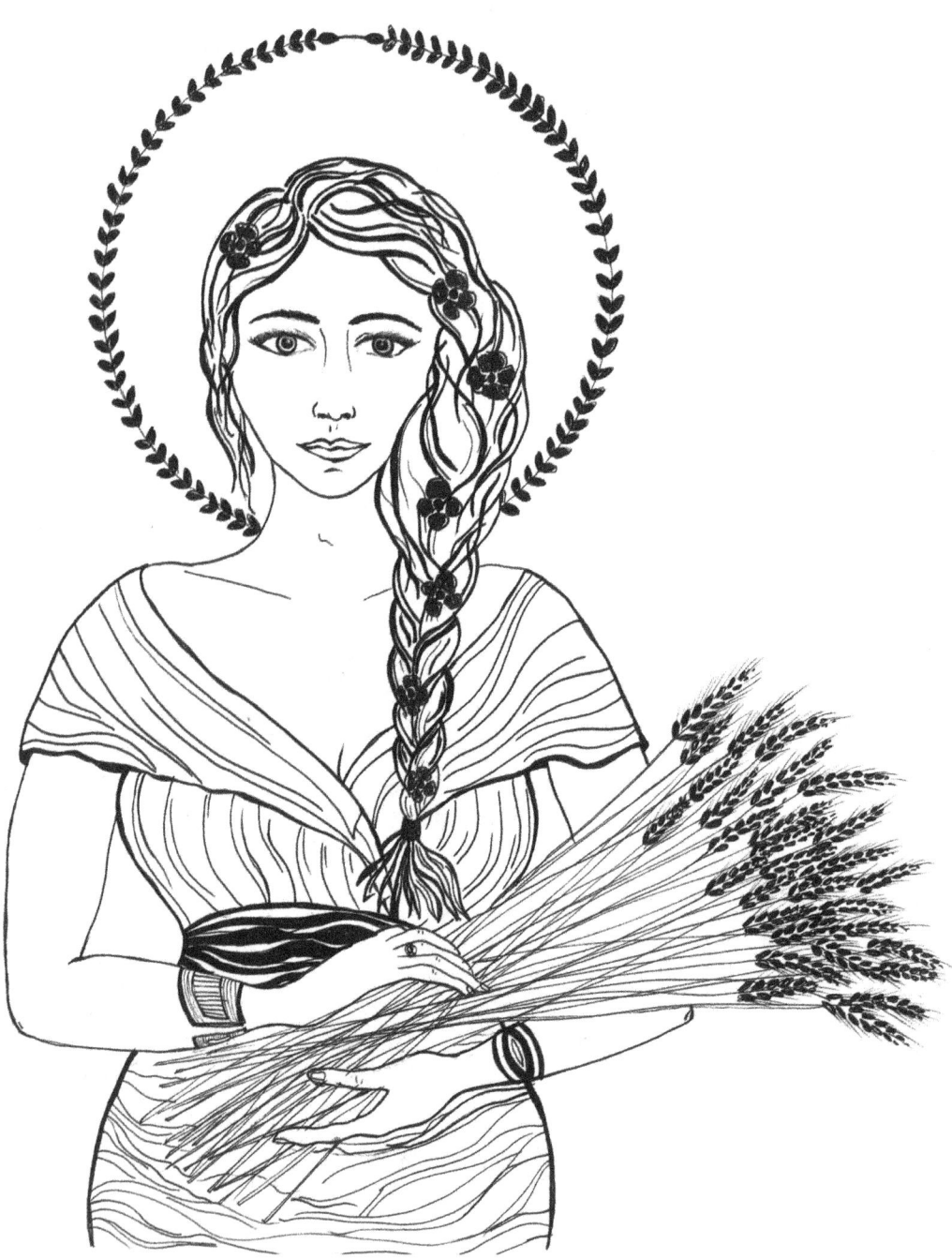

Demeter. Great Mother Goddess of fruitfulness, hope and the seed of joy.
Oats (*Avena sativa*). The great restorer who feeds the soul.

CHAPTER 3

Nutrition

Healthy eating in pregnancy

One of the most important ways to ensure a healthy pregnancy and prevent complications is to eat a nutritious diet. Good nutrition protects against many potential problems, such as anaemia, infection, pre-eclampsia, premature birth, and infant mortality, to name only a few. It helps to ensure the birth of a strong and healthy baby, whilst also laying a foundation to support a mother during breastfeeding and the precious early years of her child's life.

A healthy diet for pregnancy is made up of a varied mix of natural, nutrient-dense, preferably organic foods. In particular, pregnant women need plenty of calcium, protein, and iron in their diets, as well as essential fatty acids. Ideally, the bulk of the protein should come from fish, grains, nuts, seeds, and pulses rather than meat and dairy products. Fresh foods should be of the highest quality, organic whenever possible, or at least avoiding the 'dirty dozen' most contaminated foods, which can be found on a list released annually.[1,2] Sugar and other refined and processed foods should be avoided, along with alcohol, coffee (see 'Caffeine' below), and fizzy drinks. A comprehensive list of **Essential Nutrients in Pregnancy** can be found on pages 35–39.

Milk and dairy

For pregnant women who can digest dairy and are not allergic to it, moderate amounts of live yogurt and hard cheese can provide an easily prepared source of protein and other nutrients, particularly when produced from goat, sheep, or other non-cow dairy. I do not recommend drinking large amounts of cow's milk during pregnancy. As well as being mucus-forming and high in fat, it may also contain hormones (both naturally occurring and added with cattle feeds) plus other undesirable additives. A high consumption of cow's milk may result in excessive weight gain in the mother and this can be a disadvantage during childbirth. In herbal practice, I have seen several cases of pregnant women who consumed a large amount of milk during their pregnancies and whose children subsequently developed allergies to dairy products. While unproven, I suspect the excessive milk consumption to have been a probable causative factor.

Food allergy

All kinds of food-related patterns can originate during foetal development ranging from food preferences and sensitivities to the quality of fat cells. Pregnant women should avoid consuming any foods to which they are allergic, at the same time ensuring they are getting all their required nutrients. Sometimes the hormonal and metabolic changes of pregnancy can create new food allergies or expose pre-existing but unrecognised sensitivities. This is not the time for desensitizing programs or extreme elimination diets but it can be necessary and entirely beneficial to identify key allergens and eliminate them from the diet. It may be useful to suggest the woman keeps a food and symptom diary in order to identify suspect foods and to help track the nutrient content of her diet.

Vegetarians and vegans

Meat and dairy products are certainly not required for a healthy pregnancy, as long as a woman gets adequate nutrients from alternative sources. As well as protein, meat provides easily absorbable minerals, such as iron and zinc. Vegetarians need to ensure they are eating a nutrient rich diet that covers all the dietary requirements of pregnancy (see page 35).

Vegans need to watch their diets more carefully, especially with regard to protein, calcium, iron, vitamin B12, and vitamin D.

In pregnancy, a daily healthy vegan diet could include:[3]

> 7 servings of vegetables
> 6–11 servings of whole grains (rice, corn, wheat, millet, oats, rye, barley, and so on)
> 4 servings of cooked dried beans, peas, pulses, nuts, seeds or soya
> 3 servings of fruit
> 4 servings of calcium rich foods (see page 37)
> A source of vitamin B12 (see **Supplements** below)
>
>> *One serving* is equal to:
>> Vegetables: 75g raw, leafy greens; 100g other vegetables; 150ml tomato or vegetable juice

Grains: 1 slice bread; 25g dry cereal; 50–100g cooked cereal, rice or pasta; 100g nuts or cooked dried beans or peas, 140g tofu
Fruit: 1 medium apple, orange, banana, peach, etc.; 2 kiwis; 1 cup grapes, raspberries etc.

Vegans need to take a variety of plant proteins over the course of a day in order to ensure they are receiving the full range of the nine essential amino acids that make up complete proteins. Quinoa and chia seeds provide complete proteins, but most other vegan protein sources need to be combined, for example grains with beans or pulses, nuts or seeds with beans or pulses. Therefore, it is essential for vegans to eat a wide variety of foods. It has been shown that pregnant women on a vegan diet are at higher risk of protein deficiency, especially in the second and third trimester.[4] As well as paying attention to a healthy combination of foods, deficiency can be avoided by including additional protein in the diet, for instance 25g extra protein could be added by including 1.5 cups of lentils or 2.5 cups of soya milk daily.

Supplements (see also 'Essential Nutrients in Pregnancy', page 35)

All women are advised to take supplements of folic acid for the first twelve weeks of pregnancy to help reduce the risk of their child having a neural tube defect. Current UK government advice recommends additional thiamin and riboflavin in the last trimester and a daily supplement of vitamin D from October to March for those living at UK latitudes.[5]

In general, European and American recommended daily allowances (RNIs in the UK, RDAs in the US) tend to be low, more designed to prevent severe nutritional deficiency rather than to ensure optimum health. Together with eating the best possible diet, I often recommend pregnant women take a daily multivitamin and mineral supplement specially formulated for pregnancy and breastfeeding. A minimum requirement in a pregnancy multivitamin and mineral includes 400mcg folic acid as part of the B Complex (including B12, which is essential for vegans), zinc, vitamin C, magnesium, calcium, selenium, vitamin E, and vitamin D. See pages 35–39 for appropriate values of each nutrient. Individual formulations vary and may contain additional ingredients. The multivitamin and mineral should be combined with an essential fatty acid (Omega-3) formula providing around 400mg EPA and 200mg DHA. There are many well balanced products available, for instance, Lambert's *StrongStart for Women*, which consists of a vitamin and mineral tablet together with an omega-3 capsule and can be taken throughout pregnancy and lactation.

One precaution for supplements is to check they do not contain more than 5,000 ius or 1,500mcg of retinol, the animal form of vitamin A, since high amounts can build up in the body and may be harmful to the developing baby. Beta-carotene, a pre-cursor of vitamin A, has no such caution.

Weight gain

During pregnancy, the body becomes more efficient at absorbing energy and nutrients from the diet, for instance, the absorption of dietary calcium increases to around seventy percent of the calcium ingested, compared to the usual twenty-five percent. In the first two trimesters a woman can gain weight without increasing her food intake. For an average-weight woman, 200–300 extra calories daily are required in the third trimester. This increases to an average 500 extra calories daily while breastfeeding.

A healthy weight gain for an average weight woman lies between 11.5–16kg/25–35lb, less for an obese woman and more if underweight. Usually the appetite increases naturally, although for some women it can be normal to have a reduced appetite in the first trimester. The body of a pregnant woman will naturally build up extra fat reserves to provide a vital store of energy for breastfeeding (see Chapter 14 Lactation).

Living in a culture that equates beauty with thinness can make weight gain a challenging issue for many women and it is crucial that a woman does not limit her intake of nutrients. I encourage women to listen to their body, pay attention to signs of hunger, and learn to choose healthy foods. Where a woman is unused to doing this, for example someone with a history of an eating disorder, it can be helpful to suggest they keep a food diary of everything they eat and drink and we review this together at a consultation. Doing this increases their awareness and also provides a clear picture in order to offer guidance. Pregnancy is a time of building and nourishing. The quality of food eaten is the most important factor. If a woman is underweight, she should consume more high-calorie, nutrient-dense foods, such as fresh nuts and seeds and healthy fats.

Practitioners need to be alert to any sudden excessive weight gain after week 24, which can signal pre-eclampsia.

Cravings

In the first trimester, cravings and food aversions tend to go hand in hand. There is a widely held belief that cravings represent something a woman needs. While this can certainly be true, for instance indicating a need for green vegetables or protein, a craving can also result from sugar or carbohydrate addiction, or a woman may simply feel excessively tired and crave unhelpful stimulants like high sugar foods or coffee to provide a short-term energy lift. In these latter cases it can be helpful to advise a woman to carry healthy snacks with her such as seeds, nuts, vegetable sticks, rice cakes, hummus, or a nutritious high-protein, low-sugar energy bar.

Water

It is essential to drink plenty of water during pregnancy. Individual requirements can vary but for most women I recommend at least two litres per day, which can be taken as plain water, herb or fruit teas, diluted juices, or in other appropriate forms. For breastfeeding mothers this may need to increase to three litres or more. Some women find it a helpful reminder if they fill a large bottle (avoiding plastic) in the morning and sip it all day long. Use a high-quality water filter if using a mains water supply.

Salt

Salt should not be restricted (unless contraindicated due to kidney or heart disease). Salt is essential to maintain an expanded blood volume and to ensure sufficient placental blood supply, as well as to prevent dehydration and shock from blood loss at birth. A low salt intake has been linked to pre-eclampsia, eclampsia, miscarriage, and other complications of pregnancy.

Additional foods and substances to avoid

Tobacco and other drugs such as psychostimulants and opioids are all associated with severe risks to the health and development of the foetus and should not be used during pregnancy.

Caffeine consumed in excess amounts is linked to risk of miscarriage, low birth weight, and risk of health problems in later life. Caffeine is broken down in the liver three times more slowly than usual during pregnancy. It also reduces the absorption of nutrients and can cause the body to excrete calcium. It is best avoided altogether but at the very least limited to a maximum of 200mg daily. Approximate values in food and drinks: One mug instant coffee: 100mg, One mug filter coffee: 140mg, one mug tea 75mg (green tea can contain same amount as regular tea), one 50g bar plain chocolate: 25mg, one 50g bar milk chocolate: 10mg.

As much as possible, pregnant women should avoid exposure to household, cosmetic, industrial, and agricultural chemicals, as well as avoiding plastic food wrapping and storage containers, especially steering clear of cheese and fatty foods wrapped in cling film.

With regard to preventing infection, **basic food hygiene** is perhaps the most important factor of all. In general, the following advice may be useful:

- Wash and dry hands before and after handling meat.
- Do not use the same chopping board or utensils for uncooked meat as for fruit, vegetables, or bread.
- Surfaces and utensils should be washed thoroughly after preparing raw meat.
- Put food in the fridge as quickly as possible.
- Raw or defrosting meat should be placed on lowest shelf of refrigerator to avoid contamination of other foods.
- Cooked and uncooked meats should be covered and stored separately.
- Fruit, vegetables, and salads should be washed thoroughly before eating.
- Sprouted or green potatoes should not be eaten due to risk of solanine toxicity.

Certain other foods are often recommended to be avoided in pregnancy as they may harm the foetus or mother. Sometimes this knowledge can cause high anxiety in a pregnant woman, especially if she inadvertently eats one of the suspect foods. It is important to view the information in perspective and realise that some of the risks are exceedingly low, even if potentially serious. For some of the foods listed, other countries take a more relaxed approach, for instance in the cases of soft cheeses and pâté, which in France are regularly eaten throughout pregnancy.

Foods to avoid or take care with include:

Unpasteurised milks due to risk of bacterial infection. Milks should be pasteurised, sterilised, or UHT (ultra-heat treated). Unpasteurised milk can be boiled. Unpasteurised goat's or ewe's milk can carry toxoplasmosis-causing parasites. Toxoplasmosis rarely causes problems but if contracted for the first time in pregnancy, or a few months prior to conception, there is a slight risk that the infection can cause miscarriage, stillbirth, birth defects, or problems after the baby is born.

Certain soft and blue cheeses including mould-ripened soft cheeses (with a white rind) such as camembert, brie, and chèvre, as well as danish blue, gorgonzola, and roquefort due to a risk (low) of listeria, which can lead to miscarriage, stillbirth, or illness in newborn infants. Soft cheeses from pasteurised milk that are not mould-ripened are fine to eat, including cottage cheese, feta, ricotta, mozzarella, cream cheese, paneer, and halloumi. All hard cheeses are considered safe, including parmesan made with unpasteurised milk. This is due to the lower water content in hard cheese, making it less likely for bacteria to grow. All cheeses should be safe if they are thoroughly cooked.

Raw or partially cooked eggs due to a risk of salmonella infection, which can cause severe vomiting and diarrhoea in a pregnant woman. It is unlikely to damage a foetus. Fresh eggs from a reliable source can be considered safe. Otherwise, eggs should be cooked until whites and yolks are solid. Discard cracked eggs. Avoid foods containing raw egg such as homemade mayonnaise, chocolate mousse, and tiramisu. In the UK, Lion Code eggs (red lion logo stamped on their shell) are considered safe to be eaten raw by pregnant women.

Pâté due to a risk (low) of listeria. This is for all types, including vegetarian pâté.

Cooked and chilled poultry, ready meals due to a risk of listeria and salmonella. These foods must be heated thoroughly until piping hot.

Raw or under-cooked meats due to a risk of toxoplasmosis and salmonella. Meat and poultry must be defrosted thoroughly before cooking and cooked until the juices run clear. Avoid raw meats such as steak tartare or rare steak. Exercise caution with cold, cured, or fermented meats such as salami, prosciutto, chorizo, and pepperoni due to the risk (low) of toxoplasmosis. Cured or fermented meats can be frozen for four days before eating to reduce risk of parasites.

Game due to the risk of lead toxicity if the bird was shot with lead pellets.

Shellfish and raw fish due to a risk of bacterial or viral food poisoning from raw shellfish unless they are totally fresh and come from a reputable supplier. Cooked shellfish is fine. Raw wild fish comes with a risk of parasites, such as those found in some sushi, and should be frozen before eating.

Other fish, shark, swordfish, or marlin should not be eaten in pregnancy because of the risk of mercury toxicity, causing harm to the foetus. Tuna should also be limited to one 150g cooked weight fresh tuna steak or two 240g cans (140g drained weight) per week, due to the risk of mercury toxicity.

Liver including liver sausage, haggis, and liver pâté should only be eaten in moderation and not at all in first twelve weeks because of the risk (very low) of vitamin A overdose causing harm to foetus.

Peanuts (monkeynuts, groundnuts) carry a risk (speculated) of harm to foetus. The use of peanuts in a wide variety of convenience foods has been speculatively linked to the sharp increase in the number of children developing peanut allergies and anaphylactic responses. It is a possibility that a foetus could become sensitised to peanuts while in the womb and although there is no clear evidence to support this, it may be prudent to avoid peanut-based foods during pregnancy, especially in women with a history of food sensitivities or atopic illness.

Soft-serve ice cream carries a risk of food poisoning due to poor hygiene practices.

Essential nutrients in pregnancy

Iron—RNI (Reference Nutrient Intake[6]) 15mg (World Health Organisation recommends 30–60mg daily during pregnancy)
Iron is essential for blood formation. In the past, iron supplements were given routinely to pregnant women but it is now recognized that there is no evidence to recommend this unless a woman is already anaemic. Supplemental iron needs to be taken on an empty stomach and with vitamin C to improve absorption. Organic supplements are best. 10mg is a moderate dose to take as a supplement. See 'Anaemia' page 106.

Good sources of iron are meat and fish. Vegetable sources include bread, pulses, green leafy vegetables, nuts, seeds, and dried fruits.

Folic acid (folate, vitamin B9)—RNI 600mcg (first trimester), 300mcg (second and third trimesters)
Folic acid halves the risk of neural tube defects, such as spina bifida, and should be supplemented in pregnancy at 400mcg daily. It is best taken together with other B-complex vitamins which are crucial for the developing brain and nervous system. Choose a high strength multivitamin containing all the B vitamins, including 400mcg folic acid, around 6mcg of B12, and up to 50mg of most of the others.

Good sources of B vitamins are green leafy vegetables especially brassicas, asparagus, mushrooms, tomatoes, strawberries, and whole-wheat. Vitamin B12 is difficult to absorb from plants. Best sources are meat, dairy, and fish. B12 is also found in eggs, fortified cereals, and marmite.

Vitamin D—RNI 10–20mcg
Vitamin D is vital for the formation of bones and teeth through its role in aiding calcium absorption. It is also important for the immune system. In recent years, widespread vitamin D deficiency has been found in Ireland. Vitamin D is manufactured in the body

from exposure to sunlight. Current UK guidelines recommend supplementing around 10mcg (400 ius) daily in pregnancy. Higher levels may be appropriate in winter.

Good food sources are fatty fish, such as tuna, mackerel, and salmon, also egg yolks as well as certain fortified foods, like soya milk and cereals.

Vitamin A—RNI 700mcg
An antioxidant that is important for foetal lung and kidney development; vitamin A supplements should be no more than 5000 ius or 1.5mg daily. Beta-carotene is a safe alternative. Best sources are all yellow/orange foods and dark green fruits and vegetables. Diabetics may have trouble converting beta-carotene to vitamin A.

Vitamin C—RNI 40mg (50mg in last trimester)
Vitamin C is a powerful antioxidant with numerous important functions, including collagen formation, strengthening arteries, building white blood cells, and healthy bones. 1–2g daily can safely be taken during pregnancy. Vitamin C is best taken with bioflavonoids and can reduce the risks of pre-eclampsia and varicose veins. It should not be given to patients with haemachromatosis. Best sources are fresh fruits and vegetables. Destroyed by storage and cooking.

Vitamin E
Another valuable antioxidant that may help protect against miscarriage and pre-eclampsia. Supplement up to 400ius/270mg daily. Supplements must be d-alpha-tocopherol (known as *natural* or *natural source* vitamin E) rather than dl-alpha-tocopherol. Good sources include seeds, whole-grains and their cold-pressed oils, pulses, avocados, and olive oil. Caution in patients on warfarin or other blood thinning medication (suggested dose 100 ius).

Zinc—RNI 7mg (13mg for breastfeeding)
Zinc is a vital mineral for pregnancy, crucial for all cell growth and repair, working alongside vitamin B6. Deficiencies of zinc are linked to low birth weight babies, cleft palate, and hare lip. Supplement around 10–15mg daily, adding 1mg of copper for each 10mg of zinc, since these two minerals need to be in balance. Good sources are seeds, seafood, nuts, yeast, eggs, meat, peas, beans, and lentils.

Manganese
Helps form bone and cartilage. Supplement around 2mg daily. Good sources include whole grains, cereals, nuts, tropical fruits, blackberries, figs, and avocado.

Selenium—RNI 60mcg
Antioxidant mineral. Supports liver function. Supplement 50–100mcg daily. Toxic in excessive amounts. Good sources are seafood, brazil nuts, chicken, egg, pulses, and whole grains. Food values can be unreliable since a lot of our food is grown in soil depleted of selenium.

Magnesium

Magnesium has a role in more than 300 enzyme reactions in the body and plays a vital part in digestion, energy production, muscle contraction and relaxation, bone formation, and cell division. Known as 'nature's tranquilliser', it has a calming effect and can assist proper functioning of the heart, adrenals, kidneys, and nervous system. Magnesium can protect against pre-eclampsia, premature labour, and low birth weight babies. Supplement up to 300mg daily. Good sources include seeds (especially pumpkin seeds), nuts, peas, beans, and whole grains.

Many researchers and nutritionists now believe magnesium is more important than calcium in order to build and maintain healthy bones. In the past, most calcium and magnesium supplements contained a ratio of two parts calcium to one part magnesium based on the relative amounts of these nutrients used in the body. However, unlike calcium, which the body can store and recycle, magnesium must be replenished on a daily basis. Therefore, even though the daily need for calcium is greater, we are much more likely to become deficient in magnesium. Many nutritionists are now advising a ratio of one part calcium to two parts magnesium.

Calcium—RNI 700mg (800mg for pregnant teenagers)

As well as building bones and teeth, calcium promotes a healthy heart and nervous system and is needed for blood clotting. Calcium deficiency can predispose to pre-eclampsia.

As discussed earlier (page 32), recent research has shown that during pregnancy a woman's body absorbs dietary calcium at a much higher rate than before she was pregnant. Our bodies are truly amazing. As a result, there is not the increased requirement for calcium in the diet that was previously believed. However, it still means that women need to consume enough calcium to meet their baby's needs, but it may not be necessary to have extra during pregnancy. A good multivitamin and mineral supplement will contain calcium. Supplement around 150mg daily to achieve a balanced ratio with magnesium. Good sources–dairy products, fish with bones, nuts, seeds, poultry, almonds, and leafy green vegetables, as well as the many calcium-enriched foods available, such us calcium-enriched soya or rice milk, calcium-enriched soya yoghurt, and calcium-enriched tofu.

Cola-type drinks should be avoided. They contain excessive phosphorus, which can cause calcium to be excreted from the body and is thought to be linked to the rising incidence of osteoporosis in teenage girls.

Chromium

Chromium is vital to balance blood sugar levels, reduce cravings, and help maintain a healthy weight. Supplement 50–100mcg daily. Good sources—whole-wheat and rye, potatoes, chicken, eggs, honey, brown rice, raisins, and yeast. Caution in insulin dependent diabetics because chromium increases the effects of insulin.

Iodine—RNI 140mcg
Helps maintain thyroid function and a healthy metabolism. Rich in seafood and sea vegetables, especially kelp (granules can be cooked or sprinkled on savoury dishes). Supplement around 50mcg and obtain a further 100mcg from food.

Protein—RNI 0.75g per kg of bodyweight per day, plus an additional 6g per day for pregnant women
Proteins are the building blocks of life. Pregnant women should aim for three to four servings of protein daily, where one serving is equal to 85g meat or poultry, 100g fish, two eggs. 100g cooked dried, peas or beans, 100g nuts, 140g tofu, 100g cheese. Other good vegetarian sources include quinoa, shitake mushrooms, and brown rice.
 See page 30 for advice about combining plant proteins for vegans.

Complex carbohydrates and fibre
Fibre is crucial for a healthy digestive tract. Good sources are beans, pulses, peas, whole-grains, fruits, and vegetables.

Essential fatty acids
Essential fatty acids have a profound effect on every system of the body. They are vital for a healthy blood flow to the foetus and crucial for brain, eye, and nervous tissue development. Essential fats and related fats include linoleic acid (LA), gamma-linoleic acid (GLA), arachidonic acid (AA), eicosapentanoic acid (EPA), and decosahexanoic acid (DHA). Best sources are seeds, nuts, oily fish, and cold-pressed oils. A diet containing a variety of these foods can give a healthy balance of omega-3s, omega-6s, and omega-9s. Supplementation can be with an omega-3 fish oil capsule (1000–3000mg per day) or for vegetarians a tablespoon of ground flax seeds daily or flax seed capsules (1000–3000mg per day). It has been suggested that a diet high in omega-3 essential fatty acids in the third trimester helps prevent postpartum depression.

Antioxidants
Pregnant women should eat at least five portions of brightly coloured fruits and vegetables to protect mother and foetus from damaging free radicals. Citrus bioflavonoids can prevent miscarriage and premature labour. For some women, as well as a pregnancy multivitamin and mineral supplement and omega-3s, it may be appropriate to suggest an additional antioxidant formula, particularly for mothers over thirty years old or living in a polluted environment, highly stressed, or at high risk of pre-eclampsia.

Pre- and probiotics
The gut microbiome is crucial to both physical and mental health. Probiotics help ensure a healthy digestive tract, enhance immune function, and promote maternal and infant health. Good sources include live yogurt or fermented foods, such as sauerkraut, kimchi, and kefir.

Probiotics such as acidophilus can be taken as a supplement, in which case, they should be stored in the refrigerator and carry a guarantee of at least one billion viable organisms. Prebiotics help increase the probiotic bacteria. Prebiotic foods include onions, garlic, apple skins, leeks, cold potato, cold rice, and cider vinegar. Swedish bitters, Dandelion root and Yellow Dock can all help promote a healthy gut flora.

NOTE: all requirements increase when a woman is carrying two or more babies.

Notes

1. Pesticide Action Network UK, https://www.pan-uk.org/dirty-dozen/ [last accessed 20/7/21].
2. Environmental Working Group USA, https://www.ewg.org/foodnews/dirty-dozen.php [last accessed 14/2/20].
3. Suzannah Olivier. *Eating for a perfect pregnancy* (London: Pocket Books, 2001), 58.
4. Sebastiani, Giorgia, Ana Herranz Barbero, Cristina Borrás-Novell, Miguel Alsina Casanova, Victoria Aldecoa-Bilbao, Vicente Andreu-Fernández, Mireia Pascual Tutusaus, Silvia Ferrero Martínez, María Dolores Gómez Roig, and Oscar García-Algar. "The effects of vegetarian and vegan diet during pregnancy on the health of mothers and offspring." *Nutrients* 11, no. 3 (2019): 557. [last accessed 12/2/20].
5. British Nutrition Foundation www.nutrition.org.uk [last accessed 16/2/20].
6. Reference Nutrient Intakes (RNIs) are the estimated nutrient requirements for particular groups of the UK population. These originate from the Committee on Medical Aspects of Food and Nutrition Policy (COMA) who published their recommendations in 1991. COMA has since been superceded by the Scientific Advisory Committee on Nutrition (SACN) which is reviewing nutrients gradually, initially focusing on those about which there has been cause for concern, such as iron, folate, selenium and vitamin D, and has published reports on each of these. Although often similar, RNIs should not be confused with RDAs (Recommended Dietary Allowances). RDAs were developed by the US Food and Nutrition Board and are used primarily in the United States.

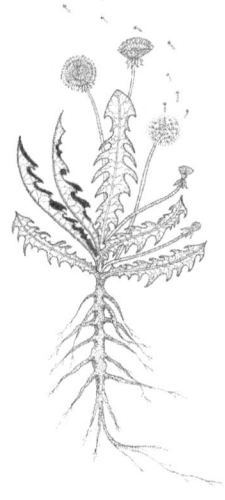

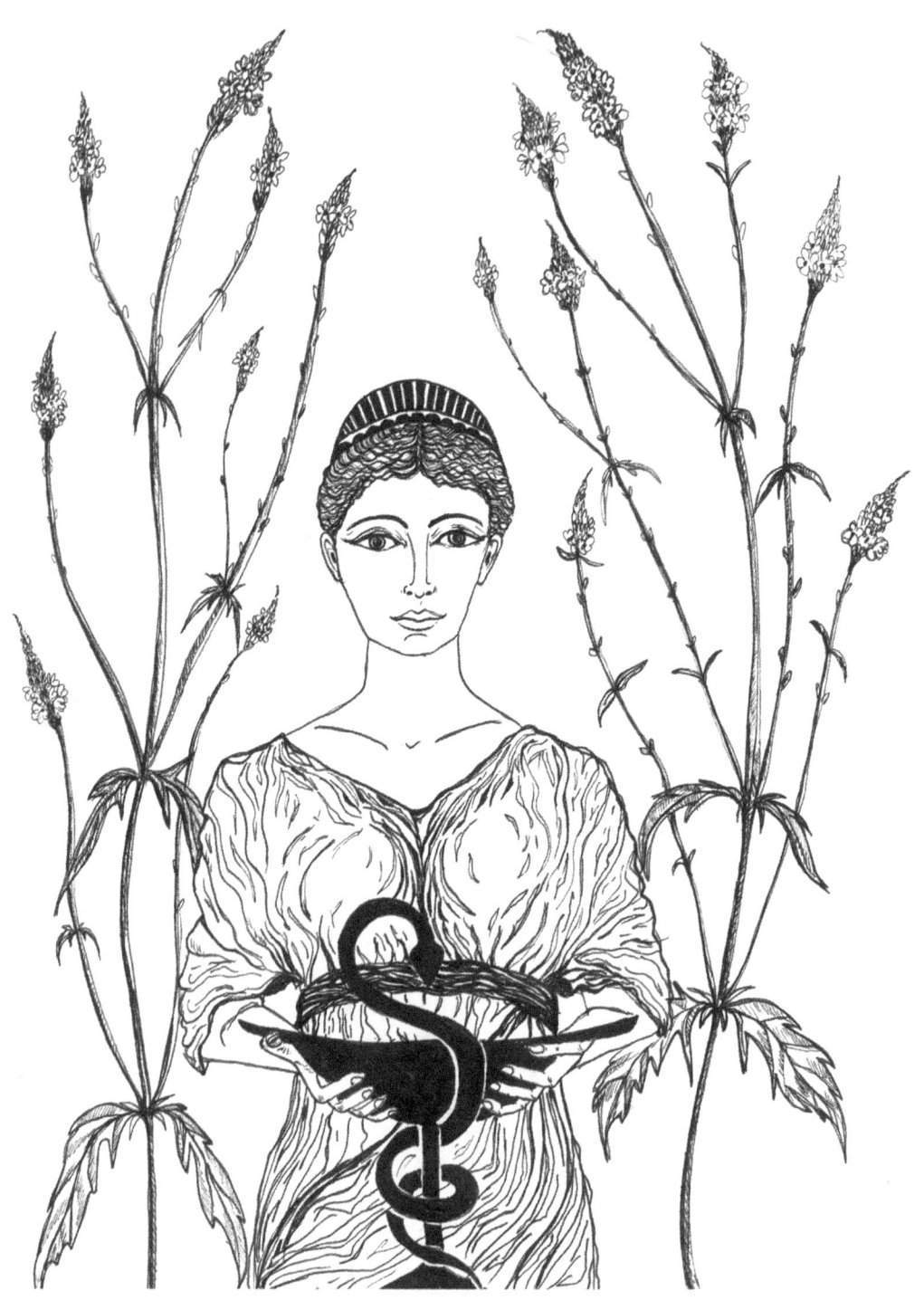

Hygeia. Goddess of good health, hygiene and preventative medicine
Vervain (*Verbena officinalis*). Magical herb of inspiration and grace.

CHAPTER 4

Exercise and lifestyle

Exercise

For a pregnant woman, exercise is as vital to health as at any other time of life. Exercise helps reduce the risk of many complications of pregnancy, including constipation, varicose veins, gestational diabetes,[1] and pre-eclampsia.[2] In addition, regular physical activity throughout pregnancy has a beneficial effect on the course and outcome of labour and delivery.

Walking in nature is one of the easiest ways for a pregnant woman to get fresh air and exercise, as well as an opportunity to connect with nature and tune into her own body. Other activities like swimming, dancing, Tai Chi, Qi Gong, and aqua aerobics can also be perfect, whatever a woman enjoys. Yoga may be particularly helpful, bringing both fitness and calmness, and offering specific exercises to relieve common discomforts of pregnancy and prepare for childbirth. Swimming or simply floating in water can be especially of benefit later in pregnancy. Some women enjoy using 'birthing balls', which can be utilised from around week 32 to help strengthen legs and open the hips, as well as providing a comfortable resting position during labour. Twenty to thirty minutes a day of moderate-intensity aerobic activity is a useful target. The key is for a woman to listen to her body. In the first trimester she may simply feel too exhausted to exercise.

It is best to avoid extreme workouts and any sports that risk a fall or a blow to the abdomen, such as skiing, horse riding, skating, or roller blading. A woman may also need to take extra care not to over-strain, for example while doing stretching exercises, weights, or aerobics. During pregnancy, the hormone relaxin relaxes smooth muscle, especially in the pelvic region, in order to allow more space and elasticity for childbirth and the growing foetus. This causes a softening of ligaments and joints, which allows the pelvis to open more easily but combined with the extra weight and body changes, may also lead to injury if a woman over-strains. For anyone not used to regular exercise, they should build up an exercise program slowly and gently. Care should be taken in women with a history of miscarriage, pre-term labour, pre-eclampsia, incompetent cervix, multiple foetuses, or a history of bleeding in pregnancy.

Pelvic floor exercises (Kegels)

Pregnancy can be a great opportunity for a woman to become familiar with and improve the health of her pelvic floor muscles. Not only can this assist her baby's delivery and prevent tearing of the perineum, it will be of lifelong benefit, both improving her sex life and preventing a whole range of female problems, such as uterine prolapse and urinary incontinence. When pelvic floor exercises are done properly and consistently, they work exceedingly well and it is of most benefit to start them during pregnancy rather than waiting until after delivery.

A simple exercise is to squeeze the vaginal muscles (the same muscles used to stop the stream of urine, although this is only some of them) and hold for a slow count of ten (ten seconds). Relax for a count of five, then repeat. Do five sets three times daily (more if a woman already has incontinence or prolapse problems). It can be helpful to do them routinely at particular times each day, for example standing at the sink, after urinating, on waking, and going to sleep. Results are usually noticeable in three to four weeks. The exercises will not work if the woman is contracting her abdominal, thigh or buttocks muscles at the same time as squeezing the vaginal area. She can check for herself by putting one or two fingers in her vagina as she squeezes. These are the only muscles that should be contracting.

Another exercise, often called the 'elevator', is to imagine the vagina as a lift shaft and gradually bring up a lift from the ground floor (the vaginal opening) to the fourth floor (high inside) simply by tightening the pelvic muscles. Then bring the lift down, floor by floor, going right down to the basement by totally relaxing the muscles. Do this ten times daily.

A variety of pelvic floor toners, probes, and other accessories are available for sale online.[3] Weighted vaginal cones can be inserted into the vagina, causing reflex muscle contraction to prevent them slipping out. Studies on the treatment of urinary incontinence have shown these to be equally as effective as pelvic floor exercises but cones have much lower patient compliance.[4] Belly dancing and regular squatting are two additional methods to strengthen the pelvic floor. If necessary, a physiotherapist can help with hands-on work, breathing and movement exercises. There are also a lot of pelvic floor apps that a woman can download to help remind her to do her pelvic floor exercises.

Sex

Sexual activity can provide another way to practice the tightening and releasing of these muscles. It is perfectly safe to have sexual intercourse while pregnant since the mucous plug protects the cervix. Some women find their libido increases at certain stages (typically the second trimester) or throughout their entire pregnancy, whereas others may lose interest in sex, especially in the first trimester. Equally, some men feel nervous having intercourse with a pregnant woman, fearing they may cause harm. Sexual activity can sometimes be used as a method to initiate labour (see page 202, Chapter 9).

Rest

It is normal to feel tired, sometimes extremely so, in early pregnancy. This is no surprise considering how much change, growth, and development is taking place. We should encourage women to listen to their bodies and rest as much as needed. The fatigue of early pregnancy usually lifts by week 15 and tiredness often recurs in the last few weeks before delivery. As a woman grows in size, it can be difficult to find a comfortable position lying down and she may find it helpful to use pillows to support her body. All sorts of shapes and sizes of maternity body pillows are commercially available, if required.

Relaxation

For many women, pregnancy is a time to reassess priorities and slow down. Rest periods can provide an ideal opportunity to learn (or be reminded of) how to relax and let go of mental stress and physical tension. This training comes in useful for the rest of a woman's life, as well as benefiting her pregnancy and birthing experience. Therefore, this can be a great time to initiate body/mind approaches and suggest appropriate relaxation exercises (for situations where a woman is affected by stress, see 'Stress-related conditions' page *120*). Depending on the individual patient and your own time and inclination, you might recommend relaxation classes (for instance, these are often combined with yoga for pregnancy) or give relaxation exercises directly to your patients. Some examples are listed below. These can be incorporated into a consultation and given on a printed handout for a patient to practice at home. They are also useful for patients with insomnia to use at night (see also 'Sleep Disorders' page *161*). Alternatively, a wide range of recorded exercises are available online or on CD. Relaxation exercises can be combined with music or the use of essential oils, such as in an oil burner. These body-mind associations can prove helpful for relaxation in childbirth, by using music or scents already associated with a relaxed state during pregnancy.

The first step to any relaxation exercise is to find a warm, comfortable place where the person will not be disturbed. They should empty their bladder and turn off their phone. All of these exercises can be done either lying down or sitting in a chair. For someone who finds it particularly difficult to settle, it can help to take a walk or do some other kind of physical exercise before trying to relax.

Focusing on the breath can be an easy way to relax. Moreover, generating a rhythmic breathing pattern causes cardiac coherence and creates physiological entrainment.[5] This promotes deep relaxation, as well as having other wide-ranging benefits for mind and body.[6] In the first exercise below, rhythm is the biggest priority and there needs to be a fixed ratio between the in-breath and the out-breath. This simple exercise brings increased calmness and builds confidence. By practising for ten minutes daily, physiological coherence can become a default pattern. Two minutes of rhythmic breathing may bring immediate relief in any situation of acute stress. To obtain most benefit, rhythm, smoothness, and location of attention are all important.

Rhythmic breathing

Close your eyes and take a deep breath in,
    breathing right down into your belly.
    Hold the breath for a moment.
    When you're ready, breathe out.
    Pause for a moment.
    Then, repeat by breathing in.
<u>Make your breathing rhythmic</u> so there is a fixed ratio of 2:1:2:1. For instance, breathe in for the count of two, hold for the count of one, breathe out for the count of two, hold for the count of one, then repeat OR breathe in for the count of six, hold for three, breathe out for six, hold for three, then repeat. Find the count that works for you. All that matters is that whatever count you choose, you maintain the ratio consistently.

While you do this, make your breathing as smooth as possible, aiming for an even rate of air flow. At the same time, focus your attention on your heart or the centre of your chest.

    Repeat for ten minutes daily, or as required.
    Come gently back to normal awareness.

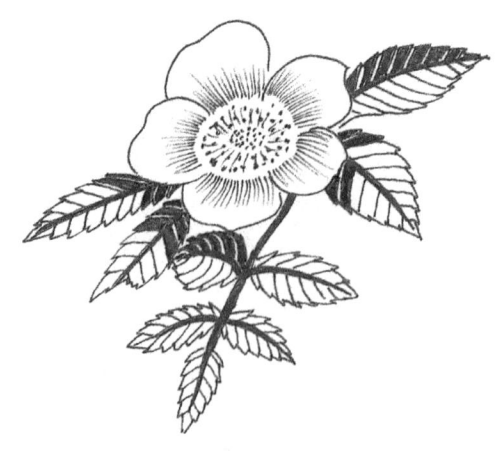

The next exercise makes use of progressive muscle relaxation, a widely used technique to increase bodily awareness and bring relaxation to the physical body, both of which are invaluable training for childbirth.

> **Progressive muscle relaxation**
>
> Close your eyes and take a few deep breaths and as you let out each breath, mentally say the word 'relax'. Continue doing this, observing your breath coming and going easily and gently.
>
> Now, take your attention to your toes. Wiggle them slightly and feel any tension they may be holding. On your next outbreath, relax your toes and feel all tension leaving them. Let the tension simply flow into the earth where it can be composted.
>
> Now, become aware of the rest of your feet and ankles, circle them around and notice any tension. On the next outbreath, let all the tension leave your feet and ankles and feel a wave of relaxation spreading through them. Your feet and ankles feel warm and relaxed.
>
> Move your attention up to your calves and lower legs, notice any tension, and then let it go. Feel a wave of relaxation spreading through your calves and lower legs.
>
> Now, move your attention to your knees. Notice any tension and then let it go, feeling relaxation spread through your knees.
>
> Move your attention to your thighs, notice any tension, let it go, and feel relaxation spreading through your thighs. Both your legs feel warm and relaxed.
>
> Work your way up through the rest of your body, repeating the previous instructions and consciously relaxing each part. Move up slowly through your pelvis and buttocks, your lower back, abdomen, upper back, and chest. Relax your shoulders and arms, elbows, and wrists, letting the tension flow down and out through your fingers. Relax your throat, neck and jaw, your cheeks and lips, and all the fine muscles around your eyes. Relax your eyebrows, forehead, scalp, and the top of your head.
>
> Enjoy this feeling of total body relaxation.
>
> If you notice your thoughts beginning to wander, gently bring them back to your body and the sensation of relaxation.
>
> Whenever you are ready, stretch your fingers and toes, and gently come back to normal awareness.

If preferred, this exercise can be done by starting at the head and working down to the feet.

Very often, a person will fall asleep before they get through the entire body. If they are still awake and would like to do more, the guided visualization below can be added at the end instead of coming straight back to normal awareness.

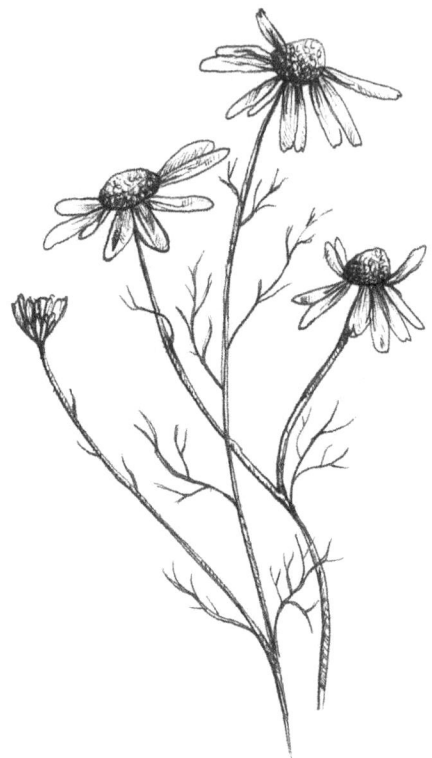

Pregnancy provides a great opportunity for a woman to tune in both to her own body as well as to the developing baby (technically an embryo at 3–8 weeks or foetus from 9 weeks until birth). The following exercise is helpful both for relaxation and to help a woman connect with her baby. It can be started at any time during the pregnancy and practised regularly. See also 'Stages of Pregnancy' page 51.

Guided visualization—connecting with one's baby

Take your attention to your breath as it comes in and out of your body.

Notice any areas of tension in your body and with each outbreath, let the tension release,

Allowing it to flow into the earth where it can be composted.

Become aware that with every in-breath you are bringing light and oxygen into your own body cells and into the baby.

Allow your body to become more and more relaxed and filled with light.

Take your awareness to the inside of your womb,

Imagine you are inside in the safety of your womb with the baby who is floating in warm amniotic fluid.

> Softly envelop and greet the baby in the reddish light of your womb.
> Feel the love you have for the baby and send loving thoughts to this perfect, delicate being.
> Allow yourself to be filled with awe and wonder at everything you see and hear in this magical place,
> The umbilical cord leading to the placenta,
> The beating of two hearts in rhythm.
> Your heart is filled with love and gratitude.
> Enfold the baby with your love,
> Knowing that he or she is held in safety and protection.
> Let your love extend to all your own body cells, your entire body.
> Simply rest in this peaceful place.
> If you have words you would like to speak to the baby, say them now.
> Take some time to enjoy this space together.
> When you are ready, bring your attention back to your breath.
> Prepare to return to ordinary reality,
> Knowing that you are in constant communication with your baby
> And can speak to them at any time.
> Stretch your fingers and toes and gently open your eyes.
> Write down any experiences you would like to record.

It is helpful to encourage a woman to connect as often as possible with her baby while in the womb, for instance by talking, singing, playing music, reading stories or poetry, or connecting by touch through their belly.

A wide range of recordings of relaxation exercises and guided meditations are available in books, CDs, and online.

Massage and essential oils

Having a massage can be a beautiful way to assist relaxation, as well as aiding the circulation, clearing congestion and stagnation, and toning muscles. This can be whole body massage, foot massage, or some other specific part of the body. Massage can help with a variety of problems including sleep issues and backache, and it is another way for a mother to connect with her own body and her baby. In many traditional cultures, a pregnant woman would receive massage as a central part of her prenatal care, often carried out by the midwife. In modern Western culture, gentle massage may be carried out by a practitioner, partner, or friend. Basic guidelines are to avoid the belly and lower back in the first trimester and avoid strong stimulation of heels, lower legs, and trapezoidal shoulder muscle in third trimester (may initiate contractions). Never massage varicosities and when massaging legs, always stroke upwards towards the heart.

As well as a component of massage oils, essential oils can be helpful in a wide variety of ways including diffusion and inhalation. See Chapter 1 for a list of essential oils used in obstetric care.

Herbal baths

Full body baths, footbaths, and handbaths are all effective methods to promote relaxation and they can be easily prepared by women at home with fresh or dried herbs. See Herbal Pharmacy page 59 and Chapters 8–15 for the treatment of specific conditions.

Notes

1. Yu, Ying, Rongrong Xie, Cainuo Shen, and Lianting Shu. "Effect of exercise during pregnancy to prevent gestational diabetes mellitus: a systematic review and meta-analysis." *The Journal of Maternal-Fetal & Neonatal Medicine* 31, no. 12 (2018): 1632–1637.
2. Chawla, Shalini, and Nick Anim-Nyame. "Advice on exercise for pregnant women with hypertensive disorders of pregnancy." *International Journal of Gynecology & Obstetrics* 128, no. 3 (2015): 275–279.
3. Kegel Exercises https://www.kegel8.co.uk/kegel8-pelvic-toners.html [last accessed 11/6/21].
4. Cammu, Hendrik, and Michelle Van Nylen. "Pelvic floor exercises versus vaginal weight cones in genuine stress incontinence." *European Journal of Obstetrics & Gynecology and Reproductive Biology* 77, no. 1 (1998): 89–93.
5. Dr Alan Watkins, *Coherence* (London: Kogan Page Ltd, 2014), 65.
6. See the work of the HeartMath Institute www.heartmath.org [last accessed 27/7/21].

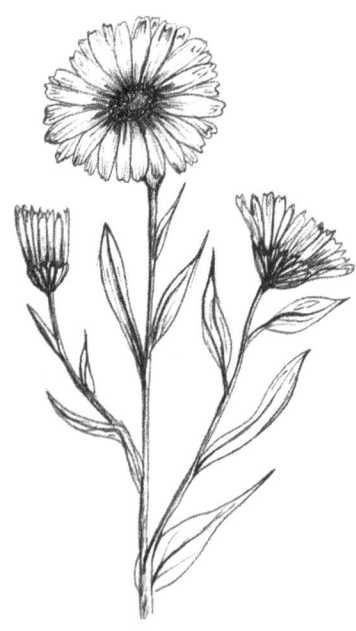

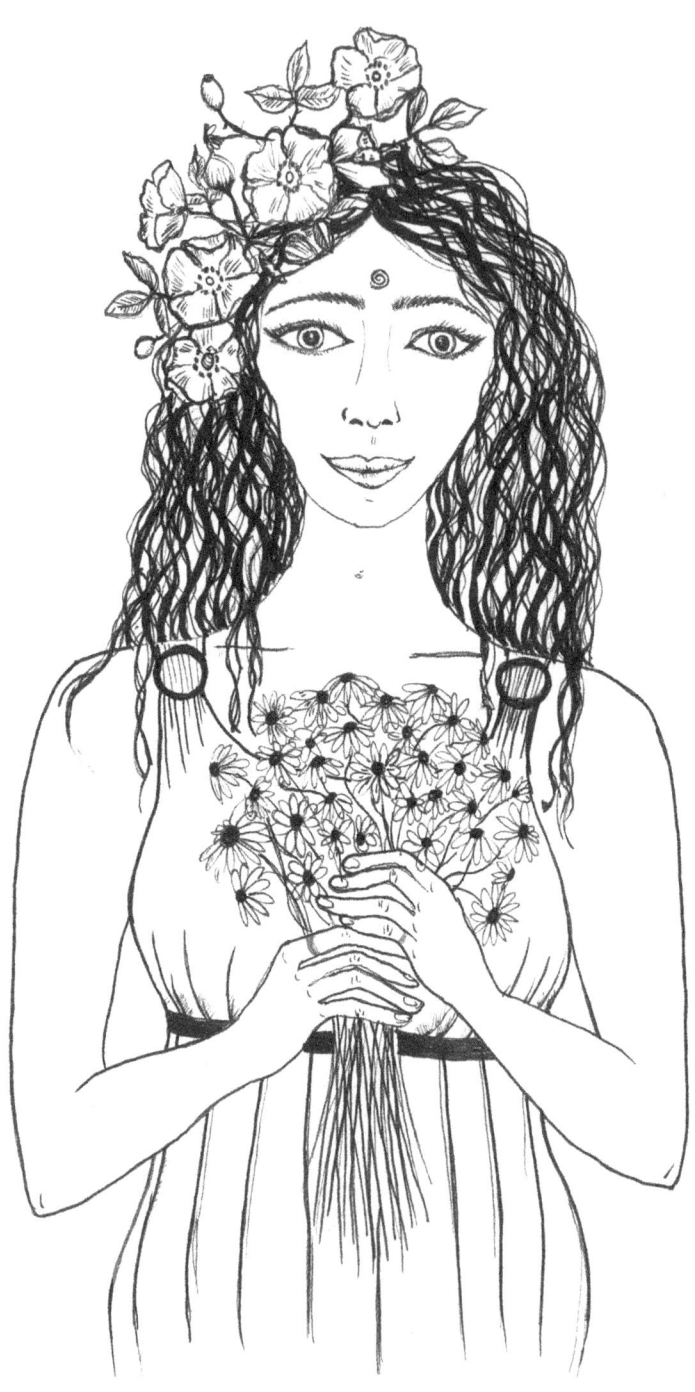

Flora. Goddess of flowers, new life and all growing things
Dog Rose (*Rosa canina*). Soother and protector of the heart. Brings unconditional love, joy, and beauty.
Daisy (*Bellis perennis*). Eases shock, brings joy and light.

CHAPTER 5

Stages of pregnancy

Conception

Conception is a magical and wondrous moment! The old stories say that the incoming soul hovers around the aura of the prospective mother for at least three months, sometimes years before conception. Sexual union is considered a powerful, sacred act and the woman's body is honoured as a representation of the Goddess. At the moment of conception, the vital essence of the mother and father unite and it is said that the etheric body[1] of the foetus is transferred to the mother, thereby setting the template for development of the physical body.

Biologically speaking, conception involves fertilsation and implantation of the embryo in the uterus. A mature egg is 0.2 mm in diameter and the largest cell in the human body. Female babies are born with up to two million eggs in their ovaries, reducing to a few hundred thousand by the time of a girl's menarche. With each menstrual cycle, usually a single egg ripens and is released at ovulation. Sperm, on the other hand, are much smaller, have a short life span and are created continuously from puberty to old age, hundreds every second. Two hundred to three hundred million will enter the vagina at ejaculation and an average three million of these will reach the uterus and fallopian tubes.

Fertilisation of the egg usually takes place in the fallopian tubes. This process is often portrayed as an army of sperm racing against each other to their target, with one triumphant winner who penetrates the egg. In fact, the latest embryological research shows conception as a beautiful collaboration between egg and sperm.[2] In a kind of reciprocal mating dance, the sperm are attracted by a mucus substance that both the egg and oviduct excrete. Hundreds of sperm cells arrive at the egg, arranging themselves around the zona pellucida (its protective coating). Substances secreted by the egg cause an acrosome reaction, where the sperm undergo physiological changes preparing them for fertilisation. There is no actual penetration by the sperm cell, instead the zona pellucida dissolves and the cell membranes of the egg and a single sperm merge. This union is followed by a time of stillness, after which the egg begins to vibrate and an 'activation' or 'ignition' takes place, which, if detected with fluorescence microscopy, appears much like a firework display.[3] What appears to happen is that calcium levels rise in the egg after merging with the sperm. The high calcium levels cause billions of zinc atoms to be released outside the egg and if these atoms are given a fluorescent tag they can be seen by human observers as a flash of light. The brighter the flash, the more viable the egg, a feature that is of interest to in vitro fertilization (IVF) researchers, since it may help them to select the optimum eggs for pregnancy. Of course, this is only one small part of the picture. Recent research suggests that bioelectric signalling may have an even more primary role than genetics and is an essential part of embryonic formation.[4]

As previously stated, this is a mysterious process! In the fertilised egg, the male and female aspects unite as one and a third point emerges into being. The egg becomes the zygote, a new organism in its own right, a unicellular manifestation of a human body.

The cells of the prospective embryo now divide rapidly, responding intelligently to their environment. This is the morula stage, a solid mass of cells that further divide to form a blastocyst made up of an inner group of cells with an outer shell. The new conceptus[5] floats gently down the fallopian tube and into the uterus for implantation. The blastocyst sends out a small gelatinous 'foot' to attach to the uterine wall. Once implanted, it releases human chorionic gonadotrophin (hCG), which enters the maternal circulation and supports the corpus luteum to produce the hormones crucial for pregnancy. At this point the woman's endocrine system is profoundly affected as mother and embryo become deeply entwined.

Human chorionic gonadotrophin can be detected in the urine as early as seven to nine days after fertilisation and is used as an indicator of pregnancy in most over-the-counter pregnancy tests. Rising levels of hCG are partly responsible for the urinary frequency of early pregnancy, since hCG causes increased elimination through the kidneys.

Implantation typically occurs around seven to fourteen days after having sex and approximately fifteen to twenty-five percent of women will experience some light implantation bleeding, which may be mistaken for a period but usually occurs earlier than menstruation is due. Implantation bleeding may involve minor spotting or it may start out pink and turn brown over one or two days. Other possible implantation symptoms include mild abdominal cramps, a prickly or tingling sensation in the abdomen, swollen breasts, swollen abdomen, and headaches.

Gestational age

Conventional practice is to measure gestational age (weeks of pregnancy) from the first day of a woman's last menstrual period, typically two weeks before fertilisation. Therefore, at ten weeks gestation the embryo is actually eight weeks old. The date of last menstruation is not always a reliable guide, especially for a woman with an irregular cycle. In many cases, a pregnant woman will have a clear sense of when she conceived.

Where dates are uncertain, an ultra-sound scan can be performed to establish gestational age. The earlier this is done (ideally between weeks 8 and 11), the more accurate it is at estimating dates. Ultrasounds performed during the first 12 weeks of pregnancy are generally within three to five days of accuracy, although this always depends upon the skill of the sonographer and quality of the equipment. Ultrasounds performed between 12 and 22 weeks are considered to be within ten days of accuracy and after this time they are generally unreliable for estimating gestational age. Examination by an experienced midwife can be a far more dependable option.

First trimester (weeks 1–12)

Pregnancy can be divided into three roughly equal time spans of three months each, called trimesters. The first trimester includes the embryonic stage and the first four weeks of foetal development.

What's happening in the body?

The embryonic stage makes up the first eight weeks of development. After implantation, the blastocyst rapidly develops into the embryo with an amniotic sac and its own support system, the placenta. By days eighteen to twenty-two after conception, the massive heart at the embryo's centre begins to beat and by eight weeks after conception the basic layout for the body is established.

During the early stages of pregnancy, the corpus luteum in the ovary is supported by hCG and continues to produce hormones, such as progesterone, oestrogens, and relaxin, all essential to support the pregnancy and to help establish the placenta.

Progesterone fulfils many vital functions at this stage:

- It promotes blood flow to the uterus by stimulating the growth of existing blood vessels.
- It stimulates glands in the endometrium to secrete nutrients that nourish the embryo.
- It stimulates growth and thickening of the endometrium to facilitate implantation.
- It helps establish the placenta.

Relaxin levels are at their highest in the first trimester. Relaxin is believed to promote implantation of the blastocyst and growth of the placenta. It also inhibits uterine contractions in early pregnancy. It regulates the mother's cardiovascular and renal systems, helping them adapt to increased foetal demands for oxygen and nutrients and the processing of waste products. It is thought to do this by relaxing the mother's blood vessels and thereby increasing blood flow to the placenta and kidneys.

Relaxin and progesterone relax muscles and ligaments, making room for the growing baby. These effects are most concentrated in the pelvic region and can lead to pain and discomfort in the pelvis and lower back. Gut motility is also reduced, which can lead to constipation.

As the placenta grows, it develops the ability to produce hormones. Once the placenta is established, it takes over production of hormones at around week 8 to 12 of pregnancy. Progesterone levels steadily rise until the birth of the baby. Placental production of hCG is at its peak between the eighth to the tenth week of gestation and tends to plateau at a lower level for the remainder of pregnancy.

Oestrogen levels are considerably lower than progesterone but also vital, for instance, oestrogen stimulates progesterone production by the placenta. In early pregnancy, oestrogen is produced and released by the corpus luteum and later, by the foetal-placental unit. This latter term refers to the interaction between the mother and conceptus to develop hormonal balance. As part of this process, the foetal liver and adrenals make oestriol and pass it to the placenta where it is converted to other oestrogens with a wide variety of actions.

The placenta produces several other hormones including human placental lactogen and cortico-trophin releasing hormone; the latter playing a role in early pregnancy in modifying a woman's immune system to allow her body to accept the growing foetus and not reject it as foreign tissue. Later in pregnancy this hormone improves blood flow between the placenta and foetus.

After the eighth week of pregnancy until birth, the developing baby is known as a foetus. With the major organs already formed during earlier embryonic development, the foetal stage is mainly one of growth, maturation, and adding details such as hair and nails.

In the first trimester it is normal for a woman to feel tired and to need more rest. Hormonal changes may cause nausea and vomiting, breast tenderness, urinary frequency, and constipation, as well as heightened emotional sensitivity, sometimes resulting in extreme mood swings and uncharacteristic emotional outbursts. See Chapter 8 for discussion and treatment of specific conditions. Sensitivity to touch, sound, and smell are often enhanced throughout pregnancy, but especially in the first trimester. Taste is usually significantly altered and may be either enhanced or decreased. Some women experience cravings for unusual foods. Balance, spatial awareness, and short-term memory may all be affected. A mother's blood volume increases while her breathing rate and metabolism speed up, so she may feel hot. Increased blood flow to the vagina causes a degree of engorgement, which can increase sexual sensitivity and pleasure for some women. There is also an increase in vaginal mucus, which is thin, milky-white, and odourless or near-odourless and may continue throughout pregnancy.

Spiritual and energetic adjustment

While hormonal shifts play a major part in causing the physiological changes and symptoms of early pregnancy, at the same time there can be a spiritual or energetic basis for these changes. For instance, both mother and child may need to adjust their vibrational frequencies in preparation for birth, meaning that the mother (particularly her uterus) needs to raise her frequency, whereas the incoming soul needs to decrease theirs. Where appropriate, vibrational essences (see Chapter 16) can be used to assist this process and can be prescribed safely and effectively, either on their own or alongside herbal medicines.

Pregnancy is an important time for women to tune into their own inner wisdom. Trusting one's inner knowing and developing a strong prenatal bond with the baby help a mother to make appropriate decisions for herself and her child, not only during pregnancy but in later years too.

Two-way communication

It is beneficial for a woman to communicate with her baby from an early stage. This is a two-way process. A mother can communicate with her baby and a baby can communicate with its mother. This may begin even before conception through dreams and extrasensory awareness. In early pregnancy, although the baby is still tiny, a woman may find it easy to connect through her hands by placing them over her belly. Throughout pregnancy many women enjoy bonding by talking to their babies, singing, or reading stories to them. It is also an opportunity to listen to and dialogue with the baby. See Guided Visualisation *Connecting with one's baby* page 46.

A mother and her baby have an intimate connection, including the sharing of their blood and nerve supplies. Everything that happens to the mother, consciously or unconsciously, happens to the embryo too. Whatever a mother feels, her child also feels and can leave a lifelong impression. Therefore a baby can sense a mother's love or rejection and it is worth encouraging a woman to consciously give thanks and welcome the new life force within. A miraculous process is taking place inside a woman's body. As far as possible, this is an appropriate time to reflect on the wonder of life and to see one's body as a temple, a sacred place inside of which a new human form is being built. Some women face enormous challenges, and it can be natural for fears and anxieties to arise at any stage of pregnancy (see 'Emotional and Stress-Related Conditions' Chapter 8 page 120). Herbal practitioners can provide a safe space for a woman to discuss her concerns, offering information, support, and calm reassurance.

Second trimester (weeks 13–26)

What's happening in the body?

Growth of the foetus is regulated by a balance of hormones throughout pregnancy.

In the second trimester progesterone levels continue to rise, playing a crucial role in foetal development. Progesterone also stimulates the growth of maternal breast tissue and helps prevent lactation until after pregnancy. It strengthens the pelvic musculature and inhibits uterine muscle contraction until the onset of labour.

Oestrogen continues to play a significant role in the development of the foetus as well as the growth and function of the placenta. It maintains, controls, and stimulates the production of other pregnancy hormones. Along with progesterone, oestrogen promotes the growth of maternal breast tissue and prepares the mother for lactation.

Cortisol levels increase throughout pregnancy and several other hormones play important roles.

At this stage of pregnancy, most women feel at the peak of their health and energy. The risk of miscarriage is reduced, and any nausea and vomiting typically subside between weeks 12 to 15. A woman's breasts may still be tender and increased melanin production can cause darkening of the areolas. The increased blood volume makes veins more visible all over the body, especially on the breasts. Hormone levels and increased blood flow to the kidneys cause a rise in urine production leading to possible urinary incontinence (see Pelvic Floor Exercises Chapter 4 page 42) and frequency (see Conditions of Pregnancy page 164). The raised hormone levels and increased blood flow to pelvic organs, breasts, and vulva can cause an increase in libido for many women.

Braxton Hicks contractions can occur through much of pregnancy but usually only become noticeable after 20 weeks. These involve a sporadic tightening of the uterus and can be viewed as preparation for labour and birth. They are occasional, irregular, nearly always painless, and lasting less than a minute.

During this trimester the mother will usually begin to feel her baby's first 'fluttering' movements in the womb (otherwise known as quickening). For primigravidae (women who are pregnant for the first time), this is often in weeks 18–20, whereas for women who have experienced previous pregnancies it may happen any time from week 15 or even earlier.

Third trimester (week 27 — end of pregnancy)

What's happening in the body?

Oestrogen and progesterone continue to rise during the third trimester, remaining high until parturition. Prolactin levels steadily increase in preparation for breastfeeding and from week 32 the mother's breasts may leak colostrum. In the last weeks of pregnancy, cortico-releasing hormone levels rise further, coinciding with a spike in cortisol levels. Corticotrophin-releasing hormone is thought to be involved in foetal maturation and in regulating the duration of pregnancy. Increased cortisol levels are considered necessary to maintain maternal and foetal wellbeing and to promote the normal progression of labour.

For the foetus, following the complex development of body systems earlier in pregnancy, the third trimester is chiefly a time of maturation and further growth. Typically, a foetus will double its weight in its final ten weeks and will usually slow down its movements by week 37 due to lack of space in the uterus.

In the later stages of pregnancy, it is normal for the mother to feel more physically tired and require more rest. Sleep disturbances can occur, especially towards the end of pregnancy when it may be hard to find a comfortable position in bed. It can be helpful to rest during the day, both for restoration and also as training for when the baby is born and a mother may need to snatch rest periods whenever the opportunity arises.

Other common symptoms at this time include heartburn, swollen ankles, vaginal discharge, breathlessness, palpitations, back ache, and other pains, carpal tunnel syndrome, leg cramps, and restless legs. See Chapter 8 for discussion and treatment of specific complaints.

It can also be normal to feel more dreamy and 'spaced out' than usual. Many women feel particularly intuitive and reflective. This is a perfect time to tune into the baby and enjoy these final unique moments of sharing one's physical body with another being.

Babies generally love to be massaged. It can be beautiful and highly beneficial for both mother and child for a pregnant woman to begin massaging her baby while it is still in the womb. Simply by putting a little vegetable oil on her hands, she can rub her belly and massage accessible parts of the baby's body.

Approaching delivery

At this stage it can be normal for the expectant mother to experience some weight loss. The head of the foetus generally drops lower in the pelvis and engages ready for birth, although some babies will only engage at the last minute and some not at all. The most common foetal position is head down, facing the mother's back, with the neck flexed forward. Around one in thirty full term deliveries is breech, in which the baby's buttocks emerge before the head. See 'Breech Presentation' page 192.

Braxton Hicks contractions may now turn into stronger 'true' contractions, becoming steadily more frequent, regular, and painful. These help to thin the cervix in readiness for childbirth. See 'Braxton Hicks contractions' page 104 and 'Stages of Labour' page 209.

Many women experience a 'nesting' instinct as they approach delivery, manifesting as a desire to clean the house and prepare a place for the baby. For the foetus, this is a time of gathering energy fore birth. In the days before delivery, the baby's movements generally slow down in preparation for labour.

For details of labour, see Chapter 12 'Herbs for Labour and Delivery'

Notes

1. The first or lowest layer of the aura or human energy field. This layer is closest to the physical body.
2. See the work of Dutch embryologist Jaap van der Wal for a spiritual perspective on embryology.
3. Duncan, Francesca E., Emily L. Que, Nan Zhang, Eve C. Feinberg, Thomas V. O'Halloran, and Teresa K. Woodruff. "The zinc spark is an inorganic signature of human egg activation." *Scientific reports* 6, no. 1 (2016): 1–8.
4. Franklyn Sills. *Foundations of Craniosacral Biodynamics* (Berkeley: North Atlantic Books, 2012), 26.
5. The conceptus describes any of the various products of conception, including the embryo, foetus, and surrounding tissue.

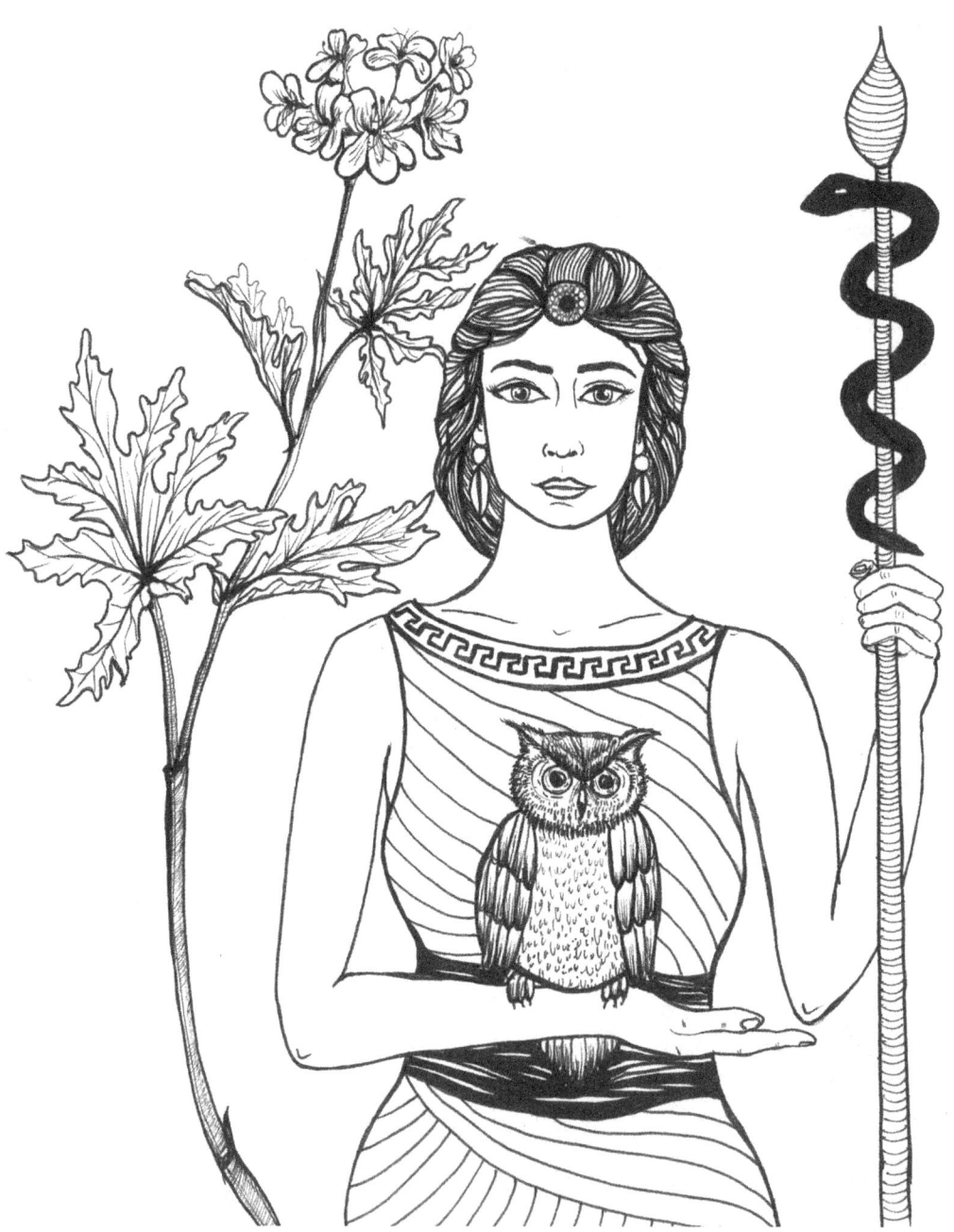

Minerva. Goddess of wisdom who teaches how to use knowledge wisely, with heart and mind as one.
Geranium (*Pelargonium graveolens*). Holder of balance, uplifting and relaxing.

CHAPTER 6

Herbal pharmacy

This chapter gives instructions for the standard preparation of herbs and herbal applications for pregnancy, lactation, and the newborn, as outlined in this book. See Chapter 1 for safety recommendations for herbs and essential oils.

See Chapters 8 through 15 for details of use in specific conditions.

See Chapter 7 'Materia Medica' for information on herbs including maximum dosage.

Standard infusions

These are hot water extracts (herbal teas or tisanes) and are generally suitable for the aerial parts of plants, such as leaves, flowers, stems, and seeds.

Method: Use up to 2g chopped dried herb/s (double for chopped fresh herbs) per 200ml boiling water, infuse in a covered container for five to fifteen minutes (or longer if a stronger infusion is required). Strain. Add honey and/or lemon juice to taste if desired. Standard dose: One 200ml cup three times daily. An infusion will keep for up to three days in a refrigerator, but has optimum potency in the first 24 hours after preparation.

The equivalent amount of herb in teaspoonfuls will vary greatly depending on the bulkiness of the herb you are using, for instance 2g can be the equivalent of one heaped teaspoon of dried Fennel seed (*Foeniculum vulgare*) or three heaped teaspoons of dried Chamomile flowerheads (*Chamomilla recutita*). In general, a full 2g may not be needed and **one heaped teaspoon of herb/s per cup is often sufficient**. You can consider 2g per cup as an upper limit, adjusted depending on the herb, the condition being treated, the constitution and taste of the patient. If more than one herb is combined in a mix, 2g represents the total herb content. Soft petals such as Rose petals can be used whole. Use ceramic, enamel, or stainless-steel vessels and a strainer, or a vessel with a built-in strainer where there is plenty of space for the water to circulate.

In some cases, cold infusions may be used. This method particularly suits mucilaginous herbs, such as Marshmallow (*Althaea off.*). It is also ideal for Valerian root (*Valeriana off.*).

To make a cold infusion: use 6g of dried herb to 600ml of cold water, steep overnight, strain, and drink over the next 1–2 days.

Standard decoctions

This method is suitable for hard, woody materials, such as roots, barks, and berries. Place 2.5g dried herb (double for fresh), finely chopped, with 330ml cold water in a saucepan (non-aluminium). Bring to the boil and simmer, uncovered, for ten to twenty minutes until reduced by a third to a half. Cover and strain. Standard dose: one 165ml cup three times daily. Will keep for up to three days in the refrigerator. For aromatic roots and barks such as Angelica (*Angelica archangelica*), cover the pan while simmering.

A reduced decoction is re-heated until it begins to steam and left uncovered on a gentle heat for a period of hours until it has reduced to less than one quarter of its original volume. This will keep for 4–5 days in a cool place or up to three weeks in a refrigerator. A reduced decoction can be preserved for a number of years by adding 500g of honey to 300ml (a pound to a half pint) of decoction (see 'Syrups' below) or by adding spirits at a proportion of 1 part alcohol to 1 part decoction.

Tinctures

A tincture is a concentrated extract, where the properties of the plant are extracted and preserved in a mixture of alcohol and water. This combination can extract more plant constituents than pure water alone. An alcohol tincture is rapidly absorbed and brings heat to the body. As long as the alcohol content is at least 20% the tincture will last for many years.

Tinctures can be made from either fresh or dried herbs. Where possible, I prefer to use fresh plant tinctures (otherwise known as 'specific tinctures'), since they tend to have more vitality and retain more of the subtle qualities of a plant.

Good quality commercial tinctures can be purchased from herbal suppliers (see 'Resources' page 313) and are available in varying strengths depending on the dilution required to extract the therapeutic constituents of a particular herb. It is crucial to seek out a reputable supplier, since the quality of medicines for general sale varies tremendously. Herbs need to be ethically sourced. Consider air miles, fair trade, and sustainable practice, as well as looking for organic or biodynamically grown. Some herbal products sold online have been found to contain completely different substances than advertised.

To make tinctures at home, professional herbalists can purchase organic ethanol from specialist suppliers and use this diluted with water at the required strength for each herb. Alcohol strengths for tinctures typically range from 25% to 60% going up to 90% in certain cases, for instance where extraction of resins is required (see 'Resources' for books giving detailed making instructions).

Home-made tinctures can also be made with a commercial (preferably organic) spirit. Vodka is often preferred, as it has little taste or smell and contains few congeners (additional biologically active chemicals). On the other hand, you might want a particular flavour or quality provided by a specific type of spirit (e.g. Lemon Balm (*Melissa off.*) blends well with tequila gold). Your chosen spirit can be used neat, in which case you will end up with a tincture of the same alcohol strength as the original spirit i.e. 40% vodka gives you a 40% tincture.[1] Using neat 40% vodka does not give you the precision of diluted ethanol but generally works well at extracting most alcohol and water based plant constituents.

To make a dried herb tincture with vodka: For a 1:4 tincture, allow 250g dried herb to one litre of vodka. Pour the vodka over the chopped herbs (or powdered if bulky) in a large jar, ensuring the plant material is completely covered. Seal the jar and leave in a dark place for two to three weeks for aerial parts, three to six weeks for fibrous or woody plant material. Shake or stir daily. Strain through muslin or other fine cloth in a strainer. Squeeze out all the liquid (known as the menstruum) and discard the herbs (known as the marc). Store in dark glass bottles, labelling the jar with a permanent pen, showing the name of the herb, the date, the % alcohol, and the weight to volume ratio.

To make a specific tincture from fresh herbs: use the same method as above but allow one part freshly picked herb to three parts vodka e.g. 250g herb to 750ml. liquid. Even though this is strictly speaking a 1:3 tincture, for prescribing purposes it is the **equivalent of a 1:4 dried herb tincture**, due to the water content of the fresh herbs. The reduction in alcohol allows for the extra water in the plant, which adds to the overall volume of menstruum. This can only be an approximation since the water content of plants is extremely variable e.g. a leafy plant like Lemon Balm (*Melissa off.*) contains far more water than a root, such as Dandelion (*Taraxacum off.*) Depending on the plant in question, more or less vodka may need to be used in order to fully cover the fresh plant material (if necessary, bulky aerial parts can be pounded down in a pestle and mortar to reduce the volume) and fresh plant tinctures may actually range from 1:2 to 1:4 or more. In clinical practice (and exercising common sense), even in pregnancy this is of little consequence and for dosage purposes, all can safely be considered as the equivalent of a 1:4 dried herb tincture. A 40% vodka specific tincture can be considered to have an estimated 25% alcohol content.

Tincture dosages given are for 1:4 dried herb tincture or 1:2 specific tincture.

Ideally, tinctures are dispensed into dark glass bottles for patient use, and should be kept away from direct heat and light. In most circumstances, they are best diluted with a little water (usually warm) before taking. Alternatively, they can be taken with a little fruit juice for taste. Dosages can vary from a few drops to 10ml three times a day although 5ml is standard.

Alcohol tinctures extract a wide range of constituents, they keep well, have good patient compliance, and are easily carried as emergency remedies. Usually, the small amount of alcohol in a tincture does not pose a problem, even in pregnancy, but alcohol tinctures may be unsuitable for sensitive people, those with stomach irritation, liver or kidney damage, and recovering alcoholics. If needed, patients can remove some of the alcohol before taking the tincture by pouring a little boiling water over it and allowing the steam to evaporate.

For further details on the use of tinctures, see Chapter 1.

Glycerites

A glycerite is the equivalent of an alcohol tincture using vegetable glycerine instead of alcohol. The herbs are extracted and preserved in glycerine—a sweet liquid derived from palm or other oil and available from pharmacies. In some cases, glycerine can provide a soothing alternative to alcohol for tincture-making but is less effective at extracting some plant constituents and a glycerite will only last around two years. You may prefer to avoid a palm-oil derivative.

Method: For fresh plant material, pour undiluted vegetable glycerine over the herbs using the same method as for tinctures, except that that the jar should be left in the sun or a warm place to infuse. If using dried herbs, mix three parts vegetable glycerine with two parts water.

A small amount of alcohol can be added to glycerites to extend their keeping qualities and to make them less sweet. You can also use glycerine to preserve fresh plant juice such as Nettle: mix plant juice and glycerine 1:1, this is known as a succus.

Vinegars

These are preparations made by macerating herbs in vinegar. In general, vinegar is weaker than alcohol at extracting plant constituents, but it is less expensive and better tolerated. Some constituents extract better in vinegar's acid medium, and vinegar is perfect for extracting minerals from herbs, as well as helping the body's acid/alkali balance and assisting digestion.

Herbal vinegars are often made from pleasant-tasting herbs and used for cooking and in salad dressings. Cider vinegar, which has many healing benefits of its own, makes an ideal choice of solvent. The addition of honey to a vinegar tincture (called an oxymel) will cut the bite of the vinegar and may traditionally be drunk as a cordial.

Vinegar tinctures should be stored in a cool, dark place and will last around two years. **Method for dried herbs:** Vinegars are usually made at 1:10 or 1:8 for dried herbs. Place 10g of finely cut herb(s) in a jar with 100ml of cider vinegar. Macerate for two to six weeks, shaking daily. Strain, bottle, and keep in a cool, dark place. **For fresh herbs:** Fill a jar with freshly picked and chopped herbs, cover with cider vinegar. Macerate for two to six weeks, shaking daily. Strain, bottle and keep in a cool, dark place.

Honeys

In addition to its preservative qualities, honey acts as a natural antibiotic and local honey can also help prevent allergies such as hay-fever. Herbs can be directly infused in honey.

Method: Fill a jar with chopped, fresh herbs and pour honey over. Seal jar and leave in sun or warm place for two to six weeks before straining. If preferred, this can be gently heated in a bain-marie (double boiler) to speed up the process. The honey will keep indefinitely.

Honey should not be given to infants under one year old.

Syrups

In a syrup, sugar or honey is used as a preservative and can also help extract the plant material. Syrups are useful in general as soothing expectorants and other cough medicines, as laxatives for dry conditions and to improve palatability, especially for children. They are particularly suitable for mucilaginous herbs, such as Marshmallow (*Althaea officinalis*). Syrups are not suitable for diabetics nor for anyone who consumes too much sugar already. A simple syrup can be made by boiling the herb(s) with sugar and water (for keeping you will need at least 500g sugar to 600ml of fluid (1lb to a pint) and straining. Alternatively, sugar or honey can be added directly to a simple infusion or decoction in order to preserve it. The maximum amount of sugar ratio is 200g sugar to 100ml water, which will preserve for a longer period, usually several years.

Method for simple syrup: Make infusion or decoction as described above, measure the liquid and return to pan adding 500g sugar or honey per 600ml tea (1lb per pint). Heat gently until sugar/honey has dissolved, bringing the syrup just up to simmering point. Allow to cool and store in sterilised bottles, preferably with screw-top lids slightly loosened.

A more robust syrup can be made by using a **reduced decoction. Method:** Make a standard decoction as described above, strain and return to a clean pan, reducing slowly to a quarter of the volume. Measure the volume and add 200g of sugar or honey to every 100ml of decoction, continuing as for simple syrup.

Herbal infused oils

Infused plant oils can be used for massage and to treat skin conditions. The plant material is infused in a good quality vegetable oil, such as sunflower, olive, or almond, and either left on a sunny windowsill or heated in a bain-marie (double boiler). The sun method is suitable for delicate flowers like St John's Wort (*Hypericum perforatum*), or Mullein (*Verbascum Thapsus*), which would be damaged by heating. The method below is suitable for most other plants, including Comfrey (*Symphytum off.*), Marigold (*Calendula off.*), and Chamomile (*Chamomilla recutita*).

To make a heated infused oil: Gather the plant on a dry day and leave it to wilt for a few hours so that some of the water content has evaporated. Put half of the chopped plant material into a heatproof container, cover with extra virgin olive oil, and place in a bain-marie or saucepan of water, ensuring that the container is covered so that water will not splash into the oil. Heat the water and simmer for three hours. Strain the oil (in this case do not press with a wooden spoon since you do not want to extract water), pour the oil back over the remaining half of plant material and repeat the process for another three hours. Strain and leave the oil to settle, then pour off the oil from any water and plant residue that has separated out to the bottom as this would cause the oil to go rancid. The oil will keep for one year.

Herbal infused oils may be used neat or, if desired, essential oils may be added (see 'Essential Oils' below for proportions). An infused oil may also be made into an ointment or liniment.

Liniments

A liniment is an external rub and may consist of extracts of herbs in oil or alcohol or both. Most of my liniments contain a mixture of herbal oil and tincture. These are easily absorbed through the skin and particularly helpful for muscular and ligament problems. The oil moisturises, protects, and facilitates massage, while the alcohol component helps to carry the herbal properties to the muscles. Mix one part herbal oil with one part herbal tincture or as specified in the text for individual conditions. Shake well before use.

Herbal ointments

The main difference between ointments and creams is their water content, creams are an emulsion of oils and water whereas the water content in ointments is minimal so they tend to be more stable, less likely to develop moulds, and (unlike creams) less likely to curdle or separate. While creams soften the skin, ointments can form a protective layer helping to prevent further damage, for instance in nappy rash. Ointments are semi-solid whereas creams are soft.

A basic ointment can be simply made by combining an infused oil with beeswax:

For every 100ml oil, you will need 10g grated beeswax. Pour the oil into a snugly fitting heatproof bowl over a pan of boiling water. Add the required amount of beeswax and melt into the oil, stirring until clear. Remove from the heat. Add essential oils if desired (see individual conditions for directions). Pour into clean jars and allow to set.

If you have the time, you can experiment with many different ingredients to make ointments. For instance, use wheatgerm oil or jojoba in your infused oil and/or use a mix of fats and waxes, such as cocoa butter, coconut butter, shea butter, and beeswax. Depending how firm you want the ointment to be, simply vary the proportion and variety of fats and waxes.

Herbal creams

Creams are lighter and more cooling than ointments and are more suitable for hot, inflamed and weepy skin conditions. They are also better for warm, damp areas of the body, such as the groin or axilla. Creams contain water or water-based extracts (herbal teas, decoctions, and tinctures) and since oil and water do not mix of their own accord, an emulsifying agent is used to combine them. Typical emulsifying agents include egg yolks (as in making mayonnaise), lanolin (also called wool fat and used in many commercial creams), and beeswax.

For reliable and high quality creams, I generally purchase them from herbal suppliers (see 'Resources') since creams are more time-consuming and not so easily made at home. Many suppliers also sell a pure base cream, to which you can simply stir in small amounts of your own tinctures, infusions, decoctions, hydrosols, or essential oils. For example, to make a soothing Chamomile cream, stir two drops of *Chamomilla recutita* essential oil into 50g of high quality base cream.

Capsules

Ready-made capsules are available from commercial suppliers (see 'Resources') or can be made at home. You can either purchase dried powdered herbs or powder the herbs yourself in an electric coffee grinder until very fine, then sieve finely. The powder can be put into vegetable gelatin capsules (size 00 holds approximately 0.5g of powder but this depends on the density of your powder, so you will need to check in order to calculate accurate dosage; 0.5g powder is the equivalent of 2ml of a 1:4 tincture). Capsules are not as quickly or easily absorbed as tinctures but may have the advantage of being more palatable, which can be a significant factor in circumstances such as giving Ginger for nausea and vomiting in early pregnancy. Capsules can also be useful if you want to avoid alcohol completely.

Vibrational Essences (see Chapter 16 'vibrational essences')

Vibrational Essences are water extracts carrying the vibrational imprint of the flower or whatever they are made from. A flower essence can be described as a vibrational expression of a flower held within the sacred space of the water. The essence holds the unique energy patterns of the flower and encapsulates the virtues that the flower brings to the world.

Vibrational essences address psychological, emotional, and spiritual issues, which in turn helps heal their resultant physical illnesses. A wide range of essences is available commercially (see 'Resources'). A few drops are all that are needed. These can be taken neat or diluted, placed on the skin, added to baths, room sprays, creams, or other medicines.

Flower waters

Flower waters or hydrosols such as Rosewater are produced by distillation and you will need a still if you want to produce your own. If you do not have distillation equipment, some good quality flower waters are available commercially (see 'Resources') and these can be purchased for use in a variety of applications including lotions, room sprays, or for internal use.

Pessaries and suppositories

Suppositories and pessaries are absorbed directly through the mucous membrane of the rectum or vagina, respectively, and can provide a quick method to get herbal medicine into the bloodstream, as well as treating local conditions—such as irritations, vaginal candida, and other infections. See individual conditions for directions.

Marigold (*Calendula off.*) pessaries can be made by melting together 2g beeswax, 10ml infused Calendula oil and 15g cocoa butter. Pour mixture into pessary moulds and leave until set. Remove and store in refrigerator until required. Alternatively, make an infused Calendula oil following the directions for a hot infused oil and using melted cocoa butter as your oil. When completed, strain and pour into moulds.

A third method is to mix finely powdered and sieved herbs into melted cocoa butter in a ratio of one part herb to three parts cocoa butter and pour into moulds.

Suppositories are made in the same way.

If you do not have a pessary or suppository mould, you can prepare a row of foil funnels of the required shape and size. Fill and store in a refrigerator, directing your patient to peel off the foil just before use.

Steam inhalations

Use of the breath is an important way to control panic and anxiety and restore calm. Using herbs or essential oils with inhalations and vaporisers can be a useful method to bring the qualities of plants into the body as well as allowing the steam to relax the airways and encourage deeper breathing. Herbal teas and essential oils (see below) are both effective, although herb teas are gentler and offer a greater range of safe plants for pregnancy.

If using herb tea, use approximately one litre of herbal tea poured into a bowl.

If using essential oils, place freshly boiled water in the bowl and add one or two drops of your chosen oil.

Instructions:

Sit comfortably, covering the head with a large cloth or towel so that no steam escapes.

Breathe in the steam for ten minutes or until the water cools.

Afterwards it is important to sit in a warm room for at least thirty minutes to allow the respiratory system to adjust to normal temperature.

Baths

Herbal baths can have powerful healing effects for all ages, including relaxing tension, lifting the spirits, and soothing itchy skin. Any herb that can be taken internally can also be used in a bath. Herbal infusions or decoctions can be added to a full bath, lighting candles in the bathroom to make this a potent ritual. Use about 600ml of well strained tea, 300ml for a baby, adding after the bath is filled. Herbs can also be placed in a bag under the hot tap when running a bath e.g. Lavender (*Lavandula angustifolia*) as a relaxant and antispasmodic, or seaweed can be placed directly in the bath to soothe the skin, detoxify, and relieve stress. Essential oils can also be very effective (see below).

Baths should not be too hot during pregnancy. Thomas Bartram, in his *Encyclopaedia of Herbal Medicine* recommends that pregnant women should not spend more than 10 minutes in a bath of more than 40°C, due to possible adverse effects on the foetus.[2]

Footbaths and handbaths

These are a powerful and pleasant way to administer herbs. Well-known French herbalist Maurice Mességué has written several books describing his highly successful practice using hand and foot baths last century.[3] Irish herbalist, Julie-Ann O'Connor, routinely offers footbaths to her patients as part of her consultations. People love the sense of care and relaxation it brings, facilitating deep levels of communication while providing effective treatment at the same time. The hands and feet are highly sensitive areas and herbal medicines can pass easily through the skin to the bloodstream. For a pregnant woman, a footbath can be a pleasurable treat to aid sleep and restore the spirits, as well as soothing weary feet after a long day of standing or walking.

Fill a small basin or bowl with 600ml of herbal tea or decoction. Add enough warm water to cover the feet or hands and to make a comfortable temperature. Relax and soak feet and/or hands for ten to twenty minutes. Dry and wrap feet afterwards to keep warm.

Sitz baths or hip baths

These are useful for many gynaecological conditions and offer significant assistance after childbirth for easing pain, facilitating healing, and restoring damaged tissues in the entire pelvic area. A large plastic bowl or baby bath can be used, ideally with enough hot water to cover the hips. The woman needs to be well wrapped up in a warm room and have several towels so she can make herself comfortable e.g. putting one under her knees. Herbs are added as for baths above. She should start with the water as hot as possible (hot but comfortable) and stay in the bath until it cools down (without getting cold). Dry and wrap up well afterwards. Sitz baths are usually best done before bed. A footbath can be done at the same time for added efficacy.

Vaginal steaming

This is the equivalent of a herb tea steam inhalation for the vagina, uterus, ovaries, and entire pelvic area. It is an ancient practice arising from many countries around the world and becoming re-popularised in the West in recent years. Otherwise known as 'vaginal fumigation' or 'yoni steaming' and effective for many gynaecological conditions.[4] For post-partum care it is usually done to cleanse the uterine membrane, including the release of trauma. Typically, the woman sits or squats above a steaming bowl of aromatic herbs. She needs a chair with open slits (wood, cane, or plastic are all suitable and specially made chairs are available) or she can sit on a regular toilet seat. The herb tea (30g dried herbs/60g fresh in 600ml water) is simmered in a covered pan for ten minutes and left to stand for five. The pot is then placed under the woman who should be clothed from the waist up and wrapped in blankets to keep the steam in. She should sit in the steam for twenty minutes, or as long as comfortable. As for sitz baths, the woman should wrap up warm after a steam and they are best done before bed.

Lotions

These can consist of a simple infusion or decoction, a tincture diluted in water or water with essential oils (see 'Essential Oils' below). Lotions may be applied externally on cotton wool for small or large areas. They are also used for compresses and washes.

Compresses

Known as fomentations when used hot, a compress consists of a flannel or piece of cloth that has been soaked in a lotion, wrung out, and applied to an affected part of the body. Cold compresses are helpful for fresh wounds, weeping rashes, headaches, varicose veins, or inflamed tissues. Hot fomentations are used to disperse, clear, and ease pain. They are helpful for conditions such as back pain, cramping, joint pain, and boils. Hot or cold, they may need replacing regularly since they tend to dry out quickly. Where heat is required, keep the fomentation warm by covering with a piece of soft polythene, such as a section of a poly plastic bag. Cover with a towel and a hot water bottle. Repeat with more hot liquid when cooling is apparent.

Poultices

These are made by placing the fresh or dried herb between two layers of gauze, muslin, or other clean cotton. Herbs are bruised, crushed, or pounded before application. Dried herbs can be mixed with hot water or herb tea to make a paste. If fresh herbs are not available, I commonly use powders such as Slippery Elm (*Ulmus rubra*), Marshmallow root, (*Althaea off.* radix), or Comfrey root (*Symphytum off.*), all of which make superb poultices. Use cooled water for high mucilage content. The powder is mixed to a firm paste and spread onto cloth. Glycerine may be added to prevent it drying out. The poultice is applied to the affected part and held in place by cotton bandage. Where heat is required, such as for drawing, the poultice may be covered with a layer of plastic and a towel, and kept warm with a hot water bottle. Poultices are replaced as often as required, depending on the condition.

Essential oils

Also known as volatile oils, these are steam-distilled or cold-expressed from various parts of aromatic plants. Essential oils (EOs) are powerful and highly concentrated.

They represent one aspect of a plant and therefore do not necessarily have the same properties as the whole herb. EOs can cross the placenta and may affect foetal growth and development. Most are best avoided in the first trimester. EOs should not be administered orally, vaginally, or rectally throughout pregnancy. They should not be applied undiluted to the skin. Certain oils can be used in pregnancy with good effect at low dilution (1%) in carrier oils for massage, ointments, creams, lotions, inhalations, room sprays, burners, and other purposes.

Particular caution is required for breastfeeding mothers and newborn infants. In labour and postpartum, EOs can be diluted up to 2%. For babies, dilute up to 1%. Use patch testing with diluted EO before using any diluted EO directly on the skin.

See Chapter 1 for details of EOs that can be safely used for pregnancy, lactation and the newborn.

Methods of application of essential oils

Adjust number of drops according to recommended % dilution

Inhalation of essential oils

1–3 drops EOs on a cotton pad, tissue, inhalant tube, or in a diffuser or burner.

Nasal inhaler tubes are readily available online. These are small, capped tubes containing a wick that EOs or blends can be dropped onto. The cap can be removed for easy inhalation and replaced to keep the scent long-lasting. The tubes easily fit in a pocket, bag, or purse.

Alternatively, EOs can be used for steam inhalation, using the method described above under 'Steam Inhalations'.

Inhalation is the usually the quickest route for anxiety, panic, and nausea.

Skin application of essential oils
(massage oils, creams, ointments, compresses, liniments)

1–2 drops EOs in 5ml carrier oil or added to cream, ointment, or liquid for a compress or liniment. Suitable carrier oils include almond, grapeseed, sunflower, or jojoba. Diluted EOs may also be applied to pulse points via a rollerball bottle, which can be a discreet method of use, especially in a hospital setting.

Massage is typically the best method for relief of physical pain.

Baths with essential oils
(whole body, sitz, foot, or hand baths)

2–8 drops EOs dissolved in 15ml of a dispersant such as cider vinegar, yoghurt, or a lotion base. This prevents concentrated oil from getting into eyes or mucosa. Regular carrier oils can be used as dispersants for sitz, foot, or hand baths, but are unsuitable for whole body baths since they make the surface of the bath slippery and unsafe.

Add mix to warm bath water, stirring the water to help circulate the oils before climbing in.

EOs are not suitable for whole body baths during labour due to risk of contact with the baby's eyes.

Baths are often best for relaxation, insomnia, and perineal healing (sitz baths).

Sprays with essential oils

Up to 10 drops in a spray bottle with 50ml hydrosol or herb tea. Add vibrational essences as desired aa 2gtt, plus 5gtt emulsifier, such as soya lecithins. Shake well, spray as required.

Sprays have an immediate effect, enhancing atmospheres, providing personal space, and infusing a person's auric field with beneficial energies.

Notes

1. In the UK, since 1980, alcohol strength is measured as a percentage of alcohol by volume (ABV) in line with the European Union. The UK now uses the ABV standard instead of alcohol proof. In the US, alcohol proof is used as a measure of alcohol content, defined as twice the percentage of alcohol by volume. For example, US 80-proof vodka contains 40% alcohol, equivalent to 40% ABV.
2. Thomas Bartram. *Encyclopedia of Herbal Medicine* (Great Britain: Robinson, 1998), 350.
3. Maurice Mességué, *Of Men and Plants* (London: Weidenfeld and Nicolson Ltd, 1972).
4. Rosita Arvigo has done pioneering work in Belize to keep this tradition alive. To learn about her work and courses with the Arvigo Institute, visit www.arvigotherapy.com. [last accessed 27/7/21].

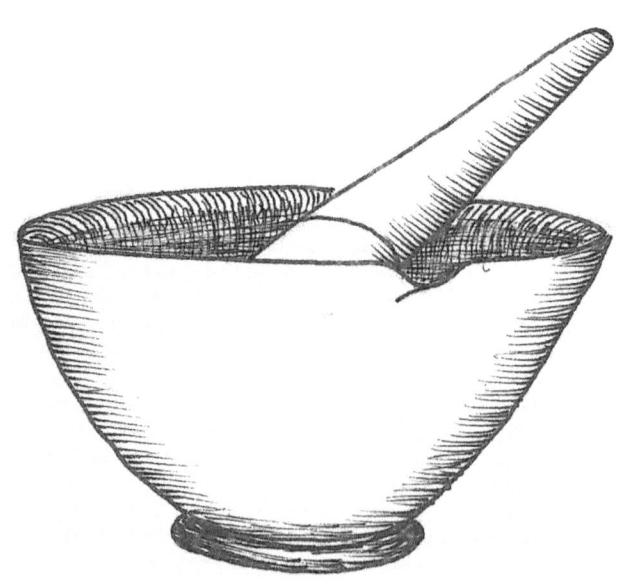

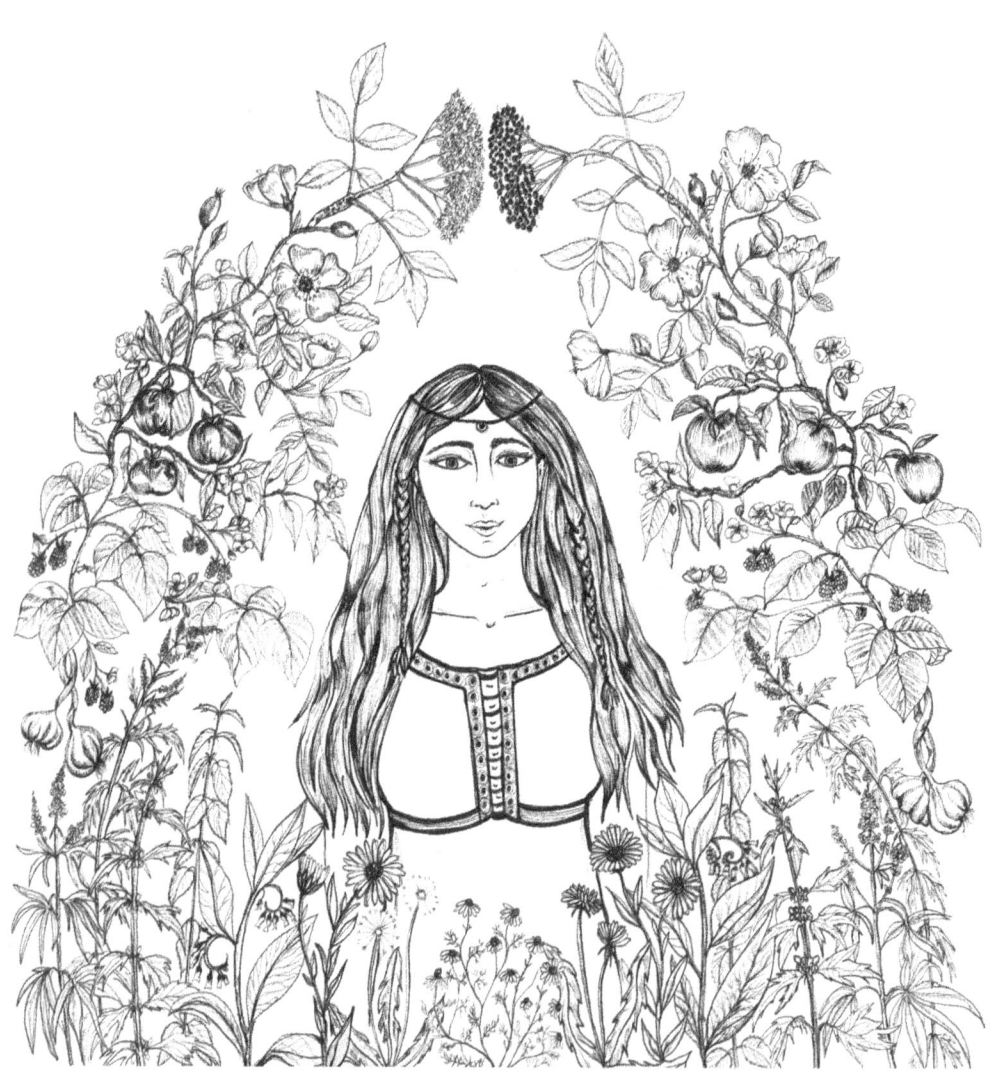

Airmid. Goddess of healing and magic. Keeper of the mysteries of herbal medicine. Airmid is surrounded by a synergistic, magical team of healing herbs, "a cure for every ill".

CHAPTER 7

Materia medica

Herbs for pregnancy, lactation, and the newborn

This Materia Medica section describes the plants referred to in the rest of the text with particular emphasis on their use for pregnancy, lactation, and the newborn. Dosages given are the typical adult dosage range considered safe for childbearing women in my practice. In the rare cases where the maximum dose can be exceeded, this is noted. Tincture dosages are for 1:4 dried herb tincture or 1:2 specific tincture unless stated otherwise. Herbs are predominately prescribed in combination and nothing is prescribed in the first trimester unless specifically indicated.

See Chapter 1 for prescribing guidelines and Chapter 6 'Herbal Pharmacy' for details of preparation.

Dosages for infants

A breastfeeding mother can take herbs and pass them on to her baby through her milk. Alternatively, infants can be given herbs directly as weak infusions. When giving herbs directly to a baby, use ¼ teaspoon dried herb per cup (double the amount for fresh), infuse 10 minutes, covered, dosage 10–30ml tds/qds, given in teaspoonful doses or added to a bottle of milk or water.

Herbs especially suitable for babies (internal use):
Agrimony (*Agrimonia eupatoria*), Aniseed (*Pimpinella anisum*), Caraway (*Carum carvi*), Catnip (*Nepeta cataria*), Chamomile (*Chamomilla recutita*), Cornsilk (*Zea mays*), Dill (*Anethum graveolens*), Elder (*Sambucus nigra*), Fennel (*Foeniculum*

vulgaris), Garlic (*Allium sativum*), Heartsease (*Viola tricolor*), Hyssop (*Hyssopus officinalis*), Limeflowers (*Tilia europaea*), Marigold, (*Calendula off.*) Marshmallow (*Althaea off.*), Nettle, (*Urtica dioica*), Red Clover (*Trifolium pratense*), Rosehips (*Rosa canina*), Slippery Elm (*Ulmus rubra*), Thyme (baths) (*Thymus vulgaris*), Yarrow (*Achillea millefolium*).

*Plants at risk or endangered in the wild at the time of writing (see Chapter 1, page 2)

20gtt = twenty drops = 1ml

Aerial parts = all the above ground parts of a plant

❦ = UK Schedule 20. Herbal Practitioner use only

Achillea millefolium (Yarrow)

Avoid in first trimester. Avoid in allergy to Compositae family. Caution with pharmaceutical anti-clotting agents.

Parts used: Leaves, flowering tops

Preparation and dosage: Infusion 1–3g/day, tincture 1–3ml/day or equivalent in capsule/powder.

Actions: Aromatic bitter, anti-inflammatory, anti-spasmodic, anti-haemorrhagic, diaphoretic (hot infusion), astringent, circulatory stimulant, uterine trophorestorative, peripheral and coronary vasodilator.

Comments: Controls excessive uterine bleeding, hypotensive esp. to diastolic pressure.

Aesculus hippocastanum (Horsechestnut)

Avoid in first trimester. Do not apply to broken or ulcerated skin.

Parts used: Seed stripped of its coat

Preparation and dosage: Decoction 1–2g/day, tincture 1–2ml/day or equivalent in capsule/powder.

Actions: Astringent, tonic to vein walls, antithrombotic.

Agrimonia eupatoria (Agrimony)

Parts used: Leaves and flowering tops

Preparation and dosage: Infusion 3–6g/day, tincture 1.5–10ml/day or equivalent in capsule/powder.

Actions: Astringent, tonic bitter. Gentle anti-diarrhoeal, cholagogue.

Comments: Promotes assimilation in babies, repairs a damaged gut lining, specific for grumbling appendix.

Agropyron repens (Couchgrass)

Part used: Rhizome

Preparation and dosage: Decoction 4–8g/day, tincture 2–15ml/day or equivalent in capsule/powder.

Actions: Demulcent, diuretic, anti-microbial.

Comments: Well tolerated. Best combined with other herbs, such as Barosma, Zea, Filipendula for urinary tract conditions.

Alchemilla vulgaris (Lady's Mantle)

Parts used: Aerial parts

Preparation and dosage: Infusion 2–4g/day, tincture 1.5–4 ml/day or equivalent in capsule/powder.

Actions: Astringent, anti-haemorrhagic, uterine and circulatory tonic, anti-inflammatory, hormone balancer with progesteronal effect, alterative.

Comments: Tones the uterus in preparation for birth. Promotes contraction during labour, prevents haemorrhage. Prevents and treats postpartum depression. Traditionally for soft, gentle women. Helps with releasing ties and bringing self-acceptance. Sitz bath for pruritis vulvae. Strong infusion as lotion to tone sagging breasts.

Allium sativum (Garlic)

Parts used: Bulb

Preparation and dosage: 3–30g/day of whole fresh bulb, juice, syrup, or tincture 2–25ml/day or equivalent in capsule/powder.

Actions: Antiseptic, antibacterial/viral/fungal, locally antiseptic in intestine, antispasmodic, diaphoretic, cholagogue, hypotensive, cholesterol lowering, anthelmintic, vascular agent reducing atheroma, anticoagulant.

Comments: 1–3 cloves daily reduces risk of pre-eclampsia.

Althaea officinalis (Marshmallow)

Parts used: Root, leaves, flowers (root is strongest demulcent)

Preparation and dosage: Cold Infusion 6–15g/day, tincture (best extracted in glycerol-water mixture) or syrup 2–30 ml/day, or equivalent in capsule/powder.

Actions: Demulcent, diuretic, emollient, vulnerary.

Comments: Macerate in cold water to extract mucilage.

Anemone pulsatilla (Pasque Flower)

Labour only. Avoid in pregnancy and lactation.

Parts used: Dried aerial parts

Preparation and dosage: Infusion/decoction 0.25g/day, tincture dried plant 1:5 max 1ml/day or equivalent in capsule/powder.

Actions: Sedative, anti-spasmodic, analgesic for reproductive system, soothes inflamed mucous membranes, relieves over-sensitivity of the vagina.

Comments: Adrenal relaxant, removes fear, apprehension, depression, hyperactive states, panic. Helps weak labour pain and mastitis. Traditionally used for fair-haired, blue-eyed women, weepy, and nervous types.

Anethum graveolens (Dill)
   Parts used: Seeds, lightly crushed
   Preparation and dosage: Infusion 1–2g/day, hydrosol 6–12ml/day, tincture 1.5–15ml/day or equivalent in capsule/powder.
   Actions: Aromatic carminative, anti-nausea, galactagogue, sedative.
   Comments: Relieves wind, hiccoughs, colic, and nausea. Specific for infant colic.

Angelica archangelica (Garden Angelica)
   Avoid in first trimester
   Parts used: Seed, root, and rhizome, leaf. Root is most powerful.
   Preparation and dosage: Infusion/decoction 1–2g/day, tincture 1–3ml/day or equivalent in capsule/powder.
   Actions: Stimulating and warming expectorant, antifungal, antibacterial, aromatic bitter tonic, diaphoretic, diuretic, anti-spasmodic, emmenagogue, oxytocic, uterine tonic.
   Comments: Cover the vessel if decocting.

Angelica sinensis (Chinese Angelica, Dong Quai)
   Avoid during pregnancy
   Parts used: Root
   Preparation and dosage: Decoction 2–4g/day, tincture 1.5–6ml/day or equivalent in capsule/powder.
   Actions: Warming and stimulating, pelvic vasodilator, increases uterine blood flow. Uterine anti-spasmodic, circulatory arterial stimulant, allays inflammation, adaptogen, sedative.
   Comments: Women's blood and energy tonic, nourishing to genito-urinary system. Helps libido. Specific as postpartum tonic, combines well with Astragalus.

Arctium Lappa (Burdock)
   Parts used: Root, leaves. Root is most powerful medicine. Leaves are a cleansing, nutritive tonic.
   Preparation and dosage: Root: infusion or decoction 2–6g/day, tincture 1–3ml/day or equivalent in capsule/powder.
   Actions: Alterative, antibacterial, diuretic, demulcent, circulatory and lymphatic stimulant, hepatic stimulant, choleretic, regulates blood sugar, tones uterus.
   Comments: Specific for chronic skin conditions with dry, scaly skin.

Arnica montana (Arnica)
   External use only.
   Parts used: Flowerheads
   Comments: Apply lotion, cream, or ointment to unbroken skin. Topical application for bruises, sprains, chilblains.

Artemisia vulgaris (Mugwort)

Avoid during pregnancy. Caution in lactation.

Parts used: Aerial parts, picked in flower

Preparation and dosage: Infusion 500mg/day, tincture 1–2ml/day or equivalent in capsule/powder.

Actions: Stimulant and bitter tonic, emmenagogue, nervine tonic, stomachic, choleretic, anthelmintic, hormone enhancer, mild sedative, antibacterial, antifungal.

Comments: Aids transitions. Used for dreaming and dream pillows, connection with 'moon forces' of the psyche. Dried herb burnt as 'smudge' for cleansing. Clears energetic blocks, helps with letting go of old and making way for change.

Astragalus membranaceus (Milk Vetch)

Avoid in acute infections

Parts used: Root

Preparation and dosage: Decoction 2–15g/day, tincture 1.5–10ml/day or equivalent in capsule/powder.

Actions: Immune enhancing tonic, adaptogen, diuretic, hypotensive, antioxidant, cardio and pulmonary tonic, hepatoprotective, hypoglycaemic, anti-neoplastic.

Comments: Indicated for pelvic organ prolapse.

Avena sativa (Oats)

Parts used: Aerial parts (Oatstraw) picked when the fruit yields 'milk' when crushed, immature milky seeds as specific tincture. Juice 10ml bd.

Preparation and dosage: Infusion 2–20g/day, tincture 1.5–15ml/day or equivalent in capsule/powder.

Actions: Nutritive, restorative nerve tonic, antidepressant, sedative, nerve anti-spasmodic.

Comments: Restores deficiency of nervous system, debility and exhaustion, strengthens bones and teeth. Eating porridge before bed promotes restful sleep by balancing blood sugar and raising serotonin levels. Combines well with Scutellaria and Hypericum for nervous debility and depression.

Ballota nigra (Black Horehound)

Parts used: Aerial parts

Preparation and dosage: Infusion 1–4g/day, tincture 1.5–15ml/day or equivalent in capsule/powder.

Actions: Anti-emetic, sedative. Mild astringent. Mild expectorant.

Comments: Combines well with Chamomile for nausea of pregnancy.

Baptisia tinctoria (Wild Indigo)

Parts used: Root

Preparation and dosage: Decoction 1–2g/day, tincture 1.5–4ml/day or equivalent in capsule/powder.

Actions: Stimulating antiseptic, allays inflammation, anti-microbial, anti-catarrhal, febrifuge.

Comments: Specific for upper respiratory tract infection and in toxic and septic conditions with ulceration. Combines well with Echinacea (*Echinacea* spp.) and Myrrh (*Commiphora molmol*) in infection, and with Galium for lymphatic infection.

*Barosma betulina (Buchu)
Avoid in first trimester
Parts used: Leaves
Preparation and dosage: Infusion 1–3g/day, tincture 1.5–5ml/day or equivalent in capsule/powder.
Actions: Genito-urinary tonic stimulant, diuretic, urinary antiseptic, antilithic, aromatic.
Comments: Soothing to pelvic nerves. Combines well with Althaea, Filipendula, and Zea in painful urinary tract conditions. Best as an infusion.

Bellis perennis (Daisy)
Parts used: Flowerheads, leaves
Preparation and dosage: Decoction 1–3g/day, tincture 1.5–4ml/day or equivalent in capsule/powder.
Actions: Astringent, tonic, anti-inflammatory, demulcent, hepatic, cardiac tonic, expectorant, leaves stimulate metabolism, anti-rheumatic, analgesic, vulnerary, anti-neoplastic.
Comments: Reduces compulsive behaviour, emotional shock. Topically: bruises.

Calendula officinalis (Marigold)
Use high alcohol tincture for optimal antiseptic action, lower alcohol for inflammation
Parts used: Flowerheads or petals (ray florets)
Preparation and dosage: Decoction 3–10g/day, tincture 1–10ml/day or equivalent in capsule/powder.
Actions: Anti-spasmodic, anti-inflammatory, promotes healing, lymphatic deobstruent, antibacterial, antifungal, antiviral, anti-neoplastic, immunostimulant, alterative, astringent, anti-haemorrhagic, improves circulation of blood and lymph in pelvis, cholagogue, vulnerary, dermatological agent, anti-haemorrhagic, healing for peptic ulcers.
Comments: Specific for enlarged or inflamed lymph nodes, inflammatory skin lesions, sebaceous cysts, blocked Fallopian tubes.

Capsella bursa pastoris (Shepherd's Purse)
Caution in labour—useful for haemorrhage but may cause hard to pass clots if given prophylactically. Tincture may lose efficacy with extended storage
Parts used: Fresh aerial parts

Preparation and dosage: Infusion 1–3g/day, tincture 1.5–10ml/day or equivalent in capsule/powder.

Actions: Astringent, anti-haemorrhagic, promotes healing, diuretic, uterine and urinary system tonic, urinary antiseptic, anti-inflammatory, hypotensive, vasodilator, antibacterial, diuretic, prostate tonic.

Capsicum minimum (Cayenne Pepper)
Parts used: Ripe fruits
Preparation and dosage: Infusion 30–120mg/day, tincture 0.1–1.5ml/day or equivalent in capsule/powder.
Actions: Pure stimulant, cardiovascular, circulatory and gastrointestinal stimulant, carminative, tonic, sialagogue, anti-spasmodic, diaphoretic, antioxidant, anti-platelet. Topically: rubefacient, antiseptic, haemostatic.
Comments: Aids parturition. Combines well with Lobelia for a more diffusive action.

Carduus marianus, Silybum marianum (Milk Thistle)
Parts used: Seed
Preparation and dosage: Decoction 1–3g/day, tincture 1.5–10ml/day or equivalent in capsule/powder.
Actions: Hepatocyte protector and trophorestorative, cholagogue, choleretic, protects the liver from damaging toxins, prevents and heals liver damage, galactagogue, demulcent, some anti-emetic action.
Comments: Combines well with Peppermint. Take warm before food.

Carum carvi (Caraway)
Parts used: Seed, lightly crushed
Preparation and dosage: Infusion 1–2g/day, hydrosol 6–12ml/day, tincture 1.5–15ml/day or equivalent in capsule/powder.
Actions: Powerful carminative, anti-spasmodic, expectorant, galactagogue, astringent, aromatic.
Comments: Combines well with Fennel seed for infant colic.

Cassia acutifolia/angustifolia spp (Senna)
Avoid with haemorrhoids or irritable bowel syndrome
Parts used: Pods
Preparation and dosage: Pods: Infusion 0.5–2g/day, tincture 1.5–6ml/day or equivalent in capsule/powder.
Actions: Laxative, acts within two to six hours.
Comments: Combine with Anethum, Foeniculum, Zingiber to prevent griping.

Caulophyllum thalictroides (Blue Cohosh)
UK: Included on general Sale List with maximum single dose of 265mg.
Unavailable for prescription in Ireland

Labour only. Traditional use in six weeks prior to delivery. Avoid in lactation

Parts used: Rhizome and roots

Preparation and dosage: Decoction 0.25–1.25g/day, tincture 1–5ml/day.

Actions: Anti-spasmodic, uterine and ovarian tonic, emmenagogue, oxytocic, anti-rheumatic.

Comments: Relieves false labour pains and prevents premature delivery. During labour: invigorates the uterus, especially in hypotonic conditions with exhaustion, relaxes a rigid os[1], co-ordinates uterine contractions, helps expel placenta. To expedite labour, combines well with Cimicifuga, equal parts, and other herbs where indicated.

Cautions: Higher doses of Caulophyllum have been linked with adverse reactions, but I have not seen ill-effects with Caulophyllum at recommended dosage (usually maximum 5ml/day in six weeks prior to delivery, and absolutely adhering to golden rule to not exceed 20ml tincture in twenty-four hours during labour, typically keeping at 9ml maximum during labour). Some herbalists caution that use in labour should cease at 5–6cm dilation due to risk of excessive dilation of blood vessels in the pelvis.

Centella/Hydrocotyle asiatica (Gotu Cola)

Parts used: Aerial parts

Preparation and dosage: Infusion 1.8g/day, tincture 3–6ml/day or equivalent in capsule/powder.

Actions: Adaptogen, alterative, mild diuretic, anti-rheumatic, dermatological agent, vulnerary.

Comments: Specific for recovery from surgery, heals without a scar. Tiredness, debility, depression.

Cetraria islandica (Iceland Moss)

Parts used: Lichen.

Preparation and dosage: Infusion 1–6g/day, tincture 3–7ml/day or equivalent in capsule/powder.

Actions: Demulcent for respiratory, gastrointestinal and urinary tracts, anti-catarrhal. Anti-emetic, expectorant, supports the thyroid.

Comments: Nutritive bitter tonic for chronic, debilitated conditions. Combines with Ballota for nausea and vomiting of pregnancy.

*Chamaelirium luteum (cultivated) (False Unicorn) AT RISK OF EXTINCTION

Parts used: Root. Small doses effective.

Preparation and dosage: Infusion or decoction 1–3g/day, tincture 1.5–5ml/day or equivalent in capsule/powder.

Actions: Safe and nourishing uterine, ovarian, and reproductive tonic, strengthens pelvic tissues and promotes pelvic nutrition, adaptogen, stimulant, mucous membrane tonic, sialagogue, bitter, aphrodisiac, hormone enhancer, enhances fertility.

Comments: Improves placental circulation, poor tone in cervix, pelvic organ prolapse and ovarian pain. Specific for threatened miscarriage and fertility problems. Supports creativity on all levels.

If Chamaelirium is unavailable, Asparagus racemosus (Shatavari) shows some promise as a substitute in certain cases, also Leonurus and *Angelica sinensis*.

Chamomilla recutita, Matricaria chamomilla/recutita (German Chamomile)
Avoid in allergy to Compositae family
Parts used: Flowerheads
Preparation and dosage: Infusion 2–6g/day, tincture 1.5–7ml/day or equivalent in capsule/powder.
Actions: Gastrointestinal carminative and anti-spasmodic, mild sedative, anti-emetic, anti-inflammatory, analgesic, neuralgesic, anti-allergic, anti-catarrhal, antiseptic, vulnerary.
Comments: Infantile colic, false labour pains, vaginal inflammation, breast disorders. Sedative for irritable, sensitive individuals and children.
Note: *Chamaemelum nobile* (Roman Chamomile) has similar properties and may be used as a substitute.

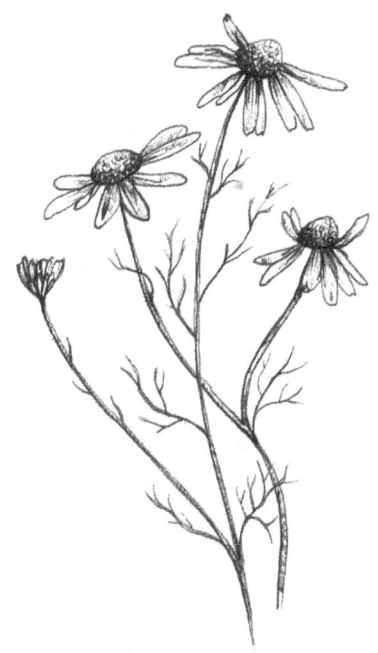

Cimicifuga racemosa (Black Cohosh)
Week 38 onwards and during labour only. Traditional use in six weeks prior to delivery. Avoid in lactation.
Parts used: Rhizome and roots
Preparation and dosage: Decoction 0.5–3g/day, tincture 1–5ml/day or equivalent in capsule/powder.
Actions: Anti-spasmodic, alterative, sedative, analgesic, emmenagogue, anti-inflammatory, nervine.

Comments: Hormone balancer with neuroendocrine effects, galactagogue. Partus preparator, eases erratic spasmodic pains and increases true contractions, relieves excessive tone, relaxes a rigid os.[1]

Cinnamonum zeylandicum/verum (Cinnamon)
Parts used: Inner bark
Preparation and dosage: Infusion 1–3g/day, tincture 1.5–4ml/day or equivalent in capsule/powder.
Actions: Anti-spasmodic, carminative, antiseptic, anti-microbial, astringent, expectorant.

Commiphora molmol, Commiphora myrrha (Myrrh)
Parts used: Resin. Best extracted as high alcohol tincture.
Preparations and dosage: Tincture 1–6ml/day or equivalent in capsule/powder.
Actions: Antiseptic, astringent, anti-inflammmatory, stimulant, anti-microbial, expectorant, anti-catarrhal, vulnerary.
Comments: Stimulates production of leucocytes. Combines well with Echinacea for systemic infection. Can help stimulate contractions and ease labour.

Crataegus monogyna/oxacanthoides (Hawthorn)
Parts used: Flowering tops, berries
Preparation and dosage: Infusion 1–6g/day, tincture 1.5–20ml/day or equivalent in capsule/powder.
Actions: Cardiotonic, trophorestorative to myocardium, coronary vasodilator, increases coronary circulation improving dyspnoea, angina and palpitations. Anti-sclerotic, relaxes tone in peripheral circulation, mild sedative, stabilizes blood pressure as cardiac function improves.
Comments: Optimum effect from taking continuously over a prolonged period.

Curcuma longa (Turmeric)
Parts used: Rhizome
Preparation and dosage: Infusion 2–9g/day, tincture 1.5–10ml/day or equivalent in capsule/powder.
Actions: Cholagogue, choleretic and hepatoprotective, anti-inflammatory, anti-oxidant, astringent, stimulant, tonic, anti-allergic, anti-microbial, stomachic, lowers cholesterol, inhibits platelet aggregation, anti-neoplastic, immunostimulant, supports adrenals.

Dioscorea villosa (Wild Yam)
Parts used: Root
Preparation and dosage: Infusion or decoction 1–6g/day, tincture 1.5–15ml/day or equivalent in capsule/powder.

Actions: Anti-spasmodic and anti-inflammatory, especially in digestive, urinary, and female reproductive systems. anti-rheumatic, cholagogue, regulates hormones, calms autonomic nervous system, parturient, oestrogenic, analgesic.

Comments: Helps prevent miscarriage.

Echinacea angustifolia, pallida, and *purpurea* (Purple Cone Flower)
Parts used: Root, whole plant, green fruit
Preparations and dosage: I use Echinacea purpurea fresh root tincture. Tinctures better than capsules or tablets.
Infusion or decoction 1–4g/day, tincture 3–40ml/day or equivalent in capsule/powder.
Actions: Immune modulator, immune enhancer, stimulating alterative for toxic conditions of blood and lymph, anti-inflammatory, vulnerary, lymphatic, sialagogue, anti-neoplastic, peripheral vasodilator.

Eleutherococcus senticosus (Siberian Ginseng)
Caution is advised in prescribing Siberian Ginseng to breastfeeding mothers in the first six weeks postpartum (see page 251 'Postpartum Care')
Parts used: Root
Preparation and dosage: Infusion or decoction 1–3g/day, tincture 5–15ml/day or equivalent in capsule/powder.
Actions: Adaptogen reducing fatigue, weakness, and stress. General restorative tonic. Tonic, anti-inflammatory, antiviral, hypoglycaemic, antidiabetic. Adrenal and thyroid trophorestorative.
Comments: Normalises hypothalamic-pituitary-adrenal function at times of stress. Improves vitality, mental ability, speed, and quality of work.

Ephedra sinica (Ma huang) ♣
Unavailable for prescription in Ireland
Short term use only during pregnancy (up to seven days followed by two-week break), not in first trimester and not during lactation. Discontinue one week prior to surgery.
Contraindications: Anxiety, hypertension, impaired cerebral circulation, heart disease, glaucoma, thyrotoxicosis, or with monoamine oxidase inhibitors.
Parts used: Young stems
Preparation and dosage: Infusion 0.5–1g/day, tincture 1–3ml/day or equivalent in capsule/powder.
Actions: Bronchodilator, relieves bronchial spasm, anti-allergic, nasal decongestant, anti-asthmatic, central nervous system stimulant, sympathomimetic.
Comments: Spray in hayfever, vasoconstrictor effect on nasal mucosa.

Equisetum arvense (Horsetail)
Parts used: Young aerial stems

Preparation and dosage: Infusion or decoction 1–4g/day, tincture 2–8ml/day or equivalent in capsule/powder.

Actions: Genito-urinary astringent, re-mineralising, tonic diuretic, stimulant, vulnerary, anti-haemorrhagic and cicatrisant to slow-healing wounds, antilithic, immune enhancer, anti-atheromatous.

Comments: Specific for healing and repair in chronic degenerative processes, such as atherosclerosis, chronic lung conditions, osteoporosis.

Euphrasia officinalis (Eyebright)
Parts used: Aerial parts.
Preparation and dosage: Infusion 2–6g/day, tincture 3–10ml/day or equivalent in capsule/powder. 10-minute decoction for eyewash.
Actions: Anti-catarrhal, astringent tonic, antihistamine, ophthalmic tonic.
Comments: Specific as anti-inflammatory lotion for eye wash and nasal douche.

Filipendula ulmaria (Meadowsweet)
Avoid in salicylate sensitivity
Parts used: Aerial parts, picked in flower
Preparation and dosage: Infusion 2–12g/day, tincture 3–15ml/day or equivalent in capsule/powder.
Actions: Tonic to digestive system, antacid, astringent, antibacterial, anti-ulcer, diuretic, mild urinary antiseptic, antilithic, anti-rheumatic, analgesic, immunostimulant, mild diaphoretic.
Comments: Gentle digestive and urinary astringent for urinary tract infection and infant diarrhoea. Combines with Ballota for vomiting of pregnancy.

Foeniculum vulgare (Fennel)
Parts used: Seeds, lightly crushed
Preparation and dosage: Infusion 1–2g/day, hydrosol 6–12ml/day, tincture 1.5–15ml/day or equivalent.
Actions: Carminative, intestinal anti-spasmodic, ophthalmic, mild expectorant for babies, aromatic, galactagogue, uterine stimulant, aphrodisiac, oestrogenic effect.
Topical: Infusion and hydrosol as eyewash for babies.
Comments: Fennel helps with seeing clearly and digesting difficult things in life.

Fucus vesiculosis (Bladder wrack)
Parts used: Whole plant
Preparation and dosage: Infusion 5–20g/day, tincture 2–20ml/day or equivalent in capsule/powder.
Actions: Lymphatic tonic alterative, anti-hypothyroid, deobstruent, anti-hypertensive, anti-rheumatic, antiobesic, rich in vitamins, minerals and trace elements.
Comments: Increase dose gradually. Helps with threatening dreams.

Galega officinalis (Goat's Rue)
   Parts used: Aerial parts (seeds also used in diabetes)
   Preparation and dosage: Infusion 2–4g/day, tincture 2–15ml/day or equivalent in capsule/powder.
   Actions: Galactagogue esp when fresh, antidiabetic, hypoglycaemic, diuretic, diaphoretic, anthelmintic.
   Comments: Combines well with Vitex and Foeniculum to stimulate milk production. Footbath for aching feet.

Galium aperine (Cleavers)
   Parts used: Aerial parts, preferably fresh
   Preparation and dosage: Infusion 2–10g/day, tincture 2–15ml/day or equivalent in capsule/powder, juice 10–20ml bd.
   Actions: Lymphatic tonic alterative, diuretic, mild astringent, demulcent, cooling, antilithic, anti-neoplastic.
   Comments: Combines well with Wild Indigo (*Baptisia tinctoria*), Calendula, and Echinacea for lymphatic conditions, with Rumex and *Arctium lappa* for skin complaints.

Gelsemium sempervirens (Yellow Jasmine) ☘
   Unavailable for prescription in Ireland
Labour only. Avoid in pregnancy and lactation.
   Parts used: Rhizome and root
   Preparation and dosage: Infusion 30mg/day, tincture 0.5ml/day or equivalent in capsule/powder.
   Actions: Sedative, analgesic for neuralgic pain, anti-spasmodic, cardiac sedative for extra systoles and functional heart disease, hypotensive.
   Comments: Combines well with Anemone to relax cervix during labour.

Gentiana lutea (Yellow Gentian)
   Parts used: Rhizome and root
   Preparation and dosage: Infusion or decoction 1–6g/day, tincture 1–10ml/day or equivalent in capsule/powder.
   Actions: Strong 'stomach' bitter, gastrointestinal tonic, stimulates gastric secretions and motility, improves gastric tone, sialogogue, anti-bilious, cholagogue.
   Comments: May aggravate stomach hyperacidity, small doses only in pregnancy. Best sipped thirty minutes before food.

Geranium robertianum (Herb Robert)
   Parts used: Leaves, flowering tops
   Preparation and dosage: Infusion 5–10g/day, tincture 2–15ml/day or equivalent in capsule/powder.

Actions: Gentle astringent, haemostatic, styptic.
Comments: Helps reduce milk supply when weaning.

Glechoma hederacea (Ground Ivy)
Parts used: Leaves, flowering tops
Preparation and dosage: Infusion 2–10g/day, tincture 1.5–15ml/day or equivalent in capsule/powder.
Actions: Anti-catarrhal, astringent, mild expectorant and anti-tussive, digestive, diuretic, vulnerary.
Comments: Combines well with Solidago for sinus catarrh.

Glycyrrhiza glabra (Liquorice)
Avoid in first trimester. Avoid in hypertension including preeclampsia, impaired cardiac or renal function, liver disease, anorexia nervosa, or with potassium depleting drugs.
Parts used: Root and stolon
Preparation and dosage: Decoction 1–3g/day, tincture 0.7–1.5ml/day or equivalent in capsule/powder.
Actions: Expectorant, demulcent, anti-spasmodic, anti-inflammatory, adrenal tonic restorative, mild laxative, hepatoprotective, anti-tumour activity.
Comments: Normaliser of the hypothalamic-pituitary-adrenocortical system. Supports ovarian function. Calms inflammation in body, mind, emotions, and spirit. Liquorice helps other herbs combine harmoniously in a mix.

Hamamelis virginiana (Witch Hazel)
Parts used: Leaves and bark
Preparation and dosage: Infusion 1–3g/day, tincture 2–5ml/day or equivalent in capsule/powder.
Actions: Astringent, gentle tonic, anti-haemorrhagic, vasoconstrictor, anti-inflammatory, ophthalmic, antiseptic, cooling, antioxidant.
Comments: Topical: Hydrosol and ointment for piles, wounds, local inflammation. Internally: Suppositories for piles.

Humulus lupulus (Hops)
Parts used: Female flowers
Preparation and dosage: Infusion 1–3g/day, tincture 0.5–3ml/day or equivalent in capsule/powder.
Actions: Sedative, hypnotic, aromatic bitter tonic, relaxant to liver and bile ducts, galactagogue, oestrogenic effect, anti-spasmodic, analgesic, cooling and sedating, especially for disturbed sleep and hyperactive states.
Comments: Combines well with Valeriana or Passiflora for insomnia. Best at low dosage.

*Hydrastis canadensis (Golden Seal)
Labour only. Avoid during pregnancy and lactation.

Parts used: Rhizome and roots

Preparation and dosage: Decoction 1–3g/day, tincture 1–7.5ml/day or equivalent in capsule/powder.

Actions: Tonic, astringent, anti-catarrhal, laxative, smooth muscle stimulant, oxytocic, bitter, stomachic, anti-haemorrhagic, choleretic, splenic tonic, immune enhancer.

Comments: Uterine tonic stimulant, promotes contractions during labour, and helps to expel placenta.

Topically: antibacterial, antifungal. Infusion of powder makes an effective eyewash.

Hypericum perforatum (St John's Wort)

Avoid in severe depression with psychosis. Discontinue three days prior to general anaesthetic. May cause photosensitization at high dose. Contraindicated with immune suppressants, digoxin, HIV medications, chemotherapeutic drugs, anticoagulants including warfarin.

Parts used: Flowers or flowering tops

Preparation and dosage: Infusion 2–8g/day, tincture 2–15ml/day or equivalent in capsule/powder.

Actions: Nervine tonic, sedative, antidepressant, psychotropic (over a period of time), astringent, anti-inflammatory, nerve trophorestorative, antiviral, vulnerary

analgesic, prolactin depressor, anti-neoplastic.

Comments: May take a few days to take effect. Combines well with Avena, Verbena, Melissa, Scutellaria.

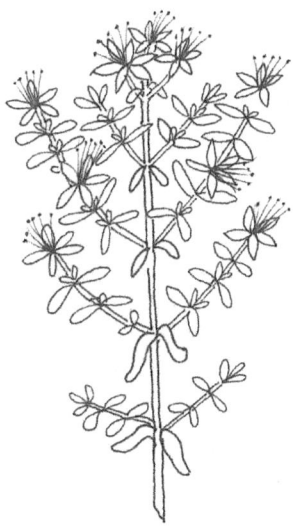

Hyssopus officinalis (Hyssop)

Parts used: Aerial parts

Preparation and dosage: Infusion 2–12g/day, tincture 1.5–12ml/day or equivalent in capsule/powder.

Actions: Carminative, expectorant, diaphoretic, sedative, anti-catarrhal, anti-tussive, anti-spasmodic.

Comments: Specific for feverish colds in babies.

Inula helenium (Elecampane)

Avoid in lactation at doses above 3g daily

Parts used: Roots and rhizomes, preferably fresh

Preparation and dosage: Decoction 2–12g/day, tincture 3–12ml/day or equivalent in capsule/powder.

Actions: Pulmonary tonic, expectorant, anti-tussive, antibacterial, diaphoretic, warming stimulant, aromatic bitter, anti-catarrhal, stomachic, hepatic, anthelmintic, vulnerary, digestive tonic.

Comments: Tones weak debilitated lungs, restores healthy immune function and sluggish capillary circulation.

Juglans cinerea (Butternut Bark)

Parts used: Bark

Preparation and dosage: Decoction 2–18g/day, tincture 2–15ml/day or equivalent in capsule/powder.

Actions: Cholagogue, laxative, alterative, stimulates peristalsis and clearing of lower bowel, relieving portal system and decongesting the liver. Hypoglycaemic, stimulates liver and pancreas.

Comments: Combines well with Arctium and *Rumex crispus* for skin diseases.

Lamium album (White Deadnettle)

Parts used: Flowering tops

Preparation and dosage: Infusion 2–10g/day, tincture 2–15ml/day or equivalent in capsule/powder.

Actions: Astringent, anti-inflammatory, anti-catarrhal, haemostatic, antiviral, demulcent, refrigerant, mild sedative, expectorant. Tonic to the urinary tract, uterus, and prostate.

Comments: Combines with Capsella for postpartum haemorrage. Specific for benign enlarged prostate. Sitz bath for vaginal candida.

Lavandula angustifolia (Lavender)

Parts used: Flowers

Preparation and dosage: Infusion 2–6g/day, tincture 2–12ml/day or equivalent in capsule/powder.

Actions: Anti-spasmodic, sedative, anxiolytic, antidepressant, carminative, astringent, anti-rheumatic, cholagogue, analgesic, antibacterial.

Comments: Best as inhalation for anti-spasmodic effect. Lavender has an affinity for conditions affecting the head, as well as depression with digestive disturbance. Combines with Rosemary for depression.

Leonurus cardiaca (Motherwort)

Parts used: Flowering tops

Preparation and dosage: Infusion 2–8g/day, tincture 2–18ml/day or equivalent in capsule/powder.

Actions: Sedative, anti-spasmodic, cardiac tonic, hypotensive, reduces nervous tension, eases palpitations from anxiety or hormonal disturbance, anti-thyroid. Gentle emmenagogue, uterine tonic and sedative, reduces pelvic irritability.

Comments: Indicated as part of treatment for threatened miscarriage or hypertonic states during labour. Specific for restless legs of pregnancy. Heals and supports the mother-child relationship on all levels.

Lobelia inflata (Lobelia) ☙

Unavailable for prescription in Ireland

External use only in pregnancy and lactation. Internal use safe for labour

Parts used: Aerial parts and seeds

Preparation and dosage: Infusion or decoction 0.6–1.8g/day, tincture 1.8–6ml/day or equivalent in capsule/powder.

Actions: Relaxant to central and autonomic nervous system and to neuromuscular action. Respiratory stimulant, anti-asthmatic, anti-spasmodic, arterial sedative, expectorant, emetic, cholagogue, hepatic.

Comments: Specific for perineal and os rigidity during labour, and in baths, rubs, and compresses to relieve tension and spasm. Combines well with Capsicum, and nervines such as Scutellaria, also Viburnum opulus as anti-spasmodic.

Medicago sativa (Alfalfa)

Parts used: Leaf, seed, sprouted seed

Preparation and dosage: Infusion 5–20g/day, tincture 2–20ml/day or equivalent in capsule/powder.

Actions: Nutritive bitter tonic, alterative, source of vitamins A, C, E, K, B1, B6, B12, and minerals such as Ca, K, Ph, Fe.

Comments: In convalescence and after weight loss.

Melissa officinalis (Lemon Balm)

Parts used: Aerial parts, picked just before flowering

Preparation and dosage: Infusion (water not quite boiling) 2–12g/day, tincture 2–15ml/day or equivalent in capsule/powder.

Actions: Carminative, anti-spasmodic, sedative, nervine, lifts mood, hypotensive, diaphoretic, thyroid stimulating hormone (TSH) antagonist. Topically: antiviral.

Comments: Specific for acute depressive states with tearfulness, 20gtt Tr prn. Topically: cream for genital herpes.

Mentha piperita (Peppermint)

Avoid in oesophageal reflux

Parts used: Leaves and flowering tops
Preparation and dosage: Infusion 2–4g/day, tincture 2–5ml/day or equivalent in capsule/powder.
Actions: Anti-spasmodic, carminative, diaphoretic, anti-emetic, stomachic, choleretic, cholagogue, cooling, sedative, anti-tussive, analgesic.
Comments: Reduces breast milk. Specific for flatulent digestive pains.

Mitchella repens (Partridge Berry)
Parts used: Aerial parts
Preparation and dosage: Infusion 2–6g/day, tincture 2–7.5ml/day or equivalent in capsule/powder.
Actions: Uterine tonic, partus preparator, diuretic, astringent, parturient, antilithic.
Comments: Tones and nourishes uterus in third trimester, strengthens during labour, helps control postpartum haemorrhage and expel placenta. Combines with Rubus and Astragalus for pelvic organ prolapse. Inspires self-confidence.

Nepeta cataria (Catnip, Catnep, Catmint)
Parts used: Leaves and flowering tops
Preparation and dosage: Infusion 2–10g/day, tincture 2–18ml/day or equivalent in capsule/powder.
Actions: Carminative, anti-spasmodic, relaxing diaphoretic, febrifuge, sedative, astringent, soothing nervine, relieves irritation, analgesic, anti-diarrhoeal.
Comments: Combines with Elder, Hyssop, and Yarrow for colds in babies, with Foeniculum for colic.

Ocimum tenuiflorum/sanctum (Tulsi/Holy Basil/Sacred Basil)
Parts used: Leaves
Preparation and dosage: Infusion 2–6g/day, tincture 1.5–5ml/day or equivalent in capsule/powder.
Actions: Adaptogenic, tonic, immune modulator, anxiolytic, antidepressant, anti-catarrhal, expectorant, anti-haemorrhagic.
Comments: Enhances stamina and endurance.

Panax Ginseng (Ginseng)
Avoid in first trimester, acute infection, acute asthma, conditions of excess heat, haemorrhaging, hypertension
Parts used: Root. Fresh white roots are perishable and turn red when preserved by steaming.
Preparation and dosage: Decoction 1–3g/day, tincture 2–12ml/day or equivalent in capsule/powder. Root chewed in labour, up to 9g.
Actions: Adaptogen, alterative tonic, antidepressant, stimulant, demulcent, anti-oxidant, increases resistance and improves physical and mental performance.
Comments: Specific for debility and exhaustion.

Parietaria judaica (Pellitory-of-the-wall)
Has caused hypersensitivity reactions in susceptible individuals: rhinitis, hay fever, rarely asthma

Parts used: Aerial parts

Preparation and dosage: Infusion 2–8g/day, tincture 2–15ml/day or equivalent in capsule/powder.

Actions: Demulcent, diuretic, kidney tonic, alterative, antilithic, vulnerary.

Comments: Combines with Althaea, Agropyron, Barosma, and Zea for genito-urinary conditions. Best given by infusion.

Passiflora incarnata (Passionflower)

Parts used: Leaves just before flowering or whole herb during fruiting

Preparation and dosage: Infusion 1–2g/day, tincture 1.5–6ml/day or equivalent in capsule/powder.

Actions: Relaxing nervine for all nervous diseases. Sedative, hypnotic, anti-spasmodic, analgesic, anxiolytic, adrenal relaxant. Relieves wakefulness, nervous excitability, restlessness, panic, and agitation.

Comments: Eases neuralgic pain, soothes adrenals after shock or stress. Combines well with Valeriana and Humulus for insomnia.

Pimpinella anisum (Aniseed)

Parts used: Seeds, lightly crushed

Preparation and dosage: Infusion 1–2g/day, hydrosol 6–12ml/day, tincture 1.5–15ml/day or equivalent.

Actions: Expectorant, anti-spasmodic, carminative, galactogogue, emmenagogue, anti-microbial.

Comments: Less strong carminative action than Caraway or Fennel, but stronger expectorant.

Plantago lanceolata/major (Plantain)

Parts used: Leaves or aerial parts

Preparation and dosage: Infusion 2–12g/day, tincture 3–12ml/day or equivalent in capsule/powder.

Action: Astringent, anti-haemorrhagic, expectorant, demulcent, anti-tussive, anti-microbial, anti-inflammatory, diuretic, pulmonary and blood tonic, antihistamine, anti-allergy, vulnerary, emollient.

Comments: Plantago psyllium gives dark psyllium seeds (my preference), light psyllium seeds are from Plantago ovata. Both are demulcent and laxative.

Quercus robur/petraea (Oak)

Parts used: Bark

Preparation and dosage: Decoction 2–6g/day, tincture 2–5ml/day or equivalent in capsule/powder.

Actions: Astringent, antibacterial, allays inflammation, haemostatic.

Comments: Topically: decoction for weeping eczema, inflammatory eye conditions, tones the nipples in lactating mothers.

Ranunculus ficaria (Lesser Celandine)
Parts used: Aerial parts
Preparation and dosage: Ointment for haemorrhoids and anal skin tags.
Actions: Astringent, anti-inflammatory.

Rhodiola rosea (Roseroot)
Parts used: Root
Preparation and dosage: Infusion 2–8g/day, tincture 2–5ml/day or equivalent in capsule/powder.
Actions: Adaptogenic tonic, stimulant, nervine tonic, antidepressant, anti-neoplastic

Ricinus communis (Castor Oil plant)
Parts used: Seeds, pressed to obtain oil
Actions: Laxative, purgative, emollient.
Comments: Traditionally, 20ml taken as laxative and to stimulate uterine contractions, often mixed with fruit juice. Topically: Castor oil packs are powerful detoxifiers, softening, and soothing inflamed surfaces while aiding elimination. Apply to navel of newborn if any difficulty healing.

Rosa species: *Rosa damascene* (Damask Rose), *Rosa canina* (Dog Rose) **Rosa gallica** (Apothecary's Rose).
Parts used: Petals when flowers newly opened
Preparation and dosage: Infusion 2–6g/day, tincture 3–12ml/day or equivalent in capsule/powder.
Actions: Astringent, antidepressant, anxiolytic, sedative, aphrodisiac, anti-inflammatory, lifts mood, calms and tones the nervous system. Topical: antiseptic, anti-inflammmatory, emollient, astringent.
Comments: Specific to soothe emotional pain in the heart, help overcome loss and feelings of low self-worth.

Rosa canina fructus (Rose hips)
Parts used: Fruits
Preparation and dosage: Infusion or decoction 2–10g/day, tincture or syrup 3–20ml/day.
Actions: Nutrient, high in vitamin C, plus small amounts A and B vitamins, astringent, mild diuretic, supports immune system, strengthens capillary fragility and connective tissue, antioxidant, mild laxative, reduces anxiety, infections, inflammation, diarrhoea, aids tissue regeneration.

Comments: Can be drunk throughout pregnancy and lactation as a nutritive tonic. Topical: seed oil for treatment of scars and tissue regeneration after surgery or injury.

Rosemarinus officinalis (Rosemary)
Parts used: Leaves and young twigs
Preparation and dosage: Infusion 2–4g/day, tincture 2–5ml/day or equivalent in capsule/powder.
Actions: Tonic for circulation and nervous system, stimulating, warming, carminative, anti-spasmodic, astringent, antidepressant, cardiac tonic, stomachic, cholagogue, hepatoprotective, anti-rheumatic, anti-microbial, improves memory and concentration. Topical: mild analgesic, parasiticide.
Comments: Rub for rheumatic conditions and neuralgia. Specific for depression with debility and hypotension. Combines well with Agrimony for depression with despondency.

Rubus fructicosus (Blackberry, Bramble)
Parts used: Leaves
Preparation and dosage: Strong decoction 10g/250ml as mouthwash.
Actions: Astringent

Rubus idaeus (Raspberry leaf, Red Raspberry leaf)
Limit to 1.5g dried/5ml tincture daily in first trimester (this caution is due to Raspberry's reputation as a uterine stimulant but is probably unwarranted)
Parts used: Leaves
Preparation and dosage: Infusion 1–24g/day, tincture 3–15ml/day or equivalent in capsule/powder.
Actions: Prime partus preparator and parturient. Uterine tonic, soothing astringent, anti-haemorrhagic, strengthens and tones pelvic muscles, relaxing at the same time. Soothes kidneys, tones mucous membranes. Nutrient-rich tonic, including vitamins C, E, A, B Complex, potassium, phosphorus, magnesium, manganese, copper, zinc, and calcium.
Comments: Indicated for pelvic organ prolapse. Emotionally: helps soften the heart and allow for greater receptivity and intuition.

Rumex crispus (Curled Dock, Yellow Dock)
Parts used: Root
Preparation and dosage: Decoction 2–6g/day, tincture 1–3ml/day or equivalent in capsule/powder.
Actions: Alterative, gentle laxative, cholagogue, iron-rich.
Comments: Provides deep cleansing of blood and tissues in chronic skin disease and chronic constipation.

Salvia officinalis (Sage, Red Sage)

Avoid during pregnancy and lactation apart from when weaning. Contraindication in pregnancy is due to concerns over toxicity of thujone content of essential oil.

Parts used: Leaves

Preparation and dosage: Infusion 1–3g/day, tincture 1–3ml/day or equivalent in capsule/powder.

Actions: Anti-spasmodic, stimulant tonic, antihidrotic, carminative, anti-microbial, astringent, adaptogen, antioxidant, adrenal (cortex) trophorestorative. Reduces milk production.

Sambucus nigra (Black Elder)

Parts used: Flowers, ripe fruits

Preparation and dosage: Flowers: Infusion 6–12g/day, tincture 3–15ml/day or equivalent in capsule/powder

Fruits: decoction 3–10g/day, tincture, syrup 3–20ml/day or equivalent in capsule/powder

Actions: Flowers: Anti-catarrhal, diaphoretic. Fruit: Diaphoretic, aperient, normalizes bowel in diarrhoea, immune enhancing.

Cautions: raw Elderberries can cause digestive upsets.

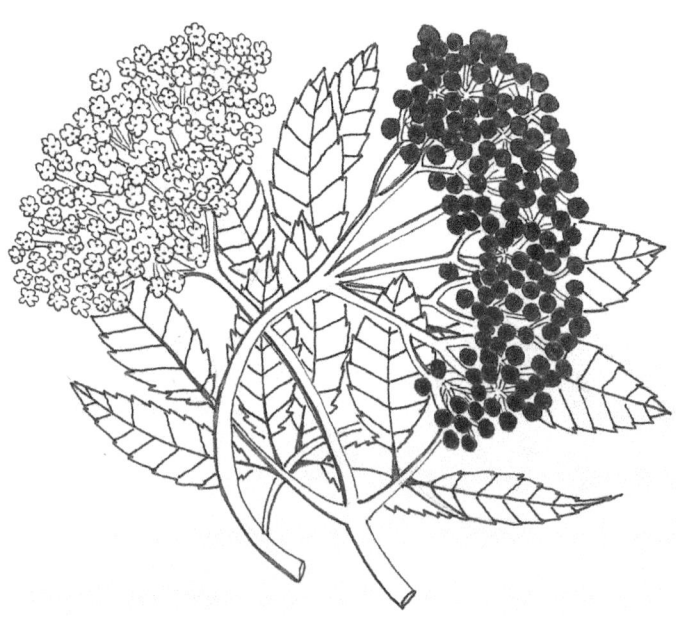

Scutellaria lateriflora (Skullcap)

Parts used: Aerial parts

Preparation and dosage: Infusion 3–6g/day, tincture 1.5–7ml/day or equivalent in capsule/powder.

Actions: Sedative, nervine tonic trophorestorative, anti-spasmodic. Relaxes nervous tension and restores an exhausted nervous system.

Comments: Combines well with Verbena, Valeriana, Passiflora, and Avena.

Serenoa repens (Saw Palmetto)

Parts used: Fruits

Preparation and dosage: Decoction 1.5–3g/day, tincture 1–4ml/day or equivalent in capsule/powder.

Actions: Diuretic, urinary antiseptic, nourishing genito-urinary and reproductive astringent tonic, adaptogen, mild sedative, warming and stimulating, aphrodisiac, endocrine stimulant, alleviates inflammation of ovaries and fallopian tubes.

Comments: Encourages intimacy and openness, learning to give and receive.

Solidago virgaurea (Goldenrod)

Parts used: Flowering tops

Preparation and dosage: Infusion 1–5g/day, tincture 1.5–3ml/day or equivalent in capsule/powder.

Actions: Anti-catarrhal, tonic, stimulating astringent diuretic, diaphoretic, antiseptic, carminative. Increases renal blood flow and glomerular filtration rate.

Comments: Specific for nasopharyngeal catarrh, acute or chronic nephritis.

Stachys betonica (Wood Betony)

Parts used: Aerial parts during flowering

Preparation and dosage: Infusion 2–6g/day, tincture 1.5–6ml/day or equivalent in capsule/powder.

Actions: Sedative, bitter tonic, astringent, stimulant, stomachic, hepatic, splenic, anti-spasmodic, choleretic.

Comments: Specific for neuralgic and ischaemic conditions affecting the head. Combines with Scutellaria for tension headache, facial neuralgia, nightmares with fearful visions, with Anemone for psychogenic head pain.

Stellaria media (Chickweed)

Parts used: Aerial parts

Preparation and dosage: Infusion 2–12g/day, tincture 3–15ml/day or equivalent in capsule/powder.

Actions: Cooling demulcent, emollient, anti-haemorrhagic, anti-rheumatic.

Comments: Specific for topical application in pruritic skin disease. Combines well with Althaea or Ulmus for ointment.

Symphytum officinale (common Comfrey)

External use only. Do NOT use Symphytum uplandicum (Russian comfrey) which is a hybrid between S. officinalis and S. asperum.

Parts used: Leaves, root, and rhizome

Actions: Topically: Demulcent, cell proliferant, astringent, anti-haemorrhagic, vulnerary, bone healing, anti-arthritic.

Indications: Ointment and infused oil specific for wound healing and tissue regeneration with reduced scar tissue formation, poultice or compress for healing bone fractures and tissue injury. Sitz bath for postpartum perineal healing.

Historical internal use for peptic ulcers, bronchial, arthritic, and ulcerative conditions.

Cautions: Comfrey contains unsaturated pyrrolizidine alkaloids (Pas) which are found in the Boraginaceae and Asteraceae (in Europe) families. Comfrey root contains higher levels than the leaf. Pas are potentially toxic but not all Pas are of the same potency, and the Pas in Symphytum are considered to be some of the mildest, albeit at relatively high levels. Targeted research is needed and out of caution, the current UK recommendation is NOT to prescribe Comfrey for oral use to pregnant or lactating women.[2] In the UK, prescribing for internal use is restricted to the leaf and for limited periods only. In Ireland, all internal use is banned.

Pas are virtually insoluble in oils, making Comfrey infused oil and ointment safe to use. Some forms of Pas are water soluble, and in pregnancy/lactation it has been suggested to use cream, poultice or lotion on unbroken skin only. Comfrey leaf (combined with Calendula) sitz baths bring invaluable and highly impressive results for postpartum perineal healing. Used once daily, for a maximum of five days postpartum, seems to me a cautious and conservative approach (not suitable for women with liver disease).

Tanacetum parthenium (Feverfew)
Labour only. Avoid in pregnancy and breastfeeding. Avoid in allergy to Compositae family.

Parts used: Leaves or flowers

Preparation and dosage: Infusion max 500mg/day, tincture 1ml/day or equivalent in capsule/powder. Twenty drops tincture hourly can be given for up to 4 hours during labour.

Actions: Anti-spasmodic, anti-inflammatory, vasodilator, bitter, carminative, emmenagogue, anti-thrombotic, mild sedative, increases uterine circulation and regularizes contractions, relaxes a rigid os.[1]

Taraxacum officinale (Dandelion)
Parts used: Leaf and root 1–2g

Preparation and dosage: Leaf: Infusion 4–30g/day, tincture 2–15ml/day or equivalent in capsule/powder.

Root: Decoction 2–24g/day, tincture 2–15ml/day or equivalent in capsule/powder.

Actions: Leaf: Diuretic, nutritive, help raise iron levels in blood

Root: Liver relaxant, cholagogue, choleretic, bitter tonic, supports liver function, gentle laxative, pancreatic, hypoglycaemic, splenic, diuretic, anti-rheumatic, anti-neoplastic.

Comments: Clears obstructions in the liver, gall bladder, and spleen. Roasted root gently stimulates digestive and eliminative organs.

Thymus vulgaris (Thyme)
Parts used: Aerial parts
Preparation and dosage: Infusion 2–12g/day, tincture 2–15ml/day or equivalent in capsule/powder.
Actions: Anti-spasmodic, carminative, anti-tussive, expectorant, antiseptic, anthelmintic, vulnerary, astringent.
Comments: Excellent calming bath for babies with catarrh, spasmodic coughs and bronchial irritation.

Tilia europaea (Common Lime/Linden Tree)
Parts used: Flowers with 'wing' attached
Preparation and dosage: Infusion 2–12g/day, tincture 1.5–7ml/day or equivalent in capsule/powder.
Actions: Diaphoretic, sedative, anti-spasmodic, nervine relaxant, diuretic, anticoagulant, enhances immunity.
Comments: Combines well with Hawthorn as a long-term tea for hypertension.

Trifolium pratense (Red Clover)
Parts used: Flowerheads and upper set of leaves
Preparation and dosage: Infusion 2–10g/day, tincture 1.5–8ml/day or equivalent in capsule/powder.
Actions: Alterative, expectorant, anti-spasmodic, dermatological agent, hormone balancer (oestrogenic effect), lymphatic cleanser, sedative, anticoagulant.
Comments: Specific for skin conditions in children, and as part of a cough mix. Helps with staying true to yourself.

Trigonella foenum graecum (Fenugreek)
Parts used: Ripe seeds
Preparation and dosage: Decoction 2–12g/day, tincture 1.5–6ml/day or equivalent in capsule/powder.
Actions: Mucilaginous demulcent, nutritive tonic, warming astringent, galactagogue, oxytocic, bitter expectorant, soothes irritable tissues, hypoglycaemic, lowers cholesterol, aids weak digestion, gentle laxative. Uterine tonic, aids fertility, increases body weight.
Comments: Specific for debility of convalescence. Helps self-nurturing.

Trillium erectum (Beth Root)
Parts used: Root and rhizome
Preparation and dosage: Decoction in water or milk 1–6g/day, tincture 1.5–8ml/day or equivalent in capsule/powder.

Actions: Astringent, anti-haemorrhagic with affinity for female reproductive system, stimulant tonic to the uterus and pelvic organs, parturient, mild expectorant.

Turnera diffusa (Damiana)
Parts used: Leaves and stem
Preparation and dosage: Infusion 2–12g/day, tincture 1.5–7ml/day or equivalent in capsule/powder.
Actions: Nervine and pelvic tonic, aphrodisiac, sexual stimulant, antidepressant, promotes well-being, laxative, diuretic, relieves anxiety, tonic to kidneys and urinary mucous membranes.
Comments: Combines well with Avena and Scutellaria as a nerve tonic.

*Ulmus rubra (Slippery Elm)
Parts used: Powdered inner bark
Preparation and dosage: Gruel drink or poultice 2–24g/day or equivalent in tablets (chewed) although these are less effective.
Actions: Demulcent, emollient, nutritive, anti-tussive, relieves inflammation, promotes healing, antacid, quietens the nervous system and aids restful sleep, soothes and lubricates the alimentary mucosa.
Comments: Specific as a gentle, nutritive food for convalescence and infants.

Urtica dioica (Nettle)
Parts used: Aerial parts
Preparation and dosage: Infusion 2–12g/day, tincture 2–20ml/day or equivalent in capsule/powder. Juice 20ml bd.
Actions: Mineral rich tonic, astringent diuretic, haemostatic, alterative, anti-allergic, circulatory stimulant, galactagogue, relieves inflammation in urinary tract, diuretic, uterine relaxant, eliminates uric acid, mildly hypoglycaemic.

Vaccinium myrtillus (Bilberry)
Parts used: Fruits
Preparation and dosage: Fresh fruit 20–50g/day, tincture 3–6ml/day or equivalent in capsule/powder. Juice 10ml bd.
Actions: Venous tonic, strengthens the micro-circulation, vasoprotective especially for eyes, astringent, allays inflammation in bladder, antioxidant, antilithic, urinary antiseptic, good source vitamin C.
Comments: Infusion of dried fruits relieves dyspepsia and diarrhoea in infants.

Valeriana officinalis (Valerian)
Caution in mania.
Parts used: Rhizome and roots
Preparation and dosage: Infusion 1–4g/day left to macerate 8–10 hours, preferably drunk cold. Tincture 3–30 ml/day, dose varying from 20 drops tds to 10–15ml hourly in acute anxiety.

Actions: Anti-spasmodic nervine, sedative, analgesic, hypnotic (without reducing concentration), carminative, hypotensive, anxiolytic, muscle relaxant.

Comments: A prime remedy for nervous system problems. Specific for nervous excitability and panic attacks. Idiosyncratic responses occur rarely (typically of stimulation), possibly due to 'sudden release of pent-up vital nerve energy'[3], give lower dose or withdraw if this happens. Said to suit small, dark haired individuals best, although I have not found this consistent. Works well as a simple, combines with Passiflora for excitability or insomnia, with Viburnum opulus for cramps.

Verbascum thapsus (Mullein)

Parts used: Leaves and flowers

Preparation and dosage: Infusion 2–16g/day, tincture 2–10ml/day or equivalent in capsule/powder. Flowers infused cold in olive oil for inflamed mucosal conditions.

Actions: Expectorant, demulcent, mild diuretic, mild sedative, anti-catarrhal (flowers), emollient, vulnerary. Soothing expectorant for acute or chronic coughs.

Comments: Flower oil specific as ear drops for painful ear conditions in infants.

Verbena officinalis (Vervain)

Parts used: Flowering spikes

Preparation and dosage: Infusion 2–12g/day, tincture 2–15ml/day or equivalent in capsule/powder.

Actions: Anti-spasmodic, nervine tonic, galactagogue, psychoneuro-endocrine and psychoneuro-immunological agent, hepatic bitter (tincture) and liver tonic, mild diaphoretic.

Comments: Infusion relaxes kidneys. Specific as a nerve tonic for over-striving, perfectionism, and obsessive behaviour. Reduces paranoia, one or two cups taken daily over a period of time. Increases spiritual understanding and psychic awareness.

Viburnum opulus (Guelder Rose, Cramp Bark)

Parts used: Bark

Preparation and dosage: Decoction 2–12g/day, tincture 1.5–20ml/day or equivalent in capsule/powder.

Actions: Powerful anti-spasmodic, weakly sedative, slightly astringent.

Comments: Prime remedy to relieve muscular tension and spasm. Combines with Dioscorea for cramp, with Valerian for hypertension.

Viburnum prunifolium (Black Haw)

Avoid in salicylate allergy

Parts used: Bark, root bark

Preparation and dosage: Infusion/decoction 2–12g/day, tincture 1.5–20ml/day or equivalent in capsule/powder.

Actions: Soothing uterine sedative, anti-spasmodic especially for pelvic organs, tonic, astringent, relaxant to uterine muscle, mild diuretic, analgesic, partus preparator, hypotensive, improves uterine and ovarian circulation, promoting pelvic nutrition.

Comments: Specific for uterine irritability and threatened miscarriage, painful conditions of pregnancy, nervous conditions affecting pregnancy or fertility. Strengthens pelvic tissues after miscarriage.

Viola tricolor (Heartsease, Pansy)
Parts used: Aerial parts
Preparation and dosage: Infusion 2–12g/day, tincture 3–7ml/day or equivalent in capsule/powder.
Actions: Dermatological agent, expectorant, diuretic, anti-inflammatory, anti-rheumatic, anti-allergy, mild laxative, alterative.
Comments: Demulcent to skin and genito-urinary tract. Topical: tea as compress for eczema.

Vitex agnus castus (Chaste Tree)
Avoid in second and third trimesters (use may extend until week 15 in rare cases).
Parts used: Berry
Preparation and dosage: Decoction 1–3g/day, tincture 1–3ml/day or equivalent in capsule/powder. This is the usual dose but there can be a wide variation depending on the person, in practice ranging from around 5gtt to 10ml tincture daily in exceptional cases. Larger doses may be required to maintain a pregnancy or in individuals with sensitive hormonal function. It is suggested that low doses increase prolactin levels while higher doses may inhibit (see page 200). Headache or nausea may indicate lack of suitability or too high a dose, discontinue immediately.
Actions: Supreme hormonal adaptogenic, galactagogue, eases inflammation, dopaminergic, indirectly progesterogenic.
Comments: Indicated for progesterone insufficiency and endocrine disorders including pituitary, ovary, adrenal, and thyroid imbalances. In pregnancy, specific for prevention of miscarriage in first trimester and as a postpartum galactagogue tonic restorative. Helps integrate different parts of self, bringing inner strength and emotional balance.

Withania somnifera (Ashwagandha, Winter Cherry)
Parts used: Root
Preparation and dosage: Decoction 1–3g/day, tincture 1–3ml/day or equivalent in capsule/powder.
Actions: Tonic nervine, adaptogen, vasotonic alterative, anti-inflammatory, controls anxiety, improves memory, anxiolytic, aphrodisiac, hypotensive.
Comments: Specific for anxiety states and debility, sexual dysfunction from exhaustion or stress.

Zea mays (Cornsilk)
Parts used: Stigmatas and styles from female flowers
Preparation and dosage: Infusion 2–15g/day, tincture 2–30ml/day or equivalent in capsule/powder.

Actions: Demulcent, diuretic, soothing and toning for all urinary and uterine conditions, antilithic, analgesic, strengthens uterine muscle tone.

Comments: Specific for acute or chronic inflammation of urinary system. Tea combines with Meadowsweet for cystitis.

**Zingiber officinalis* (Ginger)

Not always tolerated by people with sensitive stomachs and may be contraindicated with gallstones.

Parts used: Rhizome

Preparation and dosage: Infusion or decoction 0.5–2g/day, tincture 1–5ml/day or equivalent in capsule/powder.

Actions: Carminative, anti-spasmodic, diaphoretic, warming bitter, anti-emetic, circulatory and cardiovascular stimulant, peripheral vasodilator, antioxidant, sialagogue, lowers cholesterol, anti-microbial, expectorant. Improves circulation to pelvis.

Comments: Specific as anti-emetic for nausea and vomiting of pregnancy.

Notes

1. The os is the opening in the centre of the cervix, which softens and dilates in preparation for childbirth. Sometimes the os remains rigid and needs help to soften.
2. See 'Report on the safety of the oral consumption of the pyrollizidine alkaloid containing herbs *Symphytum officinale, Tussilago farfara* and *Borago officinalis*' https://nimh.org.uk/wp-content/uploads/2020/04/PA_Report2019.pdf [last accessed 6/7/21]
3. Christopher Menzies Trull. *Herbal Medicine, Keys to Physiomedicalism including Pharmacopoeia* (UK: FPHM, 2003), 889.

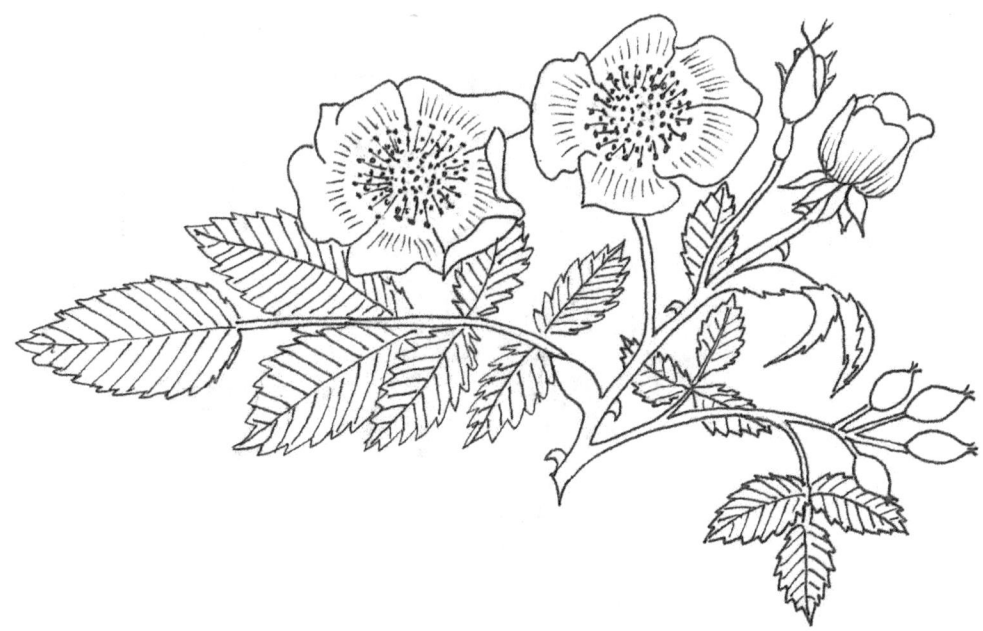

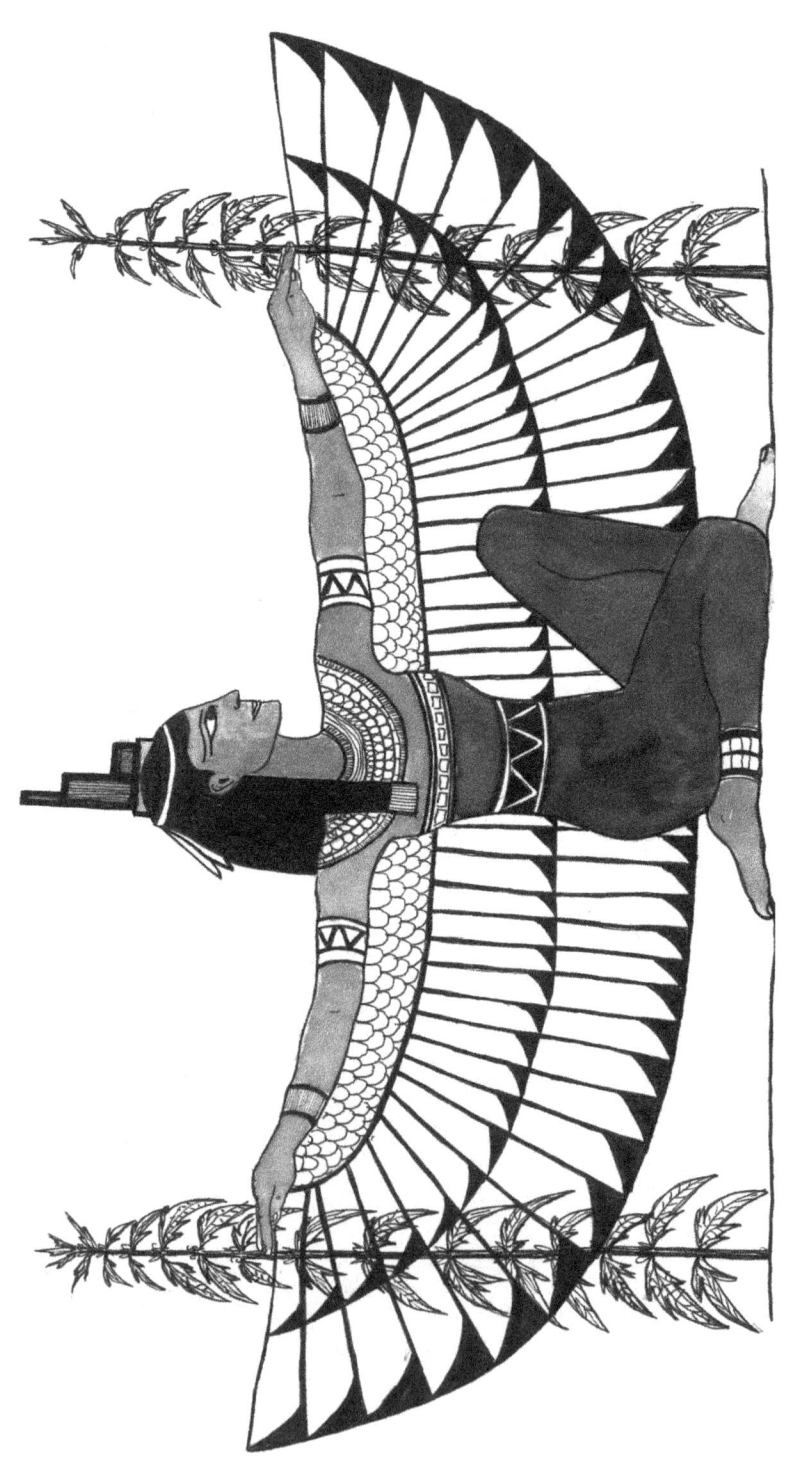

Isis. Goddess of medicine, wisdom, motherhood, fertility and magic. Giver of life. Motherwort (*Leonurus cardiaca*). The lion-hearted Mother who never gives up.

CHAPTER 8

Conditions of pregnancy

Conditions of pregnancy, an A–Z of conditions and herbal treatment

This chapter provides an A–Z of conditions that may arise in pregnancy. Some of these conditions are particularly suitable for herbal treatment, others are included for differential diagnosis and information.

Chapter 1 'Herbal Prescribing and Safety' should be read before using this A–Z.

Chapter 6 'Herbal Pharmacy' gives instructions for the standard preparation and use of herbal medicines.

Chapter 16 'Vibrational Essences' gives details for the use of essences.

NOTE: Conditions requiring urgent medical attention

Persistent vaginal bleeding: miscarriage, antepartum haemorrhage (APH), placenta praevia, placental abruption, trauma

Severe pelvic or abdominal pain

Severe headache, blurred vision or epigastric pain

Preterm/prelabour rupture of membranes prior to week 34

Regular uterine contractions prior to week 34

Cessation of foetal movement

Ectopic pregnancy

Abdominal pain and cramps

Abdominal pain in 1st trimester

Around 5 to 12 days after conception, some women experience menstrual-like cramps that may be accompanied by light spotting known as implantation bleeding, caused by the embryo attaching to the uterine wall. Cramps are usually mild (although can be intense) and spotting can last from a day to several days. Cramps (again usually mild but not always) may also occur around week 10 due to stretching of the uterine ligaments. Both of these scenarios are common and nothing to worry about. If symptoms are troublesome, they can be soothed by drinking a relaxant herbal tea such as Chamomile (*Chamomilla recutita*), Limeflowers (*Tilia europaea*), or Lemon Balm (*Melissa officinalis*)—standard infusion, up to 3 cups daily. Or apply a Chamomile compress (see page 68) as required.

Lower abdominal pain in the first trimester may also be caused by threatened miscarriage (see 'Miscarriage') or ectopic pregnancy (see 'Ectopic Pregnancy'), appendicitis, kidney inflammation or fibroid degeneration. If pain is accompanied by bleeding, this should be treated as an emergency.

Abdominal pain in 2nd and 3rd trimesters

Cramps are fairly common in the third trimester and usually no cause for alarm (see 'Braxton Hicks contractions' and 'False labour pains' in this section). Alternatively, abdominal pain in mid or late pregnancy can be referred from the spine or pelvis (see 'Back Pain, Pelvic Pain, Sciatica').

Braxton Hicks contractions

These are experienced as transitory and irregular tightenings of the uterine muscle, usually occurring any time after 20 weeks and lasting for up to a minute. They are both common and normal and are one of the ways the body prepares for labour. They do not usually require treatment. If they start to become frequent, it could be a sign of early labour, see 'Preterm labour' below, and Chapter 11 'The Process of Labour'.

False labour pains

The term 'false labour' is generally used to refer to painful uterine contractions that may seem to indicate the onset of labour, but there is no progressive dilatation[1] of the cervix.

If these contractions occur, it is typically in the last month of pregnancy, generally feeling like menstrual cramps or low backache. Clinically, they happen more often at night, but their frequency and intensity do not increase as time passes. This may simply be further preparation for eventual labour. If pains are distressing, give Motherwort, standard infusion, up to three times daily. Motherwort is an anti-spasmodic uterine sedative that calms uterine irritability. Alternatively, tincture of Motherwort may be combined in equal parts with Black Haw bark, also a uterine sedative. Take 10–20 drops of the mix, up to four times daily as required. Valerian or Chamomile tincture, 20 drops as required, may be helpful to bring relaxation, especially if sleep is disturbed or the woman is anxious.

These types of contractions will often disappear by taking a warm bath or applying a hot water bottle wrapped in a towel to the affected area. They can also be soothed by a Chamomile compress using a strong Chamomile infusion. Alternatively, you can add 1 drop each of Chamomile and Rose essential oils to 10ml of almond oil. Massage the affected area in a circular clockwise direction.

Labour

If contractions start to become frequent, it may be a sign that labour is starting (see page 211 'First Stage of Labour'). Be alert for other possible signs of labour, such as a sudden increase in the amount of vaginal discharge or sudden change in the type of discharge, a mucus show, loss of waters, a feeling of increased pressure in the pelvis or the feeling that the baby is 'pushing down'.

Preterm labour

If a woman is experiencing regular contractions (every 10 minutes or less) before 37 weeks, this may be a sign of preterm labour.

If contractions are less well-established, the woman should stay in bed and relax, staying prone to avoid gravity putting pressure on the cervix and resting on her left side to increase blood flow to the uterus. She should avoid sexual activity and vaginal examinations in order to rest the entire pelvis. Encourage her to drink plenty of water and herb teas since dehydration may be a cause, and check for a urinary tract infection (UTI, see 'Urinary Tract Conditions'), which is another cause of preterm labour. For UTIs, drink Meadowsweet (*Filipendula ulmaria*) and Cornsilk (*Zea mays*), 1 teaspoon of each dried herb per cup, four or five cups daily, and take raw garlic in the diet. Stress may be a factor (see 'Emotional and Stress-Related Conditions') and there is a greater risk of early labour in women who have already had a preterm delivery, a late miscarriage or a multiple pregnancy, or are aged under seventeen or over thirty-five.

Herbs to slow down contractions include Black Haw (*Viburnum prunifolium*) and Motherwort (*Leonurus cardiaca*). Combine tinctures in equal parts, 10–20 drops of mix every one to two hours in acute stage, then three times daily if contractions are a recurrent problem. Motherwort relaxes the central nervous system and helps nervous debility. Black Haw is specific for uterine irritability and painful conditions of pregnancy.

Wild Yam (*Dioscorea villosa*) could also be substituted as an anti-spasmodic, although the previous mix would be preferred.

Other causes of abdominal pain in late pregnancy include placental separation, ruptured uterus, ruptured stomach rectus muscle, appendicitis, or kidney inflammation. All severe pain in late pregnancy should be treated as an emergency.

Acid reflux see 'Heartburn'

Allergy

During pregnancy and lactation, the likelihood of allergy may be increased in susceptible individuals, which can mean a new allergy arising or the worsening of an existing condition (or in some cases, improvement, due to immune and hormone changes, such as increased cortisol and adrenaline). Allergy can affect any of the body systems, manifesting in symptoms such as rhinitis (see 'Rhinitis'), skin rashes, digestive disturbance, joint pains, or a host of others. If allergy occurs, proceed slowly and carefully with herbal treatment, eliminating environmental and dietary allergens as much as possible (while ensuring that adequate nutrition is maintained, see Chapter 3 'Nutrition') aiming for super-healthy gut function and administering gentle herbs appropriate to the individual. Pregnancy is not a time for extreme treatments or intense desensitisation programs.

Severe hayfever can be common, in which case favour gentle herbs, such as Elderflower (*Sambucus nigra*), Eyebright (*Euphrasia officinalis*), Nettles (*Urtica dioica*), and Chamomile (*Chamomilla recutita*). In extreme cases, small amounts of *Ephedra sinica*[2] can be given for short term use (max 3ml tincture daily for 7 days) but only after the first trimester and not while breastfeeding.

Anaemia

The World Health Organisation (WHO) defines the following haemoglobin (Hb) thresholds for pregnant women:[3]

110g/l blood in first trimester,
105g/l in second and third trimesters,
100g/l post-partum (up to six weeks post-delivery)

Any lower Hb levels are often considered to represent iron deficiency anaemia (IDA). However, a degree of anaemia in pregnancy is physiological i.e. normal, resulting from haemodilution.

Haemodilution and blood volume expansion

Blood volume increases significantly at 10 weeks gestation and continues to rise throughout pregnancy, reaching a plateau at 30–34 weeks. The total blood volume increase from pre-pregnancy levels can be as high as 100%, averaging around 50%.

Blood volume increases faster than the red blood cells can multiply, which causes haemodilution and a resultant drop in haemoglobin levels because there are less red blood cells per ml of plasma. Haemodilution is a healthy sign showing adequate blood volume expansion. Recent studies suggest that haemodilution of pregnancy has an important physiological role in improving placental microcirculation to accelerate foetal development.[4] Furthermore, women with reduced blood expansion are at higher risk of adverse reactions to bleeding.

In previous times, it was believed that a low Hb increased the risk of postpartum haemorrhage (PPH) and other problems, but there is no supporting evidence for this and it is now widely recognised as a myth although sometimes perpetuated.

Many midwives say that a woman with a lowish Hb tends to bleed less at birth, because her body automatically compensates. However, it is possible that a pre-existing iron deficiency anaemia may worsen the impact of PPH if it does occur.

Screening for anaemia

Blood testing for mean corpuscular volume (MCV) is seen as a more accurate measure of anaemia than Hb, along with mean corpuscular haemoglobin concentration (MCHC). If these are low then macrocytic and other types of anaemia (such as pernicious anaemia, thalassaemia, or sickle cell disease) need to be considered and ruled out.

In pregnancy, macrocytic anaemias are most often caused by nutritional deficiencies of folate and B12. Folic acid supplementation is rapidly effective for folate deficiency and increased B12 requirements can be met by a diet containing animal products or by B12 supplementation.

Serum ferritin, indicative of the body's iron stores, should be checked in all women at increased risk of iron deficiency, even if they are not anaemic. Women at increased risk include those with:

- Low iron stores before pregnancy (from dietary causes or from excessive blood loss, such as menorraghia)
- Previous history of deficiency
- Pre-existing blood condition (such as sickle cell, thalassaemia)
- Age <20 years
- Gut disorder (such as coeliac, IBS, previous gut surgery)
- Eating disorder
- Strict vegetarian/vegan diet

A ferritin level less than 15mg/l indicates established iron deficiency, less that 30mg/l should prompt herbal treatment.

A low haemoglobin without other evidence of iron deficiency generally requires no treatment. Of course, as well as looking at laboratory results, you will be making your own thorough assessment of a woman's health. In terms of checking how much oxygen is being carried by the blood, you can also check for pale gums, paleness under eyelids, and capillary refill when pressure is applied to the nailbed. If there is a severe Hb drop at around 33–36 weeks, it is worth considering undiagnosed twins since the foetus takes up extra iron at this time.

A high Hb level can occur for various reasons. It could be that the woman has a really good diet, because she has an iron storage disease, or because haemodilution has not occurred, which could lead to rare yet serious complications, such as pre-eclampsia/eclampsia or HELLP (haemolysis, elevated liver enzymes, and low platelets) syndrome (see 'Pre-Eclampsia/Eclampsia' page 152).

Symptoms of nutritional anaemia

The most common symptom of iron deficiency anaemia in a pregnant woman is chronic tiredness. Other symptoms include weakness, headaches, palpitations, dizziness, dyspnoea, listlessness, irritability, pallor, sore tongue, irregular heart rhythms, cracks at corners of mouth, and hair loss.

The herbalist's role

True iron deficiency anaemia poses a serious health risk for the pregnant woman and her child. As herbalists, we are in the fortunate position of being able to offer safe, and nourishing iron-rich herbs and promote absorption. By encouraging the maintenance of good iron levels throughout pregnancy we can avoid the possible need for more expensive, risky, and uncomfortable treatments. A herbalist's role includes:

- Ensuring that the woman has the required investigations. These may include full blood count, vitamin B12 and folate levels, ferritin (amount of stored iron) and transferrin saturation levels (amount of iron available to use). Be alert to any haematuria, since in rare cases of IDA (1%) the patient will have renal tract malignancy.
- Dietary advice for iron-rich foods and optimum absorption.
- Appropriate herbs. If anaemia is suspected, it is sensible to start a nourishing herbal treatment regime whilst further screening is carried out.

Herbs and dietary advice

The diet should include plenty of iron-rich foods. These include watercress, free-range eggs, beets, molasses, dark green leafy vegetables, pumpkin and sunflower seeds, dried fruit (raisins, prunes, figs, apricots), seaweeds especially Kelp, soya, parsley (not large amounts), lentils, kidney beans, butter beans, sardines, almonds, ginger, wholemeal bread, lean meat especially liver and kidney, celeriac, cottage cheese, cocoa, bananas, blackberries, blackcurrants, brown rice, cabbage, carrots, cherries, grapes, raspberries, strawberries, and sesame seeds.

Bran, tea and coffee all inhibit iron absorption and should be avoided, especially at meal times. Carbonated drinks and tobacco also limit iron uptake, as can pharmaceutical medications and antacids.

Vitamin C aids iron absorption and taking vitamin C rich foods at the same meal increases the absorption of iron from non-meat foods.

Other ways to increase absorption of nutrients include:

- Take a teaspoon of cider vinegar before meals,
- Take Gentian root tincture 10 drops before food.

Herbs excel as foods and nourishing tonics. Many herbs contain iron and other nutrients and can either be added to food or taken as teas.

Common iron-rich herbs that are easily taken as foods include Chives (*Allium schoenoprasum*), Coriander/Cilantro (*Coriandrum sativum*) leaves, Dandelion leaves (*Taraxacum off.*), Nettles (*Urtical dioica*), and Sorrel (*Rumex acetosa*).

Iron rich herbs that can be drunk as teas include Burdock leaf (*Artium lappa*), Chickweed (*Stellaria media*), Coriander leaves, Dandelion leaf and root, Elderberries (*Sambucus nigra*), Ground Ivy (*Glechoma hederacea*), Hawthorn flowering tops (*Crataegus monogyna/oxacanthoides*), Mint (*Mentha piperata*), Nettles, Raspberry leaf (*Rubus idaeus*) (max 1 cup daily in first trimester), Dog Rosehips (*Rosa canina*), Skullcap (*Scutellaria lateriflora*), Vervain (*Verbena off.*), and Yellow Dock (*Rumex crispus*).

For a simple strong iron tea, infuse 30g Nettles in 500ml boiling water for one hour, strain and drink throughout the day (can be reheated). This can be taken daily throughout pregnancy.

For treating iron-deficiency, I make the following iron tonic, which both supplies iron and facilitates absorption, as well as being delicious. This tonic is a variation of a recipe I learned from Janet Hicks and I believe was given to her originally by Scottish herbalist Brian V Lamb. It is best made in a slow cooker but can be made on top of the stove if you are careful; if so, you will need to cook on as low a heat as possible, check the pan regularly to prevent burning, top up with water if necessary and reduce cooking time by half.

Iron tonic:

1 kilo wild dried Hunza apricots (or other organic dried apricots),
1 kilo dark brown sugar
3 litres red wine
5ml/litre of each: tinctures of *Zingiber off., Gentiana lutea, Serenoa serulata, Rumex crispus, Turnera diffusa, Urtica dioica*
0.5ml/litre *Capsicum minimum*

Put apricots in slow cooker, cover with water and cook for 8 hours on a low setting.
Remove stones from apricots (if applicable).
Return apricots and liquid to slow cooker with sugar, cook 8 hours on low setting
Cool and blend in a food processor
Add 3l red wine, Stir 5–10 mins until pourable
Add tinctures, stir well and bottle.
(1kg apricots makes approximately 5l tonic. Best kept refrigerated)

Dosage: 5–10ml three times daily, on an empty stomach, one hour before meals.

This usually raises Hb about 1 point per week. In severe cases, give the 10ml dose, reducing to 5ml three times daily as Hb levels rise.

Floradix Iron + Herbs is a commercial iron tonic made from plant sources, available from health food stores. It also works well and can be taken at a double dose to raise Hb quickly.

Unlike prescribed treatments, these tonics are gentle on the stomach and do not cause constipation. For women prone to thrush (*Candida albicans*), chelated iron, from Health food stores, may be a better recommendation than Floradix, since the latter can have a tendency to ferment. If a woman is taking prescribed oral iron, ferrous citrate is preferable to ferrous sulphate, which is often poorly tolerated and absorbed.

Where someone does not respond to iron supplementation as expected, consider the possibility that there may be an underlying thyroid condition. It may be worth her having her thyroid re-tested even if screening was recently normal.

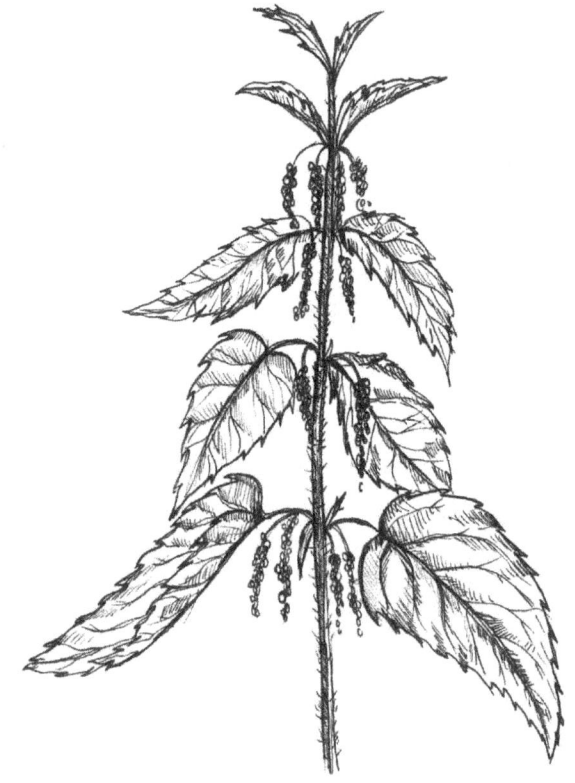

Anxiety see 'emotional and stress-related conditions'

Back pain, pelvic pain, sciatica

Back and pelvic pain and discomfort are commonly due to expansion of the pelvic joints and softening of ligaments. The weight of the baby and uterine contents puts additional strain on the lower back, which can highlight pre-existing structural issues. Pain may be related to poor posture, changes in the centre of gravity, constipation, prolonged sitting or standing, urinary tract infections, and stress on the kidneys. Women may experience pressure on the sciatic nerve giving pain in the buttocks, groin and radiating down the legs. Sometimes the loosening of ligaments allows the two sides of the sacro-iliac joint to move and rub together, which can cause intense pain in the lower back, often felt when turning over in bed or climbing stairs.

Prevention and treatment of back pain are important to avoid injury and to decrease the chance of chronic back pain. See 'Urinary Tract Conditions' for ways to support the urinary system if appropriate.

General advice for back/pelvic pain

- Pay attention to posture when sitting or standing. Avoid standing or sitting for long periods. Bend from knees rather than back.
- Establish a new centre of gravity. Flatten curve of back and bend knees slightly when standing.
- Sleep on a firm bed, lying on one side with pillows between knees for support.
- Wear flat-heeled shoes with good support.
- Do stretching exercises and exercises to strengthen the back and abdominal muscles, such as those found in prenatal yoga and pilates, taking care not to over-strain since the softening of ligaments can make injury more possible. Overstretching is a real hazard in pregnant women. Listen to the body!
- Avoid heavy lifting and moving heavy objects.
- Eat a good diet, ensuring sufficient calcium and magnesium (see page 37).
- Chiropractic adjustments, osteopathy, physiotherapy, Alexander technique, swimming and aquanatal classes may all be helpful.
- Some women find relief from wearing a maternity support belt, especially in the third trimester.
- Rest and relaxation may be needed. Breathing and relaxation exercises may be helpful if pain is stress-related.

Herbal treatment

Baths, rubs, massage oils, and other external treatments, as well as internal medicines if needed, can all be highly effective to ease back and pelvic pain.

Rubbing oils and Liniments

Comfrey leaf (*Symphytum off.*) infused oil makes a wonderful and versatile base oil to soothe pain and aid tissue repair. It can be applied on its own, mixed with appropriate essential oils (from 16 weeks) and/or essences, and made into a liniment, cream or ointment. Combine the following as a warming liniment to relax muscle spasm, relieve nerve pain, and ease deep aching: Comfrey leaf infused oil 40ml, St John's Wort (*Hypericum perforatum*) infused oil 40ml, Cramp Bark (*Viburnum opulus*) Tr 10ml, Lobelia (*Lobelia inflata*) Tr 10ml, Cayenne (*Capsicum minimum*) Tr 20 drops, Chamomile essential oil 10 drops, Bergamot essential oil 10 drops. Shake well and apply as required.

Ointments

Make an ointment with 100ml Comfrey infused oil combined with 10g beeswax and five drops each of Lavender and Bergamot essential oils (from 16 weeks). Apply as required as a healing ointment to strengthen tissues and relieve pain.

In cases of trauma, Arnica or Daisy leaf infused oil can be combined with Comfrey oil 1:1 to help clear shock. Add three drops of Arnica vibrational essence.

Massage oils

Depending on the woman's preference, select one or two essential oils from the following list (from 16 weeks): Bergamot, Chamomile, Lavender, Geranium, Ylang-ylang. Add a total of ten drops to 50ml St John's Wort or Comfrey infused oil (or use organic sesame or almond oil) and apply to affected areas as needed.

Herbal baths

Make a 30-minute infusion of Lavender or Chamomile flowers and add to bath water. Alternatively, add five drops of Lavender or Chamomile essential oil to bath water (from 16 weeks). Soak for at least 20 minutes for a relaxing bath to ease tension and aches. May be used as a footbath, if preferred.

Internal treatment

St John's Wort tea, 1g dried herb per 200ml water, three cups daily, or tincture up to 5ml three times daily or 20 drops hourly for acute conditions. St John's Wort is especially helpful to relieve nerve pain and ease anxiety and tension. Depending on the patient and severity of symptoms, I would start at 20 drops tincture three times daily, progressively going up to 5ml if needed.

Another of my favourite herbs for pain is Valerian (*Valeriana off.*). St John's Wort and Valerian combine well together in a 50:50 mix, same dosage as above.

Cramp Bark makes a useful addition for muscle spasm and cramping.

Passionflower (*Passiflora incarnata*), Skullcap (*Scutellaria lateriflora*), and Chamomile (*Chamomilla recutita*) are alternatives for back and pelvic pain.

Bleeding

For nose bleeds see 'Nose Bleeds'

A small amount of vaginal bleeding may occur in around 10 percent of pregnancies up to 28 weeks and slightly fewer after that time. It does not necessarily mean that the foetus is at risk and may be associated with implantation (see 'Abdominal Pain and Cramps' page 104), Blood loss may occur at the time of expected menstruation, or around 12 weeks when the placenta takes over hormone production from the corpus luteum.

Slight bleeding may also arise from the cervix. Due to hormone levels and the increased blood flow of pregnancy, the cervix is more engorged, softer than usual, and more friable. Therefore, it can bleed easily if touched and it can be normal to notice spotting or pink-tinged vaginal mucus after sex. Post-coital bleeding may also be caused by cervical polyps, cervicitis, or erosion.

Heavier bleeding needs immediate investigation, especially if associated with abdominal pain. If you are unsure, you should seek immediate medical assistance or send the woman to A&E. See possible causes below.

Antepartum haemorrhage (APH) is defined as bleeding from or into the genital tract, occurring from 24 weeks of pregnancy and prior to the birth of the baby. Obstetric haemorrhage is one of the major causes of maternal death in developing countries, being the cause of up to 50% of the estimated 500,000 maternal deaths that occur globally each year.[5] In the UK and Ireland, deaths from obstetric haemorrhage are uncommon. Causes of APH include; placenta praevia, placental abruption, and local causes (for example bleeding from the vulva, vagina, or cervix). It is not uncommon to fail to identify a cause for APH and it is then described as 'unexplained APH'.

Some causes of bleeding in first 20 weeks:

Implantation bleeding: can be normal, may be accompanied by sharp pelvic pains (see 'Abdominal Pain and Cramps' page 104)

Threatened miscarriage: bleeding is often the first symptom, may progress to pain like dysmenorrhoea or labour. (See 'Miscarriage' page 136)

Ectopic pregnancy: unilateral colicky pain before bleeding, progresses to generalised pelvic and/or lower abdominal pain. Can be life threatening (see 'Ectopic Pregnancy' page 119)

Abnormal development of placenta and/or foetus
Condition of cervix: erosion, cervicitis, or cervical polyps (see 'Cervix' page 117)
Infection: STD or Candidiasis (see 'Candidiasis' page 115)
Foetal death in utero
Cancer
Incompetent cervix (cervical insufficiency) (see 'Cervix' page 117)
Trauma

Some causes of bleeding later in pregnancy:

Placenta praevia: low placental implantation (varying grades) (see 'Placenta Praevia' page 151)

Placental abruption: portion of placenta is detached from uterine wall (see 'Placental Abruption' page 152)

Condition of cervix (see 'Cervix' page 117)

Intrauterine foetal death (intrauterine foetal demise)

Trauma

Uterine rupture

Preterm labour with contractions, low backache, feeling of pressure in pelvis, watery/bloody discharge (see 'Preterm labour' page 154)

Breast changes

Tender and slightly enlarged breasts can be one of the first signs of early pregnancy, even before the first missed period. Any extreme tenderness usually subsides (or at least lessens) fairly quickly, although a woman's nipples will often remain sensitive throughout pregnancy and breastfeeding.

Breasts will continue to grow during pregnancy and for large-breasted women a support bra may be helpful. The increased blood volume makes veins more visible all over the body, especially for fair-skinned women and this is often most noticeable on the breasts. Increasing melanin levels can cause enlargement and darkening of the areolas and Montgomery's tubercles (small sebaceous glands) often become visible as raised bumps around the areolas as pregnancy advances. Women with small breasts can be reassured that breast size does not affect their ability to produce sufficient milk.

As breast size increases, striations or stretch marks may appear (see 'Stretch Marks' for how to avoid). It is normal for breasts to feel more lumpy than usual due to enlargement of the alveoli. However, it is sensible to continue regular breast checks, since a significant minority of breast cancers are found during pregnancy.

Prolactin levels increase steadily in the third trimester, stimulating breast tissue to prepare for milk production. From week 32 the breast may leak colostrum, which is the nutrient-rich first food for breastfed babies (see Chapter 14 'Lactation' page 367 for information on breastfeeding). Nipple care is important during pregnancy. It can be helpful to wash nipples every day with water to remove any crusts and apply Comfrey ointment to strengthen the epithelium. Soap and abrasive agents should be avoided, since they can cause damage and predispose to cracked nipples after delivery. In late pregnancy, it helps to expose the nipples to the air.

If a woman has flat or inverted nipples, this does not affect her ability to breastfeed, but she may find it easier to establish feeding if she prepares her nipples in advance. There is no general agreement about this and some midwives believe that to diagnose inverted nipples during pregnancy will only damage a woman's confidence in being able to breastfeed. On the other hand, it can be argued that practical preparation may be helpful and effective, as well as the fact that if the issue is not mentioned, a woman may hold an unspoken fear that can equally undermine her confidence. Like so many areas, it depends on the person and requires a sensitive approach. To test a nipple for inversion, place a thumb and finger on opposite sides of the areola and gently squeeze the nipple inwards. If a nipple stands out when compressed it is not inverted. If a woman's nipples become erect in the cold or when sexually aroused then they need no preparation for breastfeeding. Where appropriate, a simple exercise to help prepare the nipples can be started in the second half of pregnancy: apply a little Comfrey ointment, almond oil or olive oil to the nipple and areola, place a thumb on either side of the nipple, press in firmly against the breast tissue and at the same time pull the thumbs apart. Unless this is painful, the exercise can be repeated daily, morning and night, moving the thumbs around the base of the nipple. If a woman has inverted nipples, it is worth her seeking advice from her midwife or a La Leche League leader. The La Leche League[6] is a respected international organisation offering a wealth of support and practical advice for breastfeeding.

Breech Presentation see Chapter 10 'Preparation for Birth' page 192.

Candidiasis, vulvovaginal, *Candida albicans*

Hormone levels of pregnancy commonly cause a proliferation of the normally benign yeast *Candida albicans* on the vaginal mucous membranes. This can develop into vaginal thrush, which occurs in around a quarter of pregnant women at some stage of their pregnancy (often asymptomatic). Occurrence may be associated with diabetes or triggered by taking antibiotics, frequently given for urinary tract infections. Symptoms of thrush include burning, itching, soreness of the labia and vulva, and a thick, white vaginal discharge. If present at birth it can be passed to the baby causing thrush in the mouth and putting extra demands on the baby's immune system (see Chapter 15 'Care of the Newborn' page 287).

Women are advised to wear loose, cotton underwear and wash the vagina with water or Marigold tea, avoiding soap, which is an irritant. Drink plenty of water and avoid yeast and sugar, which feed the candida. Foods to avoid include yeast bread and breadcrumbs, cakes, biscuits, any food or drink containing sugar, mushrooms, soy sauce and other fermented foods, sour cream, tea, coffee, alcohol, cheese, dried fruit, malted products, vinegars, smoked or preserved meat or fish, nuts that have not been freshly cracked, and concentrated fruit juices. Avoid any nutritional supplements that are not stated as yeast-free. As with any infections, candida overgrowth is more likely to occur if there is lowered resistance (see 'The Immune System in Pregnancy' page 135). Zinc and iron deficiency may predispose to candida, consider supplementation of these plus vitamin C. Take probiotics and include live yogurt in the diet. Check for systemic candida, if thrush occurs frequently.

Partners of sexually active women need concurrent treatment even if they are symptom-free. Male partners are advised to use condoms until the infection has cleared.

Herbal treatment

Include raw Garlic (*Allium sativa*) in the diet. It can be mixed with virgin olive oil and used as a spread or in a salad dressing and taken daily. Take capsules if raw is not possible, although these are generally not as effective. Other herbs to benefit the immune system include; Marigold (*Calendula off.*), Echinacea (*Echinacea* spp.), Wild Indigo (*Baptisia tinctoria*), and Thyme (*Thymus vulgaris*). Goldenrod (*Solidago virgaurea*) and Plantain (*Plantago lanceolata/major*) can be added to restore the mucous membrane.

Drink Marigold tea, one cup, three times daily (2 teaspoons petals to 200ml cup), add fresh Cleavers (*Galium aperine*) if available.

A typical mix of tinctures for vaginal candidiasis: Rx *Echinacea* spp. 40 *Baptisia tinctoria* 20, *Galium aperine* 20, *Solidago virgaurea* 20 =100ml sig 5ml tds in warm water after food.

Local treatments include Marigold cream, Aloe vera gel or live yogurt, applied to the outer genital area. If necessary, Marigold pessaries can be inserted into the vagina morning and night.

Soak a cotton pad or clean sanitary towel in a lotion made from Marigold or Lavender infusion, hydrosol or diluted tincture. Wear next to the skin, renewing every 2 hours. Alternatively, for a soothing application, mix Slippery Elm powder or Marshmallow root powder with Marigold or Chamomile tea to make a firm paste, spread on a cotton pad or sanitary towel and wear as above, renewing every 6 hours.

Carpal tunnel syndrome (CTS)

This is due to compression of the median nerve as it travels through the wrist, causing pain, tingling or numbness in the wrist, hand and fingers. It can be a common symptom of pregnancy as a result of oedema affecting the wrist (see 'Oedema'). It occurs most frequently in the third trimester and tends to be worse at night due to fluid accumulation.

Measures to ease symptoms include the avoidance of lying on arms in bed and avoiding repetitive activities that cause the wrist to bend. Elevate wrists whenever possible and, if necessary, wear a wrist splint to keep the wrist in a neutral (not bent) position.

Flexing and extending the wrist can help: Hold the arm straight out in front, with wrist and hand straight, palm facing down. Bend wrist down so that fingers point to floor, use other hand to increase the stretch, gently pulling the fingers towards the body. Hold for fifteen to thirty seconds.

For herbal relief, massage St John's Wort (*Hypericum perf.*) infused oil into the wrist, followed by the application of a cooling herbal compress or ice pack. Make a strong Cornsilk (*Zea mays*) tea (two to four teaspoons per cup, twenty minute infusion), refrigerate and use for a cold compress. Alternatively, freeze the Cornsilk infusion in an ice cube tray, crush the ice by placing in a tea towel and smashing with a rolling pin, and apply this between two layers of cloth as a cold pack around the wrist. Re-apply as needed.

Cervix, conditions of

Cervical ectopy

Also known as cervical erosion, eversion and ectropion.

This is a common condition of pregnancy where hormonal changes cause columnar epithelium to be drawn out from inside the cervical canal so that it forms a zone around the external os (the cervical opening into the vagina). The columnar epithelium excretes mucin and consequently the woman may have a heavy vaginal discharge. This is a benign condition and does not require treatment. These delicate 'soft cells' may occasionally bleed, especially after intercourse or speculum examination.

Cervical insufficiency

Also known as 'cervical incompetence' although not a useful term to use with patients.

In cervical insufficiency the cervix shortens and opens in the second trimester or early in the third trimester without any other symptoms of labour. This puts the woman at high risk of having a miscarriage (see 'miscarriage') or preterm delivery. The condition may be caused by a structural weakness; for instance, a previous cone biopsy where more than 1cm of cervical cells was removed, or cervical trauma, such as tearing of the cervix during a previous labour, an abortion performed after the week 12, or dilation and curettage (D & C). If structural weakness is suspected, the woman may be monitored via transvaginal ultrasound to check the cervix every two weeks from weeks 14–28. If she is felt to be at high risk, she is likely to be offered a transvaginal cervical 'stitch' (TVC), also known as cerclage, aiming to keep the cervix closed during pregnancy. This may be placed at the start of the second trimester, based on previous medical history, or later in the second trimester in response to cervical shortening observed by ultrasound. The stitch will normally be removed around week 37.

Less commonly, the woman's obstetrician may recommend progesterone treatment, as well as or instead of a surgical stitch. Another option is the Arabin® pessary, which is a small, soft silicon ring that is inserted through the vagina and surrounds the cervix, helping to keep the baby in the womb. This has been successfully used in Spain and the Netherlands for some time and is gaining popularity elsewhere.

Cervical polyps

A cervical polyp may form on the outside of the cervix and may cause bleeding, especially post-coitally. In the past, medical practice advised removal of cervical polyps in pregnant women but current opinion tends to favour monitoring during pregnancy as a safer approach. Individual risk assessment needs to be made.

Cervicitis

Cervicitis may give a brown or bloody discharge and is commonly caused by bacterial and viral infections, usually sexually transmitted and requiring urgent medical diagnosis and treatment. Infections include gonorrhoea, chlamydia, trichomoniasis. And genital herpes. Genital herpes is typically marked by visible painful sores or blisters on the genital skin (See 'Herpes, Genital').

Cervix, inelastic (see Chapter 12 'Herbs for Labour and Delivery' page 230)

Constipation

Constipation is a common complaint of pregnancy due to high progesterone levels, which relax the smooth muscle of the digestive tract and slow it down. It may also be caused by unsuitable diet, lack of exercise, or by taking iron tablets. In the third trimester, the growing baby and placenta put pressure on the lower bowel, which can restrict blood flow and exacerbate constipation.

Ensure the woman is eating enough fibre with plenty of fresh vegetables and fruit, unrefined carbohydrates, grains, nuts, seeds and pulses, and avoiding bran, which is an irritant. She should drink plenty of fluids, avoiding regular tea and coffee. Drinking prune juice every day may be all that is needed as a remedy. Be aware that some women drink excess amounts of milk during pregnancy and this may be constipating. Ensure healthy gut flora and eliminate food sensitivities, such as dairy or wheat. Pay attention to posture and make sure the woman is exercising. Massage or specific gentle yoga exercises may help the bowel.

Of all the organs in the body, the bowel is the biggest creature of habit. It is helpful to have a regular routine, going to the bathroom at the same time each day (ideally around 30 mins after eating breakfast), and allowing a relaxed and unhurried time for the bowel to function.

Herbal treatment

As a gentle bulking agent, Psyllium seeds or Linseeds can be recommended, 1–2 teaspoons, once or twice daily (morning and night). I find dark Psyllium seeds to be the most effective to cleanse and tone the bowel. These can be mixed with water or juice and left to stand overnight, or mixed with a little warm water so that they swell up just before taking. They may also be sprinkled on food (such as porridge or moistened breakfast cereal), in which case a full 250ml glass of water, lemon water, or herb tea needs to be drunk at the same time.

As a gentle bowel regulator, liver and digestive tonic, give Dandelion root (*Taraxacum off.* radix) decoction (once or twice daily) or tincture (10ml at night). For any stubborn cases, Butternut bark tincture (*Juglans cinerea*) 10ml at night, is my favourite stand-by and can be used at any stage of pregnancy.

Glycerol suppositories are another option (available from pharmacies). Alternatively, some women find drinking a cup of Slippery Elm (*Ulmus rubra*) before bed gives them a bowel movement in the morning.

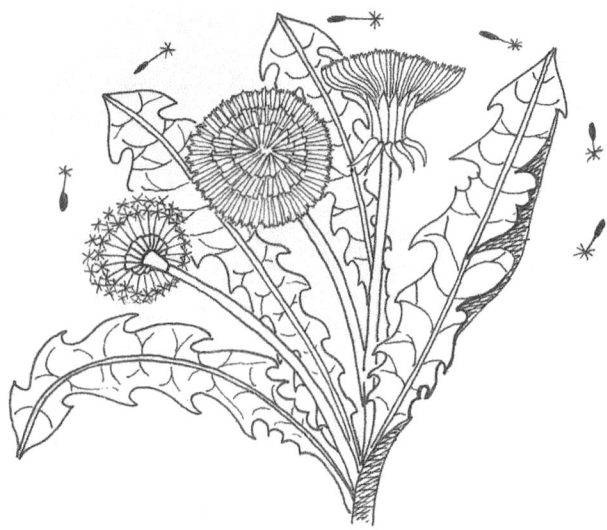

Contractions see 'Abdominal Pain and Cramps'
Depression/Low Mood/Mood swings see 'Emotional and Stress related conditions' below and Chapter 13 'Postpartum Care' 'Postpartum Depression' page 255
Diabetes see 'Gestational Diabetes'

Dizziness and fainting

Dizziness and fainting can be common in early pregnancy, especially on rising in the morning or following a hot bath or shower. Sometimes light-headedness is the first sign of pregnancy. This is usually due to hormone changes causing dilated blood vessels and a dip in blood pressure. It may also be triggered by lack of food or water, feeling queasy, or finding it hard to keep food down. The best remedy is to sit down with one's head between one's legs and generally to avoid getting up too quickly or standing for long periods. A few drops of Rescue Remedy (see page 301), neat or in water may relieve symptoms. Other possible causes include low blood sugar (see 'Hypoglycaemia') or anaemia (see 'Anaemia'). From the second trimester onwards, dizziness may be caused by lying on one's back, causing the expanding uterus to block blood flow from the lower extremities.

Eclampsia see 'Pre-eclampsia, Eclampsia'

Ectopic pregnancy

An ectopic pregnancy, where the fertilized egg implants outside of the uterus (usually in a fallopian tube), requires urgent medical attention. In most cases the pregnancy terminates between week 6 and week 10 of pregnancy either through tubal abortion or tubal rupture.

Two clinical patterns occur, the most common being subacute but occasionally acute and dramatic. A subacute presentation starts with lower abdominal pain, typically unilateral, and not necessarily easily distinguishable from threatened miscarriage. Vaginal bleeding follows the pain, usually slight, brownish in colour and continuous, with clots rarely present. This may progress to sudden acute lower abdominal pain, severe enough to cause fainting with pallor, weak pulse, and falling blood pressure. Pain may be felt in the epigastrium and referred to the shoulder. Other symptoms can include vomiting, diarrhoea, dysuria, and pain in the rectum.

An acute rupture can cause sudden collapse with little or no warning. Most usually, this develops over time, but the mild symptoms of a subacute presentation may be thought to be normal occurrences of pregnancy and mistakenly ignored. This is a medical emergency requiring urgent hospitalization and surgery. A ruptured ectopic is the most common cause of death in women in the first trimester of pregnancy.

Emotional and stress-related conditions

See also 'Sleep Disorders' below. 'Postpartum Depression' Chapter 13 page 255.

The heightened sensitivity of pregnancy can magnify both joy and sorrow. Hormonal changes act upon the brain and can cause intense mood swings, especially in the first trimester. This is part of the overall adaptation to a new state. As discussed in Chapter 5, pregnancy is a time of major transition and women may experience challenges on all levels of their being: physical, emotional, mental, and spiritual. However much a baby is wanted, pregnancy can produce a flood of conflicting emotions and it may feel overwhelming at times. Certain issues tend to arise at different stages and while many women feel better than ever during pregnancy, it can also be common to experience anxiety, dark thoughts, and irrational fears.

It is important for a woman to have a place to share her concerns. These may include the fear of labour or a particular complication of pregnancy, often influenced by past experience or family history, such as previous miscarriage or difficult birth. A woman may feel overwhelmed by the responsibility of bringing a child into the world, or she may be stressed by relationship problems, financial worries, fears around the health of the baby, of being a 'bad' mother, not fulfilling social expectations, or a host of other concerns. Along with plant medicines, we can provide a listening ear, practical advice and information as well as reassuring women that they are not alone in their fears. We can encourage a woman to listen to her own feelings, to acknowledge what is bothering her, explore where this comes from, and help her to address any underlying issues that need healing.

Pregnancy often brings up unresolved issues from the past, especially from childhood and concerning the relationship with one's own mother. This is naturally a time when women reflect on how they were raised and how they want to raise their own child. As such, it can be a wonderful opportunity to heal painful feelings from childhood and move forward into motherhood with a new perspective. Unresolved problems can lead to physical complications in pregnancy and wholistic herbal treatment needs to address whatever arises. Dealing with old emotional issues is a tangible way to help prepare a woman for birth and parenthood.

Vibrational essences can be particularly valuable in this process, encouraging a positive outlook and helping to heal deeply held emotional wounds and to change old mistaken beliefs. Selected remedies can clear dark thoughts, boost confidence and help a woman to believe in her ability to cope. For instance, Calendula essence lifts the spirits, Motherwort increases confidence, Brigid's Blessing clears self-doubt, and Chamomile relieves fear and anxiety. A few drops can be added to a herbal medicine or the essence can be taken on its own as drops or used as a room spray. See Chapter 16 page 305 for further details of suggested essences. These work well in combination with other tools, such as positive affirmations, relaxation exercises, meditation, and journaling. For deep psychological or spiritual work, you may find it helpful to refer a woman for hypnotherapy, counselling or other appropriate care.

Excellent nutrition along with adequate exercise and rest are crucial. Make sure the woman is staying hydrated and eating regularly in order to maintain stable blood sugar levels. If blood sugar needs stabilising, give Goat's Rue (*Galega off.*) tincture 20 drops three times daily or as required. This is a useful emergency bottle to carry in case of a blood sugar dip (see 'Hypoglycaemia').

At times of stress, it helps to avoid caffeine, sugar, and excess carbohydrates. Women may also benefit from frequent small meals with extra protein and high-quality fats. Zinc and magnesium rich foods are helpful to stabilise mood and a daily pregnancy formula should include B complex to support the nervous system.

Herbal treatment

Fear and anxiety

See also 'Sleep Disorders' page 161.

Any of the following sedative nervines can be used to relieve fear and anxiety in pregnancy:

Oatstraw (*Avena sativa*): tonic and restorative, especially helpful for debility and exhaustion.

Chamomile (*Chamomilla recutita*): brings softness in tense, painful conditions and where anxiety affects digestion.

Cramp bark (*Viburnum opulus*): especially if anxiety causes severe muscle tension

Lavender: anxiolytic and anti-spasmodic, gentle, and calming. Strongest antispasmodic effect is from inhalation. Inhale tea before drinking or use dried herb in a bath or footbath.

Lemon Balm (*Melissa off.*): especially helpful for weepiness, vulnerability, and where anxiety is affecting digestion.

Limeflowers (*Tilia europaea*): gentle relaxation, good for tension headaches and as a circulatory relaxant.

Motherwort (*Leonurus cardiaca*): combines well with Black Horehound to relieve anxiety and tension in third trimester.

Passionflower (*Passiflora incarnata*): for nervousness, excitability, restlessness, panic, tension affecting adrenals. Add Liquorice (*Glycyrrhiza glabra*) (5–10ml per week), if needed to support and strengthen weak or exhausted adrenals.

Skullcap (*Scutellaria lateriflora*): strengthening tonic for the nervous system, eases dark thoughts, combines well with Valerian for anxiety.

St John's Wort (*Hypericum perforatum*): helpful for anxiety, panic, and obsessive tendencies.

Valerian (*Valeriana off.*): strong sedative, hypnotic, and anti-spasmodic. Relieves pain, calms panic, soothes irritability and restlessness. If Valerian suits (see page 99), it can be used as a simple,[7] 20 drops of tincture as required (max 15 doses daily) for shock, trauma, and panic and can be carried in a woman's handbag for immediate use. Add two to three drops of 'Rescue essence' to 30ml Valerian for added efficacy. A cold infusion of Valerian can also be helpful as a lotion or added to a footbath.

Vervain (*Verbena off.*): nervous system tonic, supports the liver, relaxes the mind, eases obsessional thoughts, helps nervous exhaustion.

Baths: Strong infusions of any of the above for bath or footbath.

'Calming Waters' Herbal Bath: Equal parts Oatstraw, Chamomile, Lemon Balm, Lavender, Limeflowers. Place 10–20g of dried mix (double if fresh) in muslin bag and place under hot tap while running bath. Leave bag in bath water and relax in bath for at least 20 minutes.

Internal use: Teas or tinctures, singly or combined. Teas can be taken as standard infusions, three times daily and before bed. NOTE: Valerian is best taken as a cold infusion. Tincture dose is 5ml three times daily.

Typical anxiety mix: Rx *Valeriana officianalis, Chamomilla recutita, Scutellaria lateriflora, Passiflora incarnata, Verbena officinalis*, aa 20ml. Dosage: 5ml three times daily in warm water.

Massage oil: essential oils (from 16 weeks): Lavender, Petitgrain, Bergamot, Rose, Geranium, Chamomile, Ylang-ylang (blend between one and three oils) 1% dilution in carrier oil for relaxing foot or body massage. Pleasurable scents can be used during pregnancy to build up an association between specific smells and feelings of relaxation and enjoyment. For women prone to anxiety, the same scents can be used during childbirth (for instance in a massage oil for labour) to recreate feelings of relaxation.

Mood swings, depression

See also 'Postpartum Depression' Chapter 13 page 255.

The following herbs can help to lift depression and stabilise mood:

Oat straw—to nourish nervous system and enhance mood, nervous exhaustion.
St John's Wort—for low mood with anxiety. Combines well with Oats and Skullcap.
Lavender—lifts the spirits, calms the mind.
Lemon Balm—for grief. Useful as a simple, 20 drops as required (max 15 doses daily) for extreme low mood and tearfulness. Can be carried in a woman's handbag for immediate use.

Rosa spp.—for grief and feeling heartbroken, comforts and soothes the heart.

Skullcap—strengthens where there is deep soul unhappiness, lifts mood and enhances confidence. Combines well with Dandelion root if suppressed anger is affecting the liver.

Vervain—relaxing tonic nervine. Lifts the spirits. Combines well with Oats and Skullcap for depression with lethargy and exhaustion. Aids ability to concentrate.

Passionflower—especially helpful after chronic stress and to balance highs and lows of mood swings.

Teas: Standard infusions of the above, singly or combined. Dosage: three times daily.
'Tea of Happiness': Vervain, St John's Wort, Chamomile, Lemon Balm, Lavender
'Soothing Heart Tea': Rose petals, Lemon Balm, Motherwort

Baths: Strong infusions of any of the above for Bath or Footbath.
'Bath of Joy': Equal parts Oatstraw, Lemon Balm, Lavender, Rose petals. Place 10–20g of dried mix (double if fresh) in muslin bag and place under hot tap while running bath. Leave bag in bath water and relax in bath for 20 minutes

Tinctures: Combine five or more of the above tinctures in a mix of 100ml, dosage: up to 5ml tds aq cal.

Typical mix to lift and balance mood: Rx *Scutellaria lateriflora, Verbena officinalis, Hypericum perforatum, Avena sativa, Melissa officinalis,* aa 20ml = 100 sig 5ml tds aq cal.

Massage Oil: for emotional heart pain: essential oil Rose 1% dilution in almond oil. Apply a few drops over heart area three times daily.

Massage Oil: essential oils (from 16 weeks): Lavender, Bergamot, Geranium, Ylang-ylang (blend 1–3) 1% dilution in carrier oil for uplifting foot or body massage.

Fatigue and exhaustion

Extreme fatigue is common in early pregnancy (between weeks 6 to 15) and a woman may need much more sleep than usual. This is no surprise considering her body is busy forming a new tiny human and hormone changes are causing effects, such as smooth muscle relaxation with blood sugar and blood pressure levels reduction. A woman should be encouraged to listen to her body, cut down activities and take as much rest as needed. The fatigue can act as a useful prompt for lifestyle changes as part of the adaptation to motherhood. Relaxation exercises, yoga, meditation, and taking naps can all be helpful. Practitioners need to check for anaemia and ensure optimum nutrition. To help stabilise blood sugar, women should avoid sugar and caffeine, eat every four hours and ensure snacks are nutritious, such as fruit, nuts, seeds, and yogurt (see 'Hypoglycaemia'). Unless there are serious concomitant factors (such as pre-existing debilitation), I avoid prescribing herbs for fatigue in the first trimester.

Tiredness may recur towards the end of pregnancy when it is common for sleep to be disturbed, due to difficulties getting comfortable in bed as well as having frequent nocturia (see 'Sleep Disorders'). Again, it is important to rest as much as needed. Oatstraw tea (*Avena sativa*), three cups daily, or tincture of immature seeds, 5ml up to three times daily, is a beneficial restorative tonic to strengthen the nervous system and raise energy levels. Combine 2:1 with Skullcap (*Scutellaria lateriflora*) if there is anxiety or low mood. Overall dosage the same as for Oats above. Some women find taking Evening Primrose (*Oenothera biennis*) oil 1–3g daily helps energy levels in the third trimester.

Gestational diabetes

Gestational diabetes usually occurs in the second half of pregnancy and disappears at birth, although there is a higher than average risk of developing diabetes later in life. In gestational diabetes the mother's body becomes insulin resistant leading to an excess of glucose in the maternal blood. The excess glucose passes across the placenta to the growing foetus and can lead to a macrosomic (larger than average, regardless of gestational age) baby with other possible complications including hypoglycaemia, jaundice, and respiratory distress.

The incidence of gestational diabetes has seen a marked increase in recent years, predominantly due to rising levels of obesity and increases in maternal age. Other risk factors include a previous macrosomic baby weighing 4.5kg or above, previous gestational diabetes, first-degree relative with diabetes, or minority ethnic family origin with a high prevalence of diabetes.

Gestational diabetes may be picked up on routine urinalysis. A glycosuria of 2+ or above on one occasion or of 1+ or above on two or more occasions detected by reagent strip testing could indicate undiagnosed gestational diabetes and requires further testing to exclude it.

The condition requires careful monitoring and dietary management. A healthy eating plan should emphasise protein and high fibre complex carbohydrates, favouring foods with a low glycaemic index (GI), such as non-starchy vegetables, whole grains, and sweet potatoes. It is helpful to eat a little protein with every meal. Chromium and magnesium are closely involved in regulating blood glucose and can be included in the diet (see page 37). If a woman is taking a pregnancy multivitamin, choose one that contains 100mcg chromium along with at least 25mg of vitamin B3. All sources of sugar, honey, and refined carbohydrates should be excluded. Obese and overweight women need to limit weight gain. Regular exercise (such as walking for thirty minutes after a meal) will also improve blood glucose levels.

As long as gestational diabetes is diagnosed and well managed during pregnancy, most women have healthy pregnancies and healthy babies.

Herbal treatment

Goat's Rue (*Galega off.*) provides excellent support for the pancreas and can effectively restore healthy blood glucose regulation (along with proper diet, which is imperative).

In mild cases, dietary measures alone may be enough, but where necessary, Goat's Rue can be prescribed, up to a maximum of 35ml tincture per week, in three divided doses daily, and this can be continued as long as needed. By balancing glucose levels, this regime also helps prevent hypoglycaemic episodes. Where clinical signs disappear, in some cases it is helpful to continue Goat's Rue at a reduced dose of 10–20ml weekly as a prophylactic. Goat's Rue combines well with Burdock root (*Arctium lappa*) (10ml tincture per week). Useful adjuncts to treatment include Dandelion root and Chamomile. Passionflower may be helpful to relax the adrenals.

Prescribe with caution in patients stabilised on hypoglycaemic drugs or insulin. Close and vigilant monitoring of blood glucose is required.

Gestational trophoblastic disease

GTD; includes molar pregnancy, hydatiform mole.

This is a group of rare diseases in which abnormal trophoblast cells grow inside the uterus after conception.

Molar pregnancy (also known as hydatiform mole) is the most common form of GTD, with an incidence of about one in 500–1000 pregnancies. A molar pregnancy can be complete or partial. In a complete molar pregnancy, an anuclear empty ovum is fertilised by one or more sperm, which then duplicates its own chromosomes, with the result that the genetic material is entirely of paternal origin (Androgenic moles). There is no formation of foetal tissue and the placental tissue is abnormal and swollen, appearing to form fluid-filled cysts.

Partial molar pregnancies occur less frequently, most often due to the fertilization of an ovum by two sperm. Therefore, the embryo has 69 chromosomes instead of 46. Normal placental tissue may form along with abnormally forming placental tissue. If a foetus forms, it is usually miscarried early in the pregnancy. The incidence of a live foetus and a partial molar placenta is extremely rare and the foetus usually dies soon after birth if it survives until delivery. These pregnancies are high-risk.

Molar pregnancies occur more frequently in women in their early teens and aged over forty. They are also more common after two or more miscarriages. The condition may be diagnosed in the first trimester by high resolution ultrasound and accurate measurement of β-hCG, often before classic signs and symptoms present. The most prominent symptom of a complete molar pregnancy is dark brown to bright red vaginal bleeding in the first trimester, sometimes with the passage of grape-like cysts. Symptoms of a partial molar pregnancy include severe nausea, vomiting, and hypertension often in the first trimester. Most subsequent pregnancies following a sporadic partial or complete molar pregnancy will be full term pregnancies (1% probability of recurrence).

Accurate diagnosis is crucial since if a molar pregnancy is not treated or does not miscarry completely, it can progress to gestational trophoblastic neoplasia (GTN), the collective name for four malignant disorders, consisting of invasive mole, choriocarcinoma, placental site trophoblastic tumour (PSTT), and epithelioid trophoblastic tumour (ETT).

(see 'Miscarriage' page 141 for herbal cleansing of the uterus after miscarriage, or after medical or surgical abortion. See also Chapter 9 'Healing After Loss').

Group B streptococcus (Group B strep or GBS)

Group B Strep is a common bacterium living in the intestines and migrating to the vagina, urinary tract, and rectum. Globally, between 10–30% of pregnant women are colonised with GBS, which can be found by a swab test of the vagina and rectum, or cultured from a urine sample. Colonisation is usually harmless and patients are symptom-free, but GBS can cause urinary tract infections in mothers and GBS infections in the newborn. Many babies come in contact with GBS during labour or childbirth. This does not usually cause infection, but a small minority of babies may develop pneumonia, meningitis, or sepsis. GBS-related disease affects around 1–2 per 1000 live births and GBS has become the most frequent cause of overwhelming sepsis in neonates. Risk factors include a high density of maternal colonisation, preterm birth, prelabour rupture of membranes, maternal fever, and having previously had a baby affected by GBS infection. In extremely rare cases, GBS infection can cause miscarriage, premature labour, or stillbirth.

Pregnant women are not routinely screened for GBS in Ireland and the UK, although it is sometimes detected when tests for other infections are carried out. Conventional treatment focuses on giving intravenous (IV) antibiotics during labour to high-risk and/or colonised women to reduce GBS transmission. Antibiotics are ineffective if prescribed earlier in pregnancy. Most other high-income countries offer routine testing in late pregnancy (weeks 35–37) and in the US all colonized women are offered IV antibiotics in labour. This carries the usual risks of antibiotic over-use and side effects, such as yeast infections, diarrhoea, and dysbiosis of the gut microbiome in mother and baby.

General measures for group B strep infection

For at risk women, or if GBS is picked up through screening, herbal treatment emphasizes promoting a healthy gut and vaginal flora by eating a balanced diet, low in processed sugars and high in probiotic foods such as live yogurt, sauerkraut, kimchi, kombucha, and water kefir. Include prebiotic foods, such as onions and garlic, and take 1–2 teasp cider vinegar diluted in a cup of warm water on rising. Drink plenty of water and take 1–2g vitamin C daily. Take a good quality oral probiotic for pregnant women.

Herbal treatment

Raw garlic is powerfully effective to treat GBS and protect the newborn. Take crushed raw garlic, 1 clove three times daily, mixed with water or food. As food, raw garlic can be incorporated into a salad dressing, used as a garlic butter/oil spread, or squeezed on top of cooked food at the table. Garlic capsules can be taken if raw is not tolerated.

Dandelion root decoction (*Taraxacum off.* rad.), at least one cup daily, helps restore and maintain the microbiome.

For urinary tract infection see also 'Urinary Tract Conditions'.

For preterm birth and prelabour rupture of membranes see 'Preterm Labour/Preterm Prelabour Rupture of Membranes/Preterm Premature Rupture of Membranes (PPROM)'.

Gums, swollen, bleeding

Raised progesterone levels causes softening of the gums and increased blood flow. This can cause gingivitis with soreness, bleeding, and possible bacterial infection, which could lead to gum disease.

Herbal treatment

An astringent, antiseptic, and healing herbal mouthwash can be made from any one of the following:

Marigold flowers (*Calendula off.*) strong infusion
Blackberry leaf (*Rubus fructicosus*) strong infusion
Oak bark (*Quercus robur/petraea*) strong decoction
Tinctures: *Commiphora molmol* 20ml plus *Glycyrrhiza glabra* 10ml = 30ml. Take ten drops in half a cup of water. Swill mouth for two to three minutes, after food and before bed.

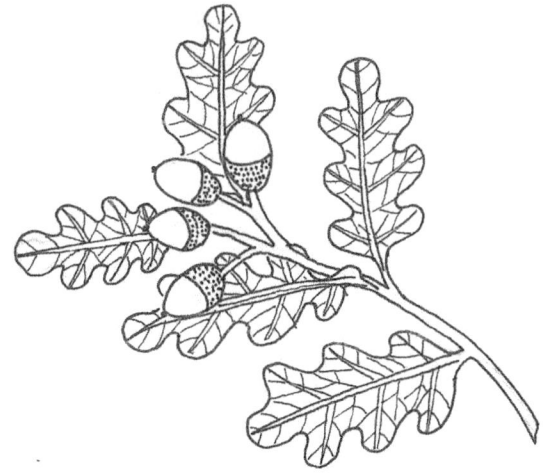

Haemorrhoids (see 'Varicose Veins')

Headaches

Head pain is not a particular feature of pregnancy but may occur for any of the usual reasons. Check for constipation, dehydration, stress, neck and back tension, blood sugar dips, food triggers, or blocked sinuses.

Herbal treatment

Suitable herbs include Chamomile (*Chamomilla recutita*), Lavender (*Lavandula off.*), Lemon Balm (*Melissa off.*), Meadowsweet (*Filipendula ulmaria*), Passionflower (*Passiflora incarnata*), Skullcap (*Scutellaria lateriflora*), Valerian (*Valeriana off.*), Wood Betony (*Stachys betonica*).

Any of the above can be taken as tea or tincture, singly or combined. Skullcap and Wood Betony are an effective combination for tension headache.

A compress of Chamomile or Lavender flowers can be applied to the affected area.

Sudden onset of headache after the fifth or sixth month could signal pre-eclampsia (see 'Pre-eclampsia').

Heartburn

Heartburn or acid reflux affects about two-thirds of all women at some stage of pregnancy. It is a so-called 'minor' disorder but can cause considerable distress and discomfort. Initially, hormone levels cause relaxation of the lower oesophageal sphincter leading to acid reflux. Later, as the baby grows, the enlarged uterus puts pressure on the digestive system which, especially in the third trimester, can bring on or further exacerbate symptoms.

Posture is an important factor and it helps to avoid bending, lying flat, or sitting hunched up. Avoid eating late at night and if necessary, prop up on extra pillows in bed. Eat small, regular, and frequent meals, chewing well, and in a relaxed and unhurried manner. Avoid drinking at mealtimes but ensure adequate fluids in between meals. Identify any personal triggers and eliminate foods or items that aggravate symptoms. Common culprits include spicy and greasy foods, coffee, sugar, alcohol, and cigarettes.

Herbal treatment

Slippery Elm (*Ulmus rubra*), is one of the most effective and soothing herbs for heartburn, ideally taken as a hot drink or Slippery Elm 'gruel'.

Method: mix a teaspoon of Slippery Elm powder to a paste with a little cold water in a cup. Gradually add hot water, stirring well as the mixture becomes a cup of thickened liquid. This nutritious drink can be drunk as often as required. It can be taken as it is or sweetened with a little honey.

Where a drink is not practical, Slippery Elm tablets can be taken instead, being well chewed before swallowing.

Helpful teas for heartburn include Chamomile (*Chamomilla recutita*), Marshmallow (*Althaea off.*), Lemon Balm (*Melissa off.*), and Meadowsweet (*Filipendula ulmaria*).

Useful formula: Chamomile 2 parts, Meadowsweet 1 part, Lemon Balm 1 part. Combine well. Make a 10-minute infusion, using 1–2 heaped teaspoon per cup, sipped as needed throughout the day.

Herpes, genital

Genital herpes is a sexually transmitted infection caused by the herpes simplex virus affecting the skin and mucosa of the genital organs and anus. Blisters appear two to twelve days after sexual contact and episodes are recurrent with redness, soreness, and itching followed by vulval blisters, which ulcerate before crusting over.

Herpes simplex infection of the newborn, acquired from the mother during delivery, is a rare but potentially serious condition. The risk of transmission from mother to baby at the time of birth is high in primary herpes infection, but very low (less than 1%) in a mother with recurrent genital herpes (including if their primary infection is in the first trimester). Viral shedding is rare in the absence of a lesion, but if a woman has an outbreak near her date of delivery, the midwife/obstetrician may consider a C-section to protect the baby against infection.

Dietary advice includes avoiding sugar and refined foods, and eating foods rich in antioxidants, such as plenty of fruit and vegetables. It can help to increase foods high in the amino-acid lysine (found in vegetables, sprouts, beans, fish, turkey, chicken, eggs, yogurt, beef, milk, cheese) since the herpes virus needs arginine to reproduce and l-lysine can block arginine absorption. Lysine supplementation (widely used by the non-pregnant population to reduce occurrences of herpes) is not recommended since its effects in pregnancy are currently unknown.

Herbal treatment

The herbalist's role is often prophylactic in order to prevent an attack in a pregnant woman with existing infection. Most flare-ups occur when a woman is run down and/or stressed, so herbal treatment involves attending to stress (see 'Emotional and Stress-Related Conditions') and supporting immune function (see 'The Immune System in Pregnancy' page 135). Nerve tonics such as Oatstraw (*Avena sativa*), Vervain (*Verbena off.*), Lavender (*Lavandula off.*), and St John's Wort (*Hypericum perforatum*) tea are helpful, one or two cups daily of one or a combination. Oatstraw and St John's Wort make a particularly beneficial blend and can be drunk throughout pregnancy, as needed. Garlic (*Allium sativum*) is indicated to support the immune system, ingest at least a clove a day, and Echinacea (*Echinacea* spp.) twenty drops of tincture daily.

To treat an outbreak of active herpes, all the above herbs are appropriate and dosage may need to be increased. Valerian (*Valeriana off.*) decoction or tincture is indicated for acute anxiety. Lemon Balm (*Melissa off.*) ointment is specific and can be applied liberally. Other useful ointments include Marigold (*Calendula off.*), Comfrey (*Symphytum off.*; unbroken skin), and Chickweed (*Stellaria media*; if itching is present). Sitz baths with herbs such as Marigold, Lemon Balm, St John's Wort, Comfrey, Chamomile, and Lavender provide local relief. Drops of Myrrh (*Commiphora molmol*) tincture, diluted in water, can be applied directly to blisters to dry them up quickly. This will sting but is highly effective.

Hydatiform mole see 'Gestational Trophoblastic Disease'

Hydramnios/oligohydramnios/polyhydramnios

Hydramnios and polyhydramnios refer to having excess amniotic fluid, whereas oligohydramnios refers to its lack and is the most common.

Oligohydramnios, lack of amniotic fluid

Oligohydramnios is a complication of approximately 4.5% of all pregnancies, with severe oligohydramnios being a complication in 0.7% of pregnancies. No age variables are recognised. It is most common in pregnancies that last beyond 41 weeks.

Amniotic fluid volume (AFV) increases throughout most of pregnancy, peaking at about one litre at 34–36 weeks gestation and decreasing to an average of 800ml at 40 weeks. In early pregnancy, the amniotic fluid is generated from maternal plasma, and passes through the foetal membranes by osmotic and hydrostatic forces. When the foetal kidneys start to function towards the end of the first trimester, foetal urine contributes to the fluid.

Amniotic fluid constantly circulates, with an estimated exchange rate as much as 3600ml/hour. In the first half of pregnancy, the highly permeable foetal skin carries out much of the fluid transfer. The foetal skin becomes keratinised at 22–25 weeks, after which foetal swallowing becomes the major pathway of amniotic fluid clearance for the last half of pregnancy. During this time, the major source of amniotic fluid is urine excreted by the foetus, with a smaller amount of fluid contributed by the foetal respiratory tract.

Oligohydramnios can occur at any time in pregnancy but is rare in the first trimester and is most commonly found in the third. It is usually secondary to either an excess loss of fluid or a decrease in foetal urine production or excretion. These two causes include a range of possible conditions, including premature rupture of membranes (PROM) and foetal malformations. In many cases, oligohydramnios indicates issues with the uteroplacental circulation, the precise details being uncertain.

As previously stated, post-term gestation is the most common occurrence. The decreased efficiency of placental function is often cited as a cause, but this has not been confirmed histologically and currently the exact cause of decreased AFV in post-term pregnancies is unknown. Decreased foetal renal blood flow and decreased foetal urine production have both been demonstrated in pregnancies involving oligohydramnios beyond 42 weeks gestation.

Maternal factors such as dehydration, pre-eclampsia, hypertension, diabetes, and chronic hypoxia all have an effect on AFV.

Signs and symptoms of oligohydramnios include uterine size smaller than normal for dates, leaking of amniotic fluid, abdominal discomfort, sudden drop in foetal heart rate, or reduced foetal movement. Mild cases are asymptomatic. Diagnosis is by ultrasound scan and prognosis depends on cause and severity. In severe cases, it can cause foetal complications or loss of the pregnancy. The baby needs to be carefully monitored with serial ultrasound scans, particularly if risk factors are present e.g. maternal diabetes, chronic high blood pressure, and use of ACE inhibitors.

Herbal treatment

Depending on cause and severity, this condition responds well to herb teas and can resolve entirely within a short time. It is important that the woman drinks plenty of fluids. The fluid balance of mother and foetus has a significant effect on AFV and increased maternal fluid intake is usually crucial. The woman also needs plenty of rest.

Cornsilk (*Zea mays*) as a 15 minute infusion, one or two teaspoons dried herb per cup, three times daily, is a specific remedy to increase amniotic fluid, presumably by supporting foetal kidney function. Other useful herbs include Pellitory-of-the-Wall (*Parietaria judaica*) and Couchgrass (*Agropyron repens*). Cornsilk is effective as a simple or it may be given as part of a blend (often easier to take) e.g. 2 parts Cornsilk, 1 part Pellitory-of-the-Wall, 1 part Couchgrass, two teaspoons per cup, infused 15 mins, 3 cups daily. If required, Hawthorn tops can be added to support the mother's circulatory system including the uteroplacental circulation. Teas are the best mode of treatment.

CASE NOTES: Irish herbalist Juliet Fishbourne, recounts the experience of one of her first patients when she was a herbal student at the Balham Training Clinic in the 1980's. A woman in her third trimester presented with abdominal discomfort and oligohydramnios. The mother was distressed and worried for the health of her baby. Chris Hedley, Juliet's tutor, encouraged Juliet to consider how the amniotic fluid arises, emphasising the significance of supporting healthy urine production in the foetus. She prescribed Cornsilk infusion, three times daily, resulting in significantly increased comfort for the woman within a few days. The woman maintained the daily Cornsilk tea for support until the birth of her healthy baby at term.[8]

Polyhydramnios, hydramnios, excess amniotic fluid

Polyhydramnios occurs in about 1% of pregnancies. Most cases are mild and not harmful to the baby. However, if levels of amniotic fluid are very high, it can trigger major complications with pregnancy and birth and pose a health risk to the baby.

The cause is often unclear, but it can be due to maternal diabetes (pre-existing or gestational), multiple pregnancy, foetal anomalies with disturbed foetal swallowing of amniotic fluid, foetal infections, and other, rarer causes.

Mild polyhydramnios can be asymptomatic, while more severe cases may be associated with shortness of breath, heartburn, constipation, swelling in the lower extremities and abdominal wall, uterine discomfort, preterm labour, and foetal malposition, such as breech presentation. If the uterus is larger than expected for gestational weeks, it may indicate excess amniotic fluid. The condition is detected by ultrasound, most commonly in the later stages of pregnancy. Prognosis depends on its cause and severity.

Herbal treatment

This depends on the underlying cause, for instance if diabetes is diagnosed, see 'Gestational diabetes' for recommendations. Where the cause is less clear, Meadowsweet tea (*Filipendula ulmaria*) will often reduce amniotic fluid volume, especially in milder cases. It is anti-inflammatory, antiseptic, and balancing for the urinary system and may help by reducing excessive foetal urine production. Make a ten to fifteen minute infusion of one heaped teaspoon dried herb per cup, taking three cups daily.

Hypertension and hypertensive disorders

Hypertension in pregnancy is referred to as 'chronic' (that precedes or coincides with pregnancy), 'gestational' (or 'pregnancy-induced hypertension') if not accompanied by proteinuria or other signs of pre-eclampsia, 'pre-eclampsia', or 'eclampsia', which leads to convulsions and/or coma (see Pre-eclampsia, Eclampsia).

Most hypertensive disorders have good outcomes for pregnancy but some can have devastating consequences. Severe hypertension is one of the leading causes of maternal mortality worldwide, with increased risk of stroke, blood clotting problems, kidney and liver damage, and severe bleeding from the placenta. It also increases the risk to the foetus of stillbirth, preterm labour, and being smaller or less developed than normal for gestational age.

Chronic hypertension and mild or moderate pregnancy-induced hypertension pose little risk for the mother or the foetus, unless they develop into severe hypertension, pre-eclampsia, or eclampsia.

Blood pressure readings associated with mild, moderate and severe hypertension are as follows:

	Systolic	**Diastolic**
Mild hypertension	140–149mmHg	90–99mmHg
Moderate hypertension	150–159mmHg	100–109mmHg
Severe hypertension	160mmHg or greater	110mmHg or greater

NOTE: normally there is a slight fall in blood pressure in early pregnancy.

Herbal measures described below can help prevent gestational hypertension and are useful aspects of a treatment plan for any type of high blood pressure in pregnancy.

A vegetarian diet can lower blood pressure, especially if based on 70–80% vegetables and fruit, including citrus fruit for vitamin C and bioflavonoids to strengthen blood vessels. Take garlic and onions. Avoid excess salt and dairy products, as well as stimulants such as caffeine, nicotine, and spicy foods.

Oily fish and omega 3 fatty acids will reduce blood pressure, and have an antiplatelet and antithrombotic effect. Calcium supplementation during pregnancy appears to reduce the risk of women developing pre-eclampsia, especially women with low dietary calcium.

Rest and relaxation are important, and women with hypertension are often advised to rest at home in bed, or they may be admitted to hospital for bed rest and surveillance. In fact, bed rest may or may not be helpful and the usefulness should be assessed on an individual basis. For some women bed rest simply creates another stress; it can be disruptive, it may result in financial or social costs, and it can introduce the additional risk of thromboembolic disease. Stress and disturbed sleep certainly need to be addressed as a priority (see 'Emotional and Stress-Related Conditions' and 'Sleep Disorders'). Regular exercise should be encouraged where appropriate.

Herbal treatment

Garlic, (look for a garlic product equivalent of up to 4g of fresh garlic and where the 'allicin potential' is preserved).

Tinctures of Crataegus (flos or fruct), Valeriana, *Viburnum opulus, Tilia europaea, Leonurus cardiaca, Passiflora incarnata, Achillea millefolium* (maximum 5–10ml per week, avoid in first trimester). Garlic *Allium sativum* tincture can also be added to a mix if needed.

Typical formula: Rx *Crataegus monogyna/oxacanthoides* 30, *Valeriana officinalis* 20, *Viburnum opulus* 20, *Leonurus cardiaca* 20, *Achillea millefolium*, 10 sig 5ml tds.

Add Skullcap and Wood Betony tea, equal parts, standard infusion, two cups daily for high blood pressure with severe tension and anxiety.

Hawthorn tops and Limeflowers, equal parts, standard infusion, up to three cups daily as long-term support for heart and circulation that can be taken throughout pregnancy to reduce tension and balance blood pressure.

Add herbs as required for kidney support and/or diuresis e.g. Dandelion leaf, Pellitory-of-the-Wall (*Parietaria judaica*), Cornsilk (*Zea mays*), Cleavers (*Galium aparine*), Couchgrass (*Agropyron repens*), Yarrow (*Achillea millefolium*; not in first trimester).

A quarter of a teaspoon of Cayenne Pepper (*Capsicum minimum*) can be taken twice daily in water to help balance blood pressure (or add *Capsicum minimum* to tincture mix, 5–10ml per 100ml)

Hypoglycaemia

A hypoglycaemic event happens when blood glucose levels drop too low and can occur as a 'hypo' in insulin dependent diabetics, often as a result of taking too much insulin or missing a meal or snack. In severe cases, hypoglycaemia can lead to seizures, coma, and even death.

During pregnancy, hypoglycaemic episodes may also be experienced in gestational diabetes (See 'Gestational Diabetes' for details), as well as in non-diabetic women.

In this latter group, the condition is termed *reactive hypoglycaemia* and responds well to dietary management and herbs. As in non-pregnant women, reactive hypoglycaemia may be associated with over-consumption of refined carbohydrates, causing a rapid rise in blood sugar and a correspondingly sharp fall, usually between one and four hours later. However, during pregnancy, it is thought that blood sugar imbalances are exacerbated or caused by hormonal factors, such as elevated maternal cortisol, with the result that women need to eat more frequently than usual in order to maintain stable blood glucose levels. Little and often is best. Other factors contributing to hypoglycaemia include stress, over-consumption of caffeine, and food allergies. Symptoms of hypoglycaemia include sweating, shakiness, blurred vision, anxiety, irritability, confusion, and dizziness. The symptoms are quickly relieved by eating, particularly sugar, although this is most unhelpful in the long run and a small amount of a protein food, such as a few nuts or seeds, is ideal.

Sugar levels can easily dip too low if a woman does not eat frequently enough or if she is eating the wrong kinds of foods. In my experience, this condition is most pronounced in early pregnancy but can occur throughout. Women should avoid refined carbohydrates and caffeine, eat a well-balanced diet consisting chiefly of protein (preferably mainly of vegetable source) and fat with some unrefined carbohydrate, at frequent intervals, taking as many as five small meals daily. This gives a sustained release of blood glucose. Alternatively, take three moderate meals daily and a snack every two hours, ensuring snacks are nutritious, such as fruit, nuts, seeds, or natural yogurt. See 'Gestational Diabetes' for further advice regarding diet and supplements.

For extra glucose control, some women find it helpful to avoid carbohydrates in the morning when cortisol is highest (cortisol peaks thirty minutes after waking) and can cause insulin to spike. Fruit and yogurt can make a suitable breakfast, favouring fruit with a low glycaemic index such as apples, dried apricots, and pears.

Herbal treatment

As described for gestational diabetes, combined with proper dietary management, Goat's Rue (*Galega off.*) is highly effective at supporting the pancreas and helping the body to regulate blood glucose levels in pregnancy. For women who are experiencing hypoglycaemic episodes (whether reactive hypoglycaemia or associated with gestational diabetes), if dietary measures alone are not sufficient, Goat's Rue is highly beneficial given as a tincture, either singly or as part of a mix (up to 35ml per week in divided doses). It is also recommended as an 'emergency' bottle to take in case of hypoglycaemic episodes, particularly at the start of treatment, before levels have stabilised, or at the end, in case of any recurrence e.g. 30ml *Galega officinalis* tincture in a dropper bottle with a dose of ten to twenty drops directly under the tongue as required to relieve hypoglycaemic symptoms and help restore overall balance.

Other useful herbs for hypoglycaemia include Burdock (*Arctium lappa*), Dandelion root (*Taraxacum officinale radix*) and Chamomile (*Chamomilla recutita*). Overworked or tense adrenals may be part of the picture. If so, Passionflower (*Passiflora incarnata*) can be added to relax the adrenals, with Liquorice (*Glycyrrhiza glabra*) to nourish and restore if the adrenals are exhausted.

Infections of pregnancy

Infections most commonly associated with pregnancy are those affecting the genito-urinary system. These are described in separate sections: see 'Candida', 'Cervicitis', 'Herpes', 'Urinary Tract Infection', 'Vaginal infection'.

The immune system in pregnancy

The immunology of pregnancy is complex. In the past, it was believed that a pregnant woman's immune system was suppressed in order for the foetus to thrive and not be rejected by the mother's body. This created a myth of pregnancy as a state of immunological weakness and therefore of increased susceptibility to infectious diseases. In fact, nature has a much better design, and although it is still little understood, the latest research indicates that a woman's immune system changes throughout pregnancy in a highly orchestrated and precise manner in order to protect both mother and child. Pregnancy is a unique immunological state where the maternal immune system interacts with the foetal–placental immune system[9] which can be considered an immunological organ in its own right. Signals originating in the placenta can modulate the way the maternal immune system behaves.

So, it is a mistake to consider pregnancy as a time of suppressed immunity or to believe that pregnant women have increased susceptibility to colds and flus, or indeed, any infectious diseases. In fact, some women have improved immunity during pregnancy. However, just as in the non-pregnant population, pregnant women can pick up normal common infections and some women may have low immune status (either pre-existing or with onset during pregnancy). Lowered resistance may be due to a number of causes such as chronic tiredness, emotional shock, poor diet, or chronic constipation, all of which need to be attended to. Treatment will often include herbs to support the immune system and achieve optimal function.

General formula for immune support: Rx *Echinacea* spp. 30, *Sambucus nigra* fructus 20, *Allium sativum* 20, *Commiphora molmol* 10, *Curcuma longa* 10, *Astragalus membranaceus* 10 sig 10–20gtt tds as a preventative, to 5–10ml tds to treat infection.

Adjust according to individual requirements e.g. add *Sambucus nigra* flos for upper respiratory infection; *Inula helenium* and/or *Thymus vulgaris* for chest complaints.

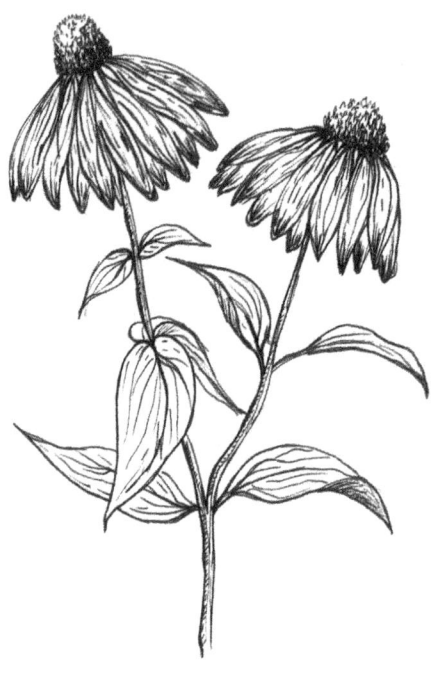

Itching see 'Pruritis'
Leg Cramps see 'Muscle cramps'

Miscarriage, threatened miscarriage

See also 'Healing After Loss' page 175.

Miscarriage is defined as the spontaneous loss of a pregnancy before the foetus is viable (week 24). It affects one in four pregnancies in the UK, with at least eighty percent occurring before 12 weeks. These are called early miscarriages. A late miscarriage is one that happens from 13 weeks to 24 weeks of pregnancy. After 24 weeks (exact number varies depending what country you live in) the loss of a baby is termed a stillbirth.

It is believed that over half the babies miscarried during the first 14 weeks of pregnancy have a chromosomal abnormality. Other causes of miscarriage include hormone deficiency, genetic incompatibility, antiphospholipid syndrome (APS), uterine abnormalities, and cervical insufficiency (see 'Cervical insufficiency'). Less common causes include poorly controlled diabetes, undiagnosed thyroid problems, and other generalised maternal illness. Very often the cause is unknown.

Low progesterone as a cause of early miscarriage

Low serum progesterone ('progesterone insufficiency') is a significant factor affecting pregnancy loss in the first trimester. In the early weeks after fertilisation, the corpus luteum is responsible for progesterone production and if this is defective ('luteal phase insufficiency' or 'luteal phase defect') it is one of the causes of implantation failure and is responsible for many cases of miscarriage as well as unsuccessful assisted reproduction.[10]

Once the placenta is established, at around week 8 to 12, it takes over production of hormones (including progesterone) and after this the risk of miscarriage from low progesterone is significantly reduced. Chaste Tree (*Vitex agnus castus*) is a prime remedy to prevent pregnancy loss from progesterone insufficiency, having the wonderful capacity to support the corpus luteum and maintain healthy levels of progesterone and HCG. If a woman has a history of early miscarriage and low progesterone is suspected, Chaste Tree (*Vitex agnus castus*) can be prescribed prophylactically at **1–3ml daily from the start of pregnancy until the end of week 12** (sometimes extending to week 15). It may be given on its own as a simple or combined with other appropriate herbs as outlined in the case study below. If an acute episode of cramping or spotting occurs, give **an emergency dose of ten to twenty drops every thirty minutes to an hour** until symptoms subside. It is beneficial to give the patient an emergency bottle at the start of treatment 'just in case'.

Spotting on week 9 is a classic and frequent sign of early miscarriage associated with low progesterone and should alert you to this possibility in a first time pregnancy. If a primigravida experiences an episode of bleeding and you suspect progesterone insufficiency, the appropriate herbs should be continued at a maintenance dose once bleeding has stopped. An example of a patient with progesterone insufficiency is given in the case study on page 138.

Women with polycystic ovary syndrome, or thyroid or prolactin disorders, are at high risk of the corpus luteum luteal phase defect, and a low progesterone environment is created iatrogenically by chemical interventions in assisted reproduction. These are instances where treatment with Chaste Tree (*Vitex agnus castus*) can be a crucial factor to help maintain a pregnancy. Assisted reproduction is a complex area and a full discussion is outside the scope of this book. Suffice to say, treatment priorities include hormonal balancing, restoring pelvic health with tonics, and supporting the liver, kidneys, and nervous system.

Acute threatened miscarriage

The main symptom of threatened miscarriage is bleeding which may be light, moderate or heavy (see 'Bleeding'). Abdominal cramping can also be present (see 'Abdominal Pain and Cramps').

Black Haw (*Viburnum prunifolium*) and False Unicorn (*Chamaelirium luteum*) root are a classic combination for threatened miscarriage and one that has proved effective time and time again. Both are powerful uterine sedatives and tonics. False Unicorn (*Chamaelirium luteum*) strengthens pelvic tissues, promotes pelvic nutrition and improves the placental circulation. During pregnancy, it is specific for sensations of downward pressure and/or lack of tone in the cervix. Black Haw (*Viburnum prunifolium*) brings the added benefit of relieving anxiety and tension, and it is considered specific for lower back pain with a sense of bearing down in the pelvis. Sadly,

False Unicorn (*Chamaelirium luteum*) root now faces extinction due to over-harvesting and other threats such as habitat loss.[11] At the time of writing, almost all of the False Unicorn on the market is being harvested, often illegally, from the wild. DO NOT USE THIS HERB UNLESS YOU KNOW IT HAS BEEN CULTIVATED.

In the past, for acute threatened miscarriage, I would combine equal parts of *Chamaelirium luteum* and *Viburnum prunifolium* tinctures, giving ten to twenty drops of the mix every fifteen minutes to an hour, depending on severity, until symptoms subside. The woman should continue to take twenty drops twice daily as a preventative for the next three days. If cramps or blood loss are recurrent, it is advisable to continue these prophylactic measures for several weeks or months, increasing the dose should any acute symptoms arise. If sustainable sources of *Chamaelirium luteum* are not available, it can be replaced by Raspberry leaf (*Rubus idaeus*), Partridge Berry (*Mitchella repens*), or Motherwort (*Leonurus cardiaca*).

CASE STUDY: woman with recurrent miscarriage and low progesterone

Sarah, a 33 year old woman, came to see me at 5 weeks pregnant, asking for help to maintain her pregnancy.

At age 26 she had experienced a miscarriage at 9 weeks gestation, followed by a 15 week miscarriage at age 28. She conceived again later that year and her doctor prescribed weekly progesterone injections from week 7 following an episode of vaginal bleeding. She had no more bleeding episodes but suffered from constant fatigue throughout the pregnancy, with frequent headaches, daily sweats, and hot flushes. Her son was born by forceps delivery at 42 weeks. Sarah's headaches and severe exhaustion had continued post-partum, and she had become hypersensitive to a range of substances, such as perfumes and sunlight, primarily causing skin reactions. She felt the progesterone treatment, while successful at maintaining her pregnancy, was the cause of her persistent fatigue, headaches, and hypersensitivity. She also suspected that the treatment had affected her son, who had exhibited a range of sensitivities since infancy. She was keen to avoid the same treatment in this pregnancy. Sarah had a history of constipation since childhood. When she presented her bowel movements were regular.

I started her on a mix of: Rx *Vitex agnus castus* 20, *Chamaelirium luteum* 20, *Viburnum prunifolium* 20, *Taraxacum officinale* radix 20, *Fucus vesiculosis* 20 = 100 sig 5ml tds pc aq cal.

Vitex agnus castus to support hormone levels, *Chamaelirium luteum* and *Viburnum prunifolium* as uterine tonic sedatives, *Taraxacum officinale* for gentle liver support and *Fucus vesiculosis* as a nutritive and gently cleansing alterative.

I also gave her a bottle of emergency drops to take in case of bleeding or cramps: Rx *Chamaelirium luteum* 30, *Vitex agnus castus* 40, *Viburnum prunifolium* 30, Rescue essence 3gtt = 100 sig 20gtt hourly prn.

Aside from manageable nausea, the next month progressed well. At 9 weeks she started getting period-type cramps, lasting for about a half hour, stopping and starting. These stopped after two days. She took the extra emergency drops when needed and this episode stopped after two days. I advised some bed rest together with relaxation and visualisation exercises and inner dialogue with her baby. I also gave Psyllium seeds, one or two teaspoons daily in water, as a gentle laxative to keep the bowel moving smoothly and avoid any reflex irritation of the uterus.

She had two milder recurrences of cramps over the next three weeks. These cleared within a few hours with the use of the emergency drops.

In this instance, Vitex agnus castus was continued until 15 weeks (partly due to her previously having had a miscarriage at that time, partly an intuitive sense—in practice, I may cease giving Vitex agnus castus anywhere between week 12 and week 15, depending on the person) at which time her prescription was adjusted as follows to give ongoing support:

Rx Chamaelirium luteum 30, Viburnum prunifolium 30, Mitchella repens 20, Rubus idaeus 20, initally at 40gtt tds pc aq cal and reduced to 20gtt bd at week 20, discontinued at week 28.

At week 28, she began drinking a mix of Raspberry leaf (*Rubus idaeus*) and Partridge Berry (*Mitchella repens*) leaf tea daily, increasing to three cups daily from week 36. Sarah went on to have a normal delivery at 40 weeks and gave birth at home to a healthy baby boy.

This example indicates the variability of responses to Chaste Tree (*Vitex agnus castus*). For most women, stopping Chaste Tree at 12 weeks is appropriate, but occasionally a woman presents who needs it for a slightly longer period and may develop signs and symptoms of threatened miscarriage if it is stopped too early. Careful attention and monitoring is required. Headache may indicate the need to reduce dosage or withdraw the herb.

Alternative prescribing

Raspberry leaf (*Rubus idaeus*) and Partridge Berry (*Mitchella repens*) are valuable uterine tonics that provide a strengthening and relaxing combination for the uterus and are extremely helpful where functional support is needed to maintain the growing foetus. They offer an alternative option to treat threatened miscarriage, and they work particularly well as preventatives. Combine equal parts of dried Raspberry leaf and Partridge Berry and drink one or two cups daily, or combine the tinctures and take from twenty drops to 5ml twice daily of a mix of tinctures to prevent miscarriage throughout pregnancy.

For acute threatened miscarriage:

Take a combination of Raspberry leaf and/or Partridge Berry with Black Haw at ten to twenty drops every fifteen minutes to an hour. If necessary, Cramp Bark (*Viburnum opulus*) can be substituted for Black Haw as an antispasmodic, although the latter has a superior action for spasmodic conditions of the pelvis. Cramp Bark is less specific for pelvic conditions but nevertheless a powerfully effective antispasmodic. Wild Yam (*Dioscorea villosa*) is another option as a uterine antispasmodic both for acute symptoms or as a preventative. Motherwort (*Leonurus cardiaca*) is an alternative uterine sedative particularly helpful for uterine cramping without blood loss. It combines well with Raspberry leaf for extra tonic action.

Partridge Berry also combines well with Oatstraw (*Avena sativa*), if there is general debility and exhaustion, and nervines such as Valerian (*Valeriana off.*), Skullcap (*Scutellaria lateriflora*) and Vervain (*Verbena off.*) may all have a role to prevent miscarriage. Vervain brings valuable kidney and liver support, while additional kidney herbs, such as Cornsilk (*Zea Mays*) can be indicated for longer term support. Milk Vetch (*Astragalus membranaceus*) may be helpful to raise the uterine energy and help to hold it.

For any threatened miscarriage, wherever possible and appropriate, encourage women to rest in bed, ideally with a pillow under the hips to elevate the pelvis. Pelvic floor exercises can be recommended (see Chapter 4 page 42), together with suitable visualisation or relaxation exercises. Vibrational essences (see page 301), such as Rescue, and/or a soothing tea of Rose petals, Lemon Balm (*Melissa off.*), Limeflowers (*Tilia europaea*), or Chamomile (*Chamomilla recutita*) can give additional support.

Threatened miscarriage is often amenable to herbal treatment, but herbs will not maintain a pregnancy where miscarriage is due to foetal abnormality or placental misplacement. Properly prescribed herbal medicine will not stop or delay an inevitable miscarriage, nor in any way endanger the patient.

Completing a miscarriage

If there is heavy, bright red bleeding accompanied by cramping, loss of the pregnancy is more likely and if bleeding does not resolve, a miscarriage (often termed a 'spontaneous abortion') may occur. Sometimes solid tissue will be passed and in a case of recurrent miscarriage, a woman may want to keep this for medical investigations. It is recommended that a scan be performed on any woman reporting fresh blood loss, especially in the second or third trimesters. This can check for retained products of conception, which may call for surgical evacuation or surgical curettage ('D and C') due to the risk of continued bleeding or infection.

For a woman with rhesus negative blood, there is a 20% chance of developing antibodies if she miscarries after 13 weeks (this may cause varying degrees of jaundice and anaemia in her next baby). Therefore, she may want to have an anti-D injection, which should be given within seventy two hours of an episode of heavy bleeding.

Note that if twins or other multiple pregnancy were a possibility (even unknown) then this may necessitate a scan or pregnancy test to know if there is still a viable foetus.

Many women prefer to allow a miscarriage to complete naturally, and in the absence of infection, haemorrhage, or other concern, herbal medicine can be given to support the process of cleansing and healing.

Shepherd's Purse (*Capsella bursa-pastoris*), White Deadnettle (*Lamium album*), Lady's Mantle (*Alchemilla vulgaris*) and Raspberry leaf (*Rubus idaeus*), singly or combined, can all help to control bleeding, taken either as cups of tea or twenty drops of tincture. These can be taken as required although caution is advised with Shepherd's Purse and White Deadnettle since strong anti-haemorrhagics may cause the formation of large clots which are hard to pass. Golden Seal (*Hydrastis canadensis*) tincture, ten drops four to six times daily is helpful both to control bleeding and for uterine cleansing.

Raw garlic, one to two cloves daily, should be taken crushed into food, to protect against infection. If bleeding either increases unexpectedly or does not settle down in a reasonable time, this may be a sign of infection requiring medical assistance. Other signs to look out for include lower abdominal pain, tenderness, offensive discharge, and fever, which is frequently an early diagnostic sign before other symptoms develop.

For cleansing the uterus after miscarriage, or after medical or surgical abortion, Mugwort (*Artemisia vulgaris*) can be helpful as a stimulant and tonic emmenagogue, also being antibacterial, antifungal, and mildly sedative. Mugwort is a herb of transitions and assists letting go. Take twenty drops of tincture or drink the infusion, two or three times daily. Black Cohosh (*Cimicifuga racemosa*) is another useful sedative and antimicrobial emmenagogue that stimulates and contracts the uterus and relieves pain. Vervain (*Verbena off.*) is helpful as part of a cleansing mix, especially if extra support is needed for the nervous system.

A typical formula to take after pregnancy loss: Rx *Artemisia vulgaris* 20, *Cimicifuga racemosa* 20, *Lamium album* 20, *Verbena off.* 20, *Leonurus cardiaca* 15, *Rosa* spp. 5. Rescue Remedy 3gtt sig 5ml tds/qds for one or two weeks, with additional herb teas at the start if needed and a longer term restorative tonic at the end, as outlined below. Vibrational essences are indicated for emotional, psychological, and spiritual support (see page 301).

Sitz baths and vaginal steaming are of benefit to cleanse and support the uterus and entire pelvic area. Once bleeding is manageable, sitz baths can be started and continued daily for thirty days after pregnancy loss. Suitable herbs include Mugwort (*Artemisia vulgaris*), Marigold (*Calendula off.*), Motherwort (*Leonurus cardiaca*), Plantain (*Plantago lanceolata*), Raspberry leaf (*Rubus idaeus*), Rose petals (*Rosa* spp.), Lady's Mantle (*Alchemilla vulgaris*), Sage (*Salvia off.*), Shepherd's Purse (*Capsella bursa-pastoris*), Lavender (*Lavandula angustifolia*). Add sea salt for additional benefit. Vaginal steaming (using any of the herbs listed for sitz baths) can be helpful, but only once bleeding has ceased. See Chapter 13 Postpartum Care page 244 for further details of sitz baths and vaginal steaming.

Iron-rich foods should be encouraged in the diet.

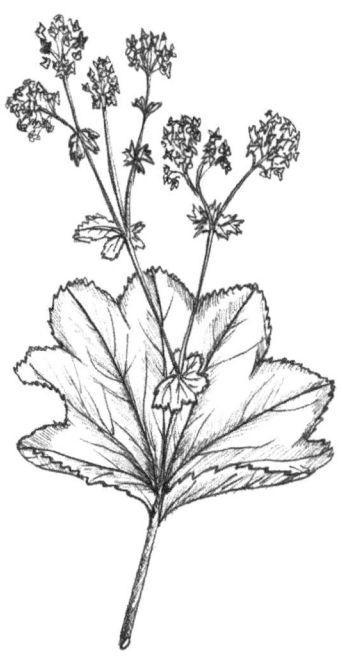

Restoration after miscarriage

From a herbal perspective it is important to strengthen the woman as much as possible before she conceives again. This entails cleansing, rebalancing, healing, and restoring, as well as addressing whatever emotional, mental, and spiritual issues are relevant (described in next chapter 'Healing After Loss').

Herbal tonics are indicated to restore healthy uterine function, together with hormone balancers, and nervines as needed. A strengthening formula can be taken for up to six months, with herbs being added or substituted as appropriate for the individual. Depending on the exact prescription, treatment may need to be stopped or adjusted before trying to conceive again. Some suggested herbs include:

Tonics to restore uterine function:
Black Haw (*Viburnum prunifolium*), Raspberry leaf (*Rubus idaeus*), Partridge Berry (*Mitchella repens*), False Unicorn (*Chamaelirium luteum*), Oatstraw (*Avena sativa*), Milk Vetch (*Astragalus membranaceus*).

Other tonics and balancers:
Chinese Angelica (*Angelica sinensis*)—women's blood tonic, nourishing, relaxing and warming nervine

Mugwort (*Artemisia vulgaris*)—emmenagogue, tonic bitter with emphasis on liver

Motherwort (*Leonurus cardiaca*)—gentle emmenagogue, uterine tonic, sedative

Dandelion root (*Taraxacum officinale* radix)—liver restorative

Vervain (*Verbena off.*)—nervine trophorestorative, tones and cleanses uterine lining

Chaste Tree (*Vitex agnus castus*)—hormone balancer and adaptogenic

Siberian Ginseng (*Eleutherococcus senticosus*)—general restorative tonic

Typical restorative formula to treat uterine weakness:
Rx *Rubus idaeus* 20, *Mitchella repens* 20, *Angelica sinensis* 20, *Astragalus membranaceus* 10, *Vitex agnus castus* 15, *Avena sativa* 15, sig 5ml tds

Chaste Tree is included for at least the first four weeks since progesterone is likely to be low following miscarriage.

Recurrent miscarriage

Recurrent pregnancy loss (RPL), or recurrent abortion, occurs in about one in one hundred pregnant women.[12] In the past, RPL was defined as three or more consecutive clinically recognised spontaneous pregnancy losses before twenty weeks gestation. Recent recommendations have reduced this to two consecutive spontaneous miscarriages when other features of pregnancy loss are present.[13] Factors that increase the risk of miscarriage include maternal age over 35, polycystic ovaries, autoimmune disorders, poorly controlled diabetes, multiple pregnancy, and having had two or more previous miscarriages. However, it should be remembered that these are simply statistical factors and herbal medicine introduces many positives that can have a significant effect on statistics. Where there is no obvious cause for miscarriage, the prognosis is generally excellent following herbal treatment and patients can be reassured that there is a high probability of successful outcome.

Women with recurrent first trimester miscarriage and all women with one or more second trimester miscarriages should have a pelvic ultrasound to assess uterine anatomy. They should also be screened for antiphospholipid antibodies. Women with a history of miscarriage or who threaten miscarriage should avoid sexual stimulation until their babies are ready to be born.

Antiphospholipid syndrome (APS)

Around 15% of women with recurrent early miscarriage have an autoimmune condition where they produce antibodies to some of their own cells (autoantibodies). This is known as antiphospholipid syndrome (APS), which describes the anti-phospholipid antibodies, lupus anticoagulant, anticardiolipin antibodies, and anti-B2-glycoprotein I antibodies. These can cause clotting in the placenta and are associated with recurrent miscarriage and other possible complications, such as preeclampsia, thrombosis, autoimmune thrombocytopenia, and foetal growth restriction. APS is an important cause of recurrent miscarriage. Recommended supplements include Flaxseed oil or fish oils, calcium (with magnesium), vitamin D, and vitamin E. Indicated herbs are Garlic (*Allium sativum*), Gingko (*Gingko biloba*), Hawthorn (*Crataegus monogyna/oxacanthoides*), Limeflowers (*Tilia europaea*), and Meadowsweet (*Filipendula ulmaria*). Heparin and low-dose aspirin, given throughout pregnancy, have been used successfully. If these are being prescribed, Garlic and Gingko should be avoided and women can drink a tea of Hawthorn and Limeflowers, two or three cups daily.

Herbal approach to recurrent miscarriage

For a woman with a history of recurrent miscarriage, restorative treatment (as described above 'Restoration after miscarriage') is recommended as soon as possible after a pregnancy loss. Depending on circumstances, a woman may come for treatment months or years after her last miscarriage, and pregnancy outcome is much improved if she presents at any time in advance of becoming pregnant. This also applies to women who have had unsuccessful pregnancy attempts using assisted reproductive technologies, such as *in vitro fertilisation* (IVF). The length of time required for preparatory herbal treatment varies, but a general recommendation is to start between three to six months in advance of trying to get pregnant. This allows for dietary and lifestyle changes to be addressed and for the diagnosis and treatment of specific conditions. A thorough assessment of both partners is required since they both may need treatment. Just as after a miscarriage (and in many cases you may be both restoring and preparing a patient at the same time), herbal preparation focuses on cleansing, nourishing, balancing, and repair, as well as any assistance needed for mental, emotional, and spiritual well-being. Unhelpful tissue memory may have a role in unexplained recurrent miscarriage and this is discussed in the next chapter (see 'Scar tissue' page 259).

In preparation for another pregnancy, much benefit may be gained by including tonics, such as Black Haw (*Viburnum prunifolium*), which can significantly promote fertility. Other simple preparatory measures include the avoidance of coffee, alcohol, and tobacco, the clearing of toxicity and correction of dietary deficiencies, paying particular attention to folic acid, B12, B6, zinc, magnesium, copper, and essential fatty acids. Coenzyme Q10 supplementation may also be helpful to decrease the chance of pregnancy loss.

Naturally, as in the case history on page 138, not every woman comes to us in advance of becoming pregnant and we work with whatever scenario is put before us.

For a woman who has had recurrent miscarriages, conception and pregnancy are understandably anxious times. As herbalists, we have an important role in encouraging a positive outlook and discouraging blame and obsessive thoughts. We need to offer gentle supportive care, doing our best to encourage hope and acceptance at the same time.

See next chapter for dealing with emotional and psychological disturbance after loss

Mood Swings see 'Emotional and Stress-Related Conditions'
Morning Sickness see 'Nausea and Vomiting in Pregnancy'

Multiple pregnancy

Twins occur in one in eighty spontaneous pregnancies and are more common in assisted reproduction techniques like IVF. Most of the complications of pregnancy are more likely the higher number of babies a woman is carrying and women having multiple pregnancies may need additional support to help them with the emotional, practical, and financial demands of pregnancy and planning for more than one baby. Promoting confidence can be crucial. Women are more likely to have interventions of all kinds, but this does not mean that the experience of pregnancy has to be totally medicalised, nor does it necessarily mean a birth by caesarean section.

Muscle cramps, leg cramps

For abdominal cramps, see 'Abdominal Pain and Cramps'.

Recurring leg cramps (painful spasms of the calf muscles and sometimes the feet) are experienced to some extent by nearly half of all pregnant women, especially in the last trimester. These tend to occur at night and can cause considerable distress. Sometimes they are associated with an uncontrollable desire to move the legs (see 'Restless Legs Syndrome').

Dehydration can be a factor and it is important to encourage women to drink plenty of water (or appropriate herb teas), which is crucial to maintain a healthy balance of electrolytes, particularly potassium, sodium, magnesium, and calcium. Magnesium is a key nutrient and deficiency may be a cause of cramping. Good dietary sources include seeds (especially pumpkin seeds), nuts, peas, beans, and whole grains, and magnesium can be supplemented at up to 300mg daily.

Calcium salts are widely prescribed but there is no evidence of benefit beyond placebo. In a hot climate or in women on a low salt diet, it is possible for cramps to be linked to salt deficiency, in which case, adequate hydration and eating something salty before bed can be an effective preventative.

Cramps may be related to poor circulation, varicose veins, nervous tension, and deficiency of vitamins B and D. Practical measures for reducing cramping include raising the end of the bed (or putting pillows under the mattress) in order to lift the woman's feet above the level of her heart and assist the return circulation. Wear bed socks to keep the feet warm and do ankle exercises to stretch the calf muscles before bed every night. Circling the ankles in both directions and stretching the foot forward and back are simple and effective, and can also be used in case of an attack of cramping. For quick relief of leg cramps, grab the toes and pull them towards the knees. For foot cramps, roll the foot over a bottle about eight centimetres (three inches) diameter. Avoid curling the toes as this can bring on an attack.

Massaging the legs and feet will improve circulation and relax tense muscles. Make a relaxing massage oil selecting from one to three essential oils from the following list (use from 16 weeks) to make a 1% dilution in carrier oil: Lavender (*Lavandula angustifolia*), Bergamot (*Citrus bergamia*), Chamomile (*Chamomilla recutita/Chamaemelum nobile*), Geranium (*Pelargonium graveolens*), Ylang-ylang (*Cananga odorata*). Vigorous massage (avoiding any varicosities) can be done at bedtime before doing the ankle exercises above.

Alternatively, a foot bath can be taken before bed, adding five drops of Lavender essential oil to an infusion of Chamomile, Oatstraw (*Avena sativa*) or Limeflowers (*Tilia europaea*), singly or combined.

As internal medicine, Cramp Bark (*Viburnum opulus*) and Hawthorn (*Crataegus monogyna/oxacanthoides*), berries or flowering tops, are specific for this condition, acting as a powerful anti-spasmodic and circulatory tonic respectively. Combine in equal parts, either as a decoction, two cups daily and one at night, or in tincture form, taking 5ml twice daily and 5ml at night. A small amount of Ginger (*Zingiber off.*) can be added if required as an extra boost to the circulation.

Horsetail (*Equisetum arvense*) infusion can also be effective (2 cups daily), perhaps due to its deobstruent capacity. Teas of Chamomile, Oatstraw, Limeflowers, and Motherwort (*Leonurus cardiaca*) are indicated if nervous tension is particularly high. Garlic (*Allium sativum*), fish oils, and vitamin E can be helpful to promote blood flow to the muscles. If poor digestive absorption is suspected, give 1 teaspoon of cider vinegar before meals or ten drops of Gentian (*Gentiana lutea*).

Nausea & vomiting in pregnancy (NVP) and hyperemesis gravidarum

Nausea and vomiting are perhaps the most frequent and troublesome symptoms of early pregnancy. Almost three-quarters of all pregnant women suffer from nausea and for one in ten the condition persists beyond the first trimester. Despite being known as 'morning sickness', symptoms can occur at any time of day or night, usually starting around week 5 to 6 and in most cases subsiding by week 12 to 16, although for some women symptoms continue throughout pregnancy, or disappear and recur later. For women with a multiple pregnancy, the condition is likely to be more severe and longer lasting.

The exact causes are largely unknown, but it is thought that the rapid rise in hormone levels is responsible, perhaps by irritating the vomit centre in the brain. There are countless theories as to cause, but it is often considered an indication of healthy hormone levels. Some see it as nature's way of encouraging a woman to rest and eat healthy foods, a good preparation for healthy pregnancy. In some spiritual traditions, nausea, as well as dizziness and other common symptoms of early pregnancy, are perceived as part of the process of energetic adjustment as the mother and incoming soul fine-tune their vibrational frequency, working in partnership towards childbirth.

In the past, nausea and vomiting in its most severe form (*hyperemesis gravidarum*) was a serious threat to both mother and child, but with modern medical advances, outcomes have improved dramatically. However, women with severe vomiting may still need to be admitted to hospital for treatment. Fortunately, most cases of nausea and vomiting are less severe. Many women experience fairly mild nausea, which often arises first thing in the morning or in the evening. It can manifest as waves of sickness throughout the day, frequently accompanied by fatigue and an aversion to strong smells. A metallic taste in the mouth and excess salivation (ptyalism or *sialorrhoea gravidarum*) are other common symptoms that may be part of the picture.

Nausea and vomiting of early pregnancy is very often linked to low blood sugar, especially when it occurs in the early morning and is relieved by eating. It helps to keep a dry cracker and a thermos of tea by the bed to take on waking. Avoid getting out of bed too quickly and eat little and often, having small snacks every two to three hours. Choose high protein, unprocessed carbohydrates, and easy-to digest foods such as oatcakes with tahini, almond butter on rice cakes, yogurt with fruit, soup, steamed fish, and vegetables. Large meals and excess sugar can make symptoms much worse. A late-night snack of tea and crackers before bed will help in some cases. Avoid bending forward, greasy foods, alcohol, tobacco, regular tea, coffee, and strong odours. Tea can inhibit iron absorption and caffeine in both tea and coffee may bring on nausea and headaches. Encourage women to listen to their bodies whenever possible and rest as much as needed. Fresh air and exercise are generally therapeutic, and if a woman is not too exhausted, a brisk walk may alleviate nausea. B complex can help ease symptoms and reduce the frequency of persistent nausea. It may help to wear wrist bands for travel sickness or have acupressure on the wrist (the Nei Guan point P6).

If a woman has been losing weight from vomiting, recommend high calorie, nutrient dense food, such as nuts, seeds, oils from oily fish, avocados, cold-pressed olive oil, walnut oil, sesame oil, and dried fruit. Hydration and adequate protein are crucial.

Herbal treatment

Teas can be ideal in early pregnancy, taken either singly or combined. Herbs that are pleasant tasting for a woman can be included in order to flavour a blend and ease the drinking, and women may find it easier to sip a tea every so often instead of drinking whole cupfuls. Alternatively, teas can be given as footbaths or, if warmth is not needed, another option is to freeze the infusion in an ice cube tray and suck the ice cubes. However, when a woman is nauseous she may not be able to face a tea in any form, and sometimes the aroma alone could cause her to vomit. A few drops of tincture, taken as appropriate, may work better, or the dried powdered herb taken in capsule form.

Dynamic changes are taking place in the body, and symptoms and response to herbs can vary on a daily basis. Some women appear to quickly develop a tolerance to a remedy with the result that it temporarily ceases to be effective after a relatively short time. If this happens, it can work well to give remedies in rotation, and it may be necessary to dispense small amounts of several medicines so that a woman can alternate remedies as appropriate (sometimes even on a daily basis). Depending on the woman's history, I usually start by giving a single remedy as a simple and stay in regular contact to monitor progress and make changes or additions as needed.

Ginger (*Zingiber off.*) root is one of the most well-known and widely used remedies for nausea and vomiting of pregnancy. It can be sipped as a tea of fresh or dried root, powdered and taken in capsule form (max 2g powdered root daily), or taken as 1:2 tincture 5 drops in water every hour as required. In mild cases of nausea it can be sufficient to add ginger to cooking or to take it in ginger biscuits, ginger beer, or as crystallised ginger.

Black Horehound (*Ballota nigra*) is another classic remedy for nausea and vomiting of pregnancy. The aerial parts are anti-emetic and sedative. Black Horehound combines well with Chamomile (*Chamomilla recutita*) and is effective either singly or combined, as a tea, up to 3 cups daily, tincture, from 5 drops hourly up to 5ml tds, or in capsules.

Irish herbalist Juliet Fishbourne recommends the following formula, which I have found to be effective:

Rx *Ballota nigra* 2 parts, *Filipendula ulmaria* 2 parts, *Chamomilla recutita* 1 part, *Gentiana lutea* 1 part, take 5 drops in water as required.

Raspberry leaf can also relieve nausea and vomiting. The tea can be sipped throughout the day, 1 teaspoon per cup of 10 min infusion, taking the equivalent of one and a half cups daily, or 10–20 drops tincture hourly (up to 5ml daily).

Nausea and vomiting may show up a pre-existing digestive weakness and can highlight food allergies that may not have been evident before pregnancy. Considering that so much of the body's vital energy is directed towards the uterus and pelvic tissues, there may be less available energy for digestive function and any existing weakness will be accentuated. A woman with weak digestion may be tired and pale with a weak pulse, pale tongue and watery vomit. She will often be drawn to hot drinks and may find relief from warming teas, such as Ginger or Cinnamon (*Cinnamomum verum*) to warm the stomach. Chamomile tea and Slippery Elm (*Ulmas rubra*) can also be helpful to soothe and restore the digestion. Slippery Elm may be sipped as a warm drink or chewed in tablet form. Other suitable herbs for digestive weakness include Lemon Balm (*Melissa off.*), Meadowsweet (*Filipendula ulmaria*), Iceland Moss (*Cetraria islandica*), Gentian (*Gentiana lutea*), and Peppermint (*Mentha piperita*)—avoid these last two if the digestive tract is inflamed. Fennel (*Foeniculum vulgare*) and Aniseed (*Pimpinella anisum*) are also useful, especially if there is a lot of gas. Some women find relief by taking a teaspoon of cider vinegar on waking.

A metallic taste in the mouth may be a sign of liver imbalance. Mouthwashes of Fennel, Myrrh (*Commiphora molmol*), Liquorice (*Glycyrrhiza glabra*), or Thyme (*Thymus vulgaris*) can all provide relief while systemic treatment addresses the cause. Liver weakness or imbalance may be associated with high thirst, tiredness, depression, a red tongue with yellow coating, and bitter or sour vomit. Dandelion root (*Taraxacum officinale radix*) is a prime remedy to support liver function. Give a decoction to be sipped as required or tincture 20 drops tds. Other helpful remedies to enhance liver and digestive function include Gentian, Black Horehound (*Ballota nigra*), and Wild Yam (*Dioscorea villosa*). Milk Thistle (*Silybum marianum*) is helpful if detoxification is needed.

As a hormone balancer, small doses (2–5gtt up to qds) of Chaste Tree (*Vitex agnus castus*) can relieve nausea in some cases. If symptoms are linked to anxiety and tension, any of the following are indicated: Chamomile, Lavender, Catnip (*Nepeta cataria*), Wild Yam, and Lemon Balm (especially before bed).

If excess salivation is a problem, this can be eased by taking small sips of weak Peppermint tea.

Essential oils

Use of most essential oils is not recommended in the first trimester. However, Lemon and Ginger are considered safe and effective as inhalations for nausea and vomiting. Lemon also provides emotional support. Mix one drop of Lemon or Ginger essential oil in 5ml carrier oil (1% dilution), place on a cotton pad for inhalation as needed.

Two drops of essential oil of Lemon or Ginger may also be added to a 50ml room spray.

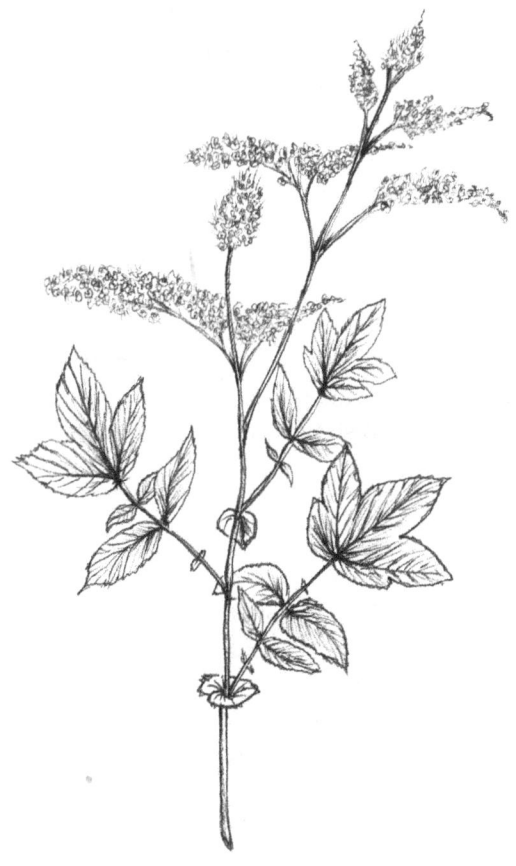

Nose bleeds, Epistaxis (see also rhinitis)

Nose bleeds are common in pregnancy, secondary to increased nasal mucosa vascularity. These are not usually severe. Tincture of fresh Shepherd's Purse (*Capsella bursa-pastoris*) on cotton wool or a tissue can be used to plug the nostril and quickly stop bleeding.

Oedema

A certain amount of oedema of legs, hands and feet is normal in the second and third trimesters due to hormone levels, increased fluid volume, and the demands of the baby. This can manifest as swollen ankles and feet, swollen fingers, hands, and face. It is worse later in the day, in hot weather, with prolonged standing, and in women who are overweight. Resting usually brings relief, especially if the feet are raised. Moderate oedema of gradual onset is not usually of concern, but if it is rapid onset, combined with headaches and visual disturbance, these can be signs of pre-eclampsia needing urgent medical attention (see 'Pre-eclampsia'). The oedema of pre-eclampsia typically starts in the calves or ankles, spreading to the hands and face, and is present on waking rather than worsening throughout the day. Check for pitting oedema, which can indicate overburdened kidneys. Oedema may also be related to poor circulation and varicose veins (see 'Varicose veins'). If there is a build-up of fluid in the tissues of the wrist, this can cause carpal tunnel syndrome causing tingling, pain, and numbness in the wrist and hand (see 'Carpal Tunnel Syndrome').

Measures to ease oedema include putting feet up as often as possible and raising the foot of the bed. Drink plenty of water and be as active as possible. Avoid wearing tight jewellery on arms and wrists, remove rings, and wear comfortable shoes and socks. Avoid standing for long periods and avoid crossing legs. Foot exercises can help reduce foot and ankle swelling; bend and stretch each foot up and down thirty times. Rotate foot eight times in each direction.

If oedema causes severe discomfort, lymphatic drainage may be stimulated by applying pressure to a point in the muscle above each breast, proximal to the axilla. Feel around the area and locate the spot that is particularly tender, simultaneously pressing and rubbing for thirty to sixty seconds. Performed correctly, this can reduce oedema when done on a daily basis.

Herbal treatment

Massaging the limbs provides effective relief for oedema, using long, flowing movements towards the heart. From week 16 onwards, select from essential oils of Lavender (*Lavandula angustifolia*), Lemon (*Citrus limonum*), Chamomile (*Chamomilla recutita/ Chamaemelum nobile*), Petitgrain (*Citrus aurantium*), Bergamot (*Citrus bergamia*) and Geranium (*Pelargonium graveolens*), making a 1% dilution in a carrier oil such as almond.

For internal use, gentle diuretics will help remove excess fluid via the kidneys: Cornsilk (*Zea mays*), Dandelion (*Taraxacum off.*) leaf, Couchgrass (*Agropyron repens*), Cleavers (*Galium aparine*) and Horsetail (*Equisetum arvense*), singly or in combination, two teaspoons per cup, drinking one cup three or four times daily, or sipped regularly throughout the day.

Cold compresses can be applied to ease swollen hands, fingers, feet and ankles. Select from the diuretic herbs above and make a hot 20-minute infusion. Strain and allow to cool before using as a compress on affected areas.

The late Thomas Bartram, UK herbalist, recommended Cornsilk as a simple for oedema of pregnancy: 1oz to 1pt, simmered gently down to half a pint. Drink half to one cup, three times daily.[14]

Oligohydramnios (see 'Hydramnios')

Palpitations

Palpitations and arrhythmias are common during pregnancy, particularly in the third trimester. Usually these are harmless, being primarily due to the increased blood volume causing a faster resting heart rate and leading to tachycardia and ectopic beats. In rare cases, palpitations may need further investigations to rule out heart disease or systemic disorders such as hyperthyroid or anaemia.

Women can be advised to avoid over-exertion and dehydration, both of which can trigger or worsen palpitations. Eat a healthy diet to ensure hypoglycaemia is not a factor (see 'Hypoglycaemia'), consider breathing exercises, relaxation, or meditation if palpitations are exacerbated by or causing stress (see Chapter 3 page 45).

If herbs are required, Motherwort (*Leonurus cardiaca*) is specific for palpitations of pregnancy, supporting the heart and easing nervous tension. Ten to twenty drops, taken as required. Valerian (*Valeriana off.*) is indicated if there is a lot of anxiety or restlessness. Passionflower (*Passiflora incarnata*) for palpitations associated with shock or nervous excitability.

Pelvic girdle pain (PGP), pelvic instability

See 'Back Pain, Pelvic Pain, Sciatica'.

Pregnancy-related pelvic girdle pain, formerly known as symphysis pubis dysfunction (SPD) is pain felt around the pelvic joints, lower back, hips, and thighs. It affects approximately 1 in 4 pregnant women to varying degrees of severity. See 'Back Pain' for suitable treatments.

Perineal Care (see Chapter 10 'Preparation for Birth' page 196)

Placenta praevia

Placenta praevia occurs when a placenta is situated wholly or partially over the lower pole of the uterus, thereby blocking the cervix to some degree. Routine ultrasound in the early second trimester reveals around 5–6% of placentae as low lying. More than 90% of these resolve spontaneously, becoming normally situated as the uterus expands later in pregnancy. In rare cases, the cervix remains completely or partially covered and placenta praevia can be an important cause of vaginal bleeding, possibly due to a defective attachment to the uterine wall, as well as damage occurring as the baby's presenting part moves into the lower uterine segment in preparation for labour. Prior caesarean section is a major risk factor. Placenta praevia classically presents as painless, bright red bleeding in the second or third trimester, varying between spotting to massive haemorrhage. Bleeding can be spontaneous or provoked by mild trauma, such as vaginal examination. There may be pain if the woman is in labour. This is a medical emergency requiring immediate hospitalisation.

Placental abruption

Placental abruption, or retroplacental haemorrhage, occurs in around 1% of pregnancies and is a major cause of vaginal bleeding after 20 weeks.

Abruption is the early separation of a placenta from the lining of the uterus and may occur at any stage of pregnancy but is most commonly diagnosed around 25 weeks or later. An abruption may be 'revealed' resulting in bright red vaginal bleeding, or 'concealed' where the bleeding remains within the uterus, and typically forms a clot retroplacentally. In the latter case, the bleeding is not visible but can be severe enough to cause systemic shock. The exact aetiology is unknown. Symptoms can include lower abdominal pain, and examination may reveal a tense and painful uterus. Abruption varies from asymptomatic to severe. Moderate and severe cases present considerable risk for mother and child. In mild cases, the patient may be allowed home after a period of observation in hospital. Herbal care of mild cases depends on individual needs, focusing on strengthening and repair with pelvic tonics and anti-haemorrhagics such as Raspberry leaf (*Rubus idaeus*), Partridge Berry (*Mitchella repens*), Black Haw (*Viburnum prunifolium*), and Nettle (*Urtica dioica*).

Polyhydramnios (see 'Hydramnios')
Posterior Presentation (see Chapter 11 'The Process of Labour' page 220)

Pre-eclampsia/eclampsia (formerly known as toxaemia)

Pre-eclampsia is considered a serious hypertensive disorder of pregnancy (see also 'Hypertension'). The diagnosis of pre-eclampsia was formerly defined as the new onset of elevated blood pressure and proteinuria after 20 weeks gestation. In recent years, this has been redefined and proteinuria is no longer a rigid diagnostic requirement. Pre-eclampsia can now be diagnosed by hypertension[15] that develops during pregnancy or post-partum and may be associated with proteinuria or with the new development of thrombocytopaenia, kidney or liver dysfunction, pulmonary oedema, ankle oedema (pitting), cerebral or visual disturbances. This is based on evidence showing that liver and kidney problems can occur without signs of protein, and that the amount of proteinuria does not predict how severely the disease will progress.

Pre-eclampsia is frequently asymptomatic, and diagnosis depends on clinical history and careful assessment of blood pressure, proteinuria, and other clinical signs. Additional signs and symptoms of pre-eclampsia include generalised oedema, extreme weight gain, headaches, nausea, vomiting, epigastric or right upper quadrant abdominal pain, shortness of breath, burning behind the sternum, confusion, heightened anxiety, and visual disturbances, such as oversensitivity to light or blurred vision. Onset can be gradual or sudden. It is sometimes associated with unaccustomed snoring at night.

Pre-eclampsia can appear at any time during pregnancy, delivery, and up to six weeks post-partum, although it is most common in the third trimester and usually resolves within forty-eight hours of delivery. It occurs primarily in first pregnancies (unless with a different partner), affecting between 2–8% of pregnancies worldwide, and a significant global cause of maternal morbidity and mortality.[16] A woman who has had pre-eclampsia in a previous pregnancy is seven times more likely to develop pre-eclampsia in a later pregnancy. Additional risk factors include chronic hypertension or renal disease, hypertensive disorder in a previous pregnancy, multiple pregnancy, IVF, family history of pre-eclampsia, Type I or Type II diabetes mellitus, obesity, autoimmune disease such as systemic lupus erythematosus or anti-phospholipid syndrome, a maternal age of more than forty or less than twenty, and history of thrombophilia.

With proper care, most women with pre-eclampsia will deliver healthy babies and make a full recovery. However, in some women the condition progresses to severe pre-eclampsia (this can happen rapidly), with complications that are life-threatening for both mother and foetus.

The exact pathogenesis of pre-eclampsia is uncertain, although the condition is often seen as a disturbance of the healthy adaptation to pregnancy. Aetiology is thought to be immunological, with abnormalities in the maternal immune system and insufficiency of gestational immune tolerance. Studies have shown that the incidence of pre-eclampsia is reduced in women who have frequent exposure to their partner's semen before conception, leading to the suggestion that pre-eclampsia may be linked to the body's attempts to select a reliable and available father for the foetus.[17] Either way, the placenta plays a key role and women with pre-eclampsia are found to have atypical placentae, characterised by poor trophoblastic invasion[18] and the abnormal formation of blood vessels, thought to lead to oxidative stress, hypoxia, and other problems.

Treatment relies on thorough medical assessment and depends on severity of the condition, ranging from surveillance, pharmaceutical medication, hospitalisation, and preterm delivery by induction or caesarean section. Bed rest has not been found to be useful and is not routinely recommended, although it may help some women.

HELLP syndrome is a rare but dangerous variant of pre-eclampsia, characterised by haemolysis, elevated liver enzymes, and low platelet count, and can result in permanent liver or renal damage. Symptoms include headache, vomiting, hypertension, proteinuria, epigastric, or right upper quadrant pain.

Eclampsia is defined as seizures occurring in pregnancy or after pregnancy that are linked to high blood pressure. This may develop as a complication of pre-eclampsia but it can be unheralded. It is a dangerous obstetric emergency, characterised by one or more seizures during pregnancy or in the post-partum period. In developed countries, eclampsia is rare and usually treatable if appropriate intervention is promptly sought. Left untreated, eclamptic seizures can result in stroke, coma, brain damage, and maternal or infant death, accounting for 12% of maternal deaths in the developed world.

Preventative treatment is best

This is an area where preventative measures work wonders. Respected American midwife, Ina May Gaskin, emphasises the importance of good nutrition and believes that most cases of pre-eclampsia can be prevented with good diet. In a published study of 775 pregnant women from the community where she worked, only one woman developed a mild case of pre-eclampsia and she was able to give birth vaginally.[19] In Ina May's book *Ina May's Guide to Childbirth*, she also cites a study in a low-income area of San Francisco involving over seven thousand mothers. The women received extensive nutritional counselling during pregnancy and the incidence of pre-eclampsia was reduced from 20–35% down to only 0.5%, with no cases of convulsive eclampsia.[20] Ina May recommends a high protein, vegetarian diet with plenty of fresh vegetables and whole grains, and water as the main beverage.

There is no doubt that poor diet and general poor health are significant contributory factors to pre-eclampsia and eclampsia. Ensure a high protein diet with adequate salt, avoiding sugar, hydrogenated fats, refined carbohydrates, and alcohol (see Chapter 3 'Nutrition' page 29). Useful supplements that are particularly linked to helping pre-eclampsia include vitamin B12, Starflower (*Borago off.*) oil or Evening Primrose (*Oenothera biennis*) oil, Flax seed oil or fish oils, vitamins C and E, and magnesium with calcium. Daily beetroot juice makes a nourishing addition to the diet and can help to lower blood pressure and improve blood circulation.

Herbal treatment

Along with good diet, nourishment can be provided by regularly drinking herb teas such as Nettle (*Urtica dioica*), Raspberry (*Rubus idaeus*) leaf, and Dandelion (*Taraxacum off.*) leaf as a rich source of potassium and support for the kidneys.

If proteinuria is discovered and/or there is a suspicion of pre-eclampsia developing, False Unicorn (*Chamaelirium luteum*) (or substitute Black Haw (*Viburnum prunifolium*) and Echinacea (*Echinacea* spp.), a mix of equal parts, is specific as a preventative. Take twenty drops three times daily, ensuring concurrent medical assessments are being made and promptly acted upon. In a mild case, if a woman is sent home from hospital for continued surveillance, herbs can be given to improve placental circulation and function: Garlic (*Alium sativum*), Cornsilk (*Zea mays*), Hawthorn (*Crataegus monogyna/oxacanthoides*), and Black Haw may all be helpful (avoid Garlic if aspirin has been prescribed), plus additional anti-hypertensives, such as Limeflowers (*Tilia europaea*), Motherwort (*Leonurus cardiaca*), Valerian (*Valeriana off.*), and Cramp Bark (*Viburnum opulus*) if required to keep blood pressure down.

Preterm labour/preterm prelabour rupture of membranes/ preterm premature rupture of membranes (PPROM)

Preterm is defined as before 37 weeks of pregnancy. Worldwide, it is estimated that fifteen million babies are born preterm every year, with significantly higher numbers in low and medium income countries. Preterm birth is the single biggest cause of neonatal mortality and morbidity in the UK, with neurodevelopmental disability being the most frequent long-term consequence for babies who survive birth. Risk of mortality increases as gestational age decreases, being highest for babies born at less than 28 weeks, less for those born between 28 and 31 weeks, and least for those born between 32 and 36 weeks.[21]

Causes of preterm birth are complex and the pathophysiology is largely unknown, although predisposing factors include antepartum haemorrhage or abruption, mechanical factors, such as cervical incompetence or uterine over-distension, hormonal changes, bacterial infection, and inflammation. Multiple pregnancies are more likely to lead to preterm delivery due to spontaneous labour or premature rupture of membranes (PROM), or as a result of maternal conditions such as pre-eclampsia or foetal disorders. Women with a history of preterm birth should avoid sexual stimulation and arousal until their babies are ready to be born.

If regular contractions (every 10 minutes or less) start before 37 weeks, the woman needs hospital admission as soon as possible since premature labour can be rapid and the baby may need specialist attention. In these circumstances, on the way to the maternity unit, it may be possible to slow labour by adopting a knee-chest position with the pelvis raised and head on crossed arms. Take Motherwort (*Leonurus cardiaca*) and Black Haw (*Viburnum prunifolium*) tinctures combined, twenty drops every hour, to slow down contractions.

Where contractions are less well-established, it is possible to prevent progression to labour. See 'Abdominal Pain and Cramps' for methods of prevention.

Preterm prelabour rupture of membranes (PPROM)

If the membranes rupture before the onset of labour this is known as prelabour/premature rupture of membranes or PPROM. In most cases, this occurs near to term (see Chapter 12 Herbs for Labour and Delivery page 210). If rupture happens before 37 weeks of pregnancy, it is called preterm prelabour/premature rupture of membranes and requires immediate hospital attention in order to assess the risk of intrauterine infection, the role of prophylactic antibiotics, steroids, and tocolytic agents, and the optimum gestation for delivery. In some cases, women will be monitored at home following a period of inpatient observation. Prophylactic Echinacea (*Echinacea* spp.), up to 5ml tds, can be given (concurrent with antibiotics if necessary), to help prevent intrauterine infection. Eating raw Garlic (*Allium sativum*) is also recommended.

Pruritis

See also 'Skin Disorders' and 'Restless Leg Syndrome'.

Pruritis is a common and often distressing symptom of pregnancy, occurring in around one third of pregnant women, most marked in the third trimester, and sometimes causing significant sleep disturbance and exhaustion. Itching is most likely to affect the abdomen and trunk but can be all over the body.

Pruritus may accompany some specific dermatoses[22] of pregnancy (see 'Skin Disorders' for details of these), including intrahepatic cholestasis of pregnancy (ICP or obstetric cholestasis), which carries serious risks to the foetus. That said, the majority of cases of pruritus occur without any obvious underlying disease, possibly linked to a variety of factors including hormonal, immunological, and metabolic.

For women suffering from pruritis from any cause, symptoms may be eased by general measures such as wearing loose cotton clothing, avoiding synthetic materials or wool, and the use of unperfumed soap, avoiding strong perfumes, overly spicy food, alcohol, and caffeine.

Herbal treatment

Cooling herbs tend to be most effective to relieve itching, best taken in the form of herb teas, not drunk too hot. A strong infusion of fresh Chickweed (*Stellaria media*), when available, is both antipruritic and cooling. Other recommended herbs, used fresh or dried, include Heartsease (*Viola tricolor*), Red Clover (*Trifolium pratense*), Lavender (*Lavandula* spp.), Chamomile (*Chamomilla recutita*), Marigold (*Calendula off.*), and Nettle (*Urtica dioica*). Drink up to three cups daily of one or a blend and/or add to a cool bath or footbath. For itchy skin conditions, cool baths are generally most helpful but may not suit everyone. Two cupfuls of cider vinegar can be added to a full bath for increased anti-pruritic action. Seaweed baths can also alleviate itch. Soak for twenty minutes.

Any of the above herb teas can be left to cool and used as a lotion, applied on cotton wool or a cloth. The frequent application of emollients will calm and soothe. Chickweed is a prime remedy, typically as a cream, although the infused oil or ointment is helpful if skin is very dry. Marigold cream is indicated if there is inflammation or damage from scratching.

For localised itching and inflamed skin, make a poultice of oatmeal with fresh Chickweed and Plantain (*Plantago lanceolata*). Pound all together, adding a little hot water if needed, to make a firm paste. Spread between two layers of muslin and apply to affected area, holding in place with bandage as required.

If itch is associated with nervous tension or anxiety, Skullcap (*Scutellaria lateriflora*), Oats (*Avena sativa*), Heartsease, and Lavender can be given as tea (singly or combined), to be enjoyed as a drink and/or added to a bath before bed. Oats can be placed in a muslin bag under the hot tap and two or three drops of Lavender oil can be added to the bath (not first trimester). Itch may also be associated with candida (see 'Candidiasis').

Generalised itching can indicate a degree of underlying toxicity requiring support for liver, kidneys, and/or bowel. If appropriate, Dandelion root (*Taraxacum officinale* radix.) and Milk Thistle seed (*Silybum marianum*) are helpful to promote healthy liver function, with Dandelion providing a gentle laxative action. Nettle, Goldenrod (*Solidago virgaurea*) and Cornsilk (*Zea mays*) can all assist cleansing through the kidneys. Red Clover and Marigold may be indicated as blood and lymphatic cleansers. For pruritis, all of these are best taken in the form of teas.

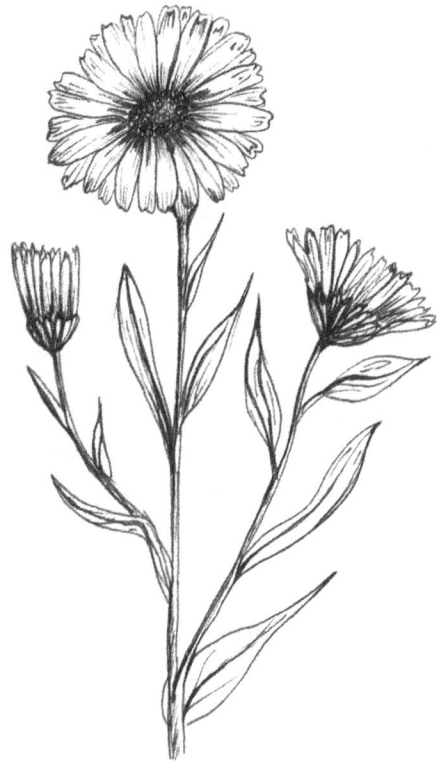

Restless legs syndrome

Restless legs syndrome (RLS), also known as Willis-Ekbom disease (WED), is a common neurosensory disorder that causes an overwhelming urge to move the legs, especially when lying down at night. It is often accompanied by an uncomfortable paraesthesia in the legs, with sensations such as tingling, burning, itching, cramps, or twitches. RLS can affect up to a third of pregnant women, with symptoms of widely varying severity, generally worse in the third trimester. Most cases that start in pregnancy will clear on delivery. While it does not pose a serious risk to the health of mother or foetus, RLS can cause significant sleep disruption, anxiety, and depressive symptoms.

The pathophysiology is unclear but it is thought to be linked to genetic factors, iron or folate deficiency, hormone levels, central dopaminergic pathways, and stretching of nerves in pregnancy.[23,24] It can be caused or exacerbated by certain pharmaceutical medications, such as beta blockers, antihistamines, antidepressants, and some anti-epileptic drugs.

Moderate regular exercise is important in treatment, for instance walking, swimming, yoga, and stretching. Relaxation exercises can be encouraged at bedtime. Other general measures include the avoidance of alcohol, caffeine, smoking, and eating late in the day. Extra magnesium may be helpful in the diet or as a supplement (200mg daily, taken an hour before bed).

Herbal treatment

See 'Sleep Disorders' for further discussion of herbs to aid sleep.

External treatments

Motherwort (*Leonurus cardiaca*), Cramp Bark (*Viburnum opulus*), Ginger (*Zingiber off.*), Lemon Balm (*Melissa off.*), and Chamomile (*Chamomilla recutita*) can be used as teas to make a hot fomentation and apply on a cloth to the lower legs before bed. Alternatively, take a moderately hot bath, either a full body bath or footbath, containing a strong infusion of Lavender (*Lavandula* spp.), Valerian (*Valeriana off.*), St John's Wort (*Hypericum perforatum*), Skullcap (*Scutellaria lateriflora*) or any of the fomentation herbs. In general, hot baths work best but for some women a cool bath is more effective. Ask the woman what most appeals. Add a handful of Epsom salts for extra potency. Three drops of essential oil of Bergamot (*Citrus bergamia*), Lavender, or Lemon (*Citrus limonum*) can be added to the bath (not in first trimester).

Massaging the legs and/or feet before bed is beneficial. Make a massage oil by selecting between one and three essential oils (not in first trimester) from Ginger, Lemon Balm, Black Pepper (*Piper nigrum*), Ylang-ylang (*Cananga odorata*), Lavender, and Chamomile, and making a 1% dilution in St John's Wort or Comfrey (*Symphytum off.*) oil. The massage oil can be used as it is or made into a liniment by combining 50:50 with tincture of *Leonurus cardiaca* or *Viburnum opulus* (or a mix of both). Use as a foot and leg rub.

Internal medicines

I consider Motherwort to be specific for RLS of pregnancy. Depending on the severity of symptoms, this can be taken as a simple, twenty drops of tincture before bed, or combined with other herbs to assist healthy neuronal activity and support circulatory function. Other effective herbs include Cramp Bark, Wild Yam (*Dioscorea villosa*), and Ginger. Passionflower (*Passiflora incarnata*) is particularly helpful if there is general restlessness and irritability; St John's Wort and Skullcap for nervousness, anxiety or low mood. Lavender and Valerian may also be suitable.

Typical mix for RLS with anxiety, insomnia and exhaustion: Rx *Leonurus cardiaca* 20, *Viburnum opulus* 20, *Hypericum perforatum* 20, *Scutellaria lateriflora* 20, *Avena sativa* 20, *Zingiber off.* 20gtt sig 5ml bd/tds

Rhinitis

Also known as vasomotor rhinitis of pregnancy or gestational rhinitis.

Pregnancy rhinitis is defined as nasal congestion present during the last six or more weeks of pregnancy, without other signs of respiratory tract infection and with no known allergic cause, disappearing completely within two weeks after delivery.

It needs to be differentiated from the common cold, sinusitis, and allergic rhinitis. Pregnancy rhinitis is common in the second and third trimesters, estimated to affect up to 40% of pregnant women to some degree. It is characterised by inflammation and swelling of the nasal mucous membranes, with symptoms that include runny nose, congestion, sneezing, and postnasal drip. Secretions vary from watery to a thick consistency. Pregnancy rhinitis may lead to secondary sinus infection, and due to the increased vascularity of the nasal mucosa, it may also be associated with nosebleeds (see 'Nosebleeds'). The exact aetiology is uncertain but it is presumed to arise from the hormone changes of pregnancy. Smoking and sensitisation to house dust mites are probable risk factors. Women sometimes worry that a blocked up nose will interfere with breathing during labour, but this rarely happens since it appears that the hormones of labour clear the nasal passages.

Measures to bring relief include:

Use a humidifier or vaporiser to add moisture to the air and alleviate congestion. This can be particularly helpful at night to get a restful sleep and awake refreshed. Add up to 3 drops of essential oils (from 16 weeks) of Lavender (*Lavandula* spp.), Lemon (*Citrus limonum*), Neroli (*Citrus aurantium bigarade*), Petitgrain (*Citrus aurantium*), or Bergamot (*Citrus bergamia*) to a vaporiser;

Drink plenty of fluids to stay hydrated;

Elevate the head when lying down;

Avoid inhaling irritants such as tobacco smoke, paint fumes, and anything that causes or exacerbates symptoms;

Take regular moderate exercise, but avoid exercising outside if there is high air pollution;

Use steam to soothe the mucous membranes and relieve symptoms. Take a warm shower and spend time in a steamy bathroom, or do steam inhalations with herb teas, such as Elderflower (*Sambucus nigra*) or Chamomile (*Chamomilla recutita*).

Elderflower or Chamomile as a tea or flower water (hydrosol) is effective as a nasal wash to rinse out the nasal passages, or given as a nasal spray. Elderflower tea can be drunk up to three times daily to cleanse and tone the mucous membranes, and reduce excess mucus. Eyebright (*Euphrasia off.*) is another useful tonic astringent for the nasal and conjunctival mucous membranes, used as a wash or taken as tea. These are symptomatic treatments that will not affect the underlying hormonal cause but may relieve congestion to some degree and help prevent secondary infection. If infected sinusitis is suspected, ingesting raw garlic is an excellent treatment. In the case of co-existing allergy, Elderflower tea may be combined with Nettle (*Urtica dioica*).

Skin disorders

See also 'Pruritus'.

Skin and hair can undergo a variety of changes during pregnancy. Many women experience enhanced hair and nail growth, while hair loss may occur for others. A dark line (the 'linea nigra') can appear going up the belly from the top of the pubic hairline to the navel, nipples may darken, and moles and freckles can become more pronounced. See also 'Stretch Marks'.

Melasma or chloasma (the 'mask of pregnancy') is a common skin discolouration that affects 50–70% of pregnant women. Symmetrical hyperpigmented patches appear on the face (cheeks, upper lip, chin, nose, and forehead can all be affected), believed to be triggered by increased hormone levels that stimulate melanin production. It is more common in women with a darker skin tone and may worsen after sun exposure. The hyperpigmentation usually fades postpartum. Progression can be minimised by wearing sunblock and a wide-brimmed hat when in the sun. It is suggested that chloasma is linked to deficiencies of folic acid and PABA (part of B Complex, found in brewer's yeast, wheatgerm, whole grains, mushrooms, spinach, liver, and other organ meats) and these can be supplemented if needed. A decoction of Daisy (*Bellis perennis*) flowerheads can be used as a lotion to help reduce the darkening.

Dry, itchy skin, brittle nails and poor hair condition may be a sign of insufficient fatty acids in the diet which can be helped by taking a tablespoon of cold-pressed Flax seed oil daily.

Many skin diseases can occur in pregnant women but pregnancy is not a time for radical cleansing. Local applications and attention to diet and lifestyle are often all that are indicated. If internal remedies are given, they need to be gentle, soothing, and supportive.

Hormone levels of pregnancy can trigger or exacerbate acne, especially in the first two trimesters. Raised androgen levels cause increased sebum production which may lead to clogged pores, bacterial infection, and inflammation. A lotion for acne can be made from distilled Witch Hazel (*Hamamelis virginiana*) 170ml, Glycerol 30ml, essential oils of Lemon (*Citrus limonum*) and Lavender (*Lavadula* spp.) aa 5gtt. Shake well before use and apply on cotton wool as required.

A few dermatological conditions are unique to pregnancy. These specific dermatoses of pregnancy comprise a diverse group of pruritic inflammatory skin diseases that occur exclusively during pregnancy and/or immediately postpartum. They include the following conditions; atopic eruption of pregnancy (eczema in pregnancy, prurigo of pregnancy, pruritic folliculitis of pregnancy), polymorphic eruption of pregnancy (PEP; also known as pruritic urticarial papules and plaques of pregnancy [PUPPP]), pemphigoid gestationis, intrahepatic cholestasis of pregnancy.

Of these, the most frequently occurring is atopic eczema/dermatitis, which can worsen or present for the first time during pregnancy. The herbal approach in pregnancy is gentle, following the same basic principles as the treatment of atopic eczema in the general population, a full discussion of which is outside the scope of this book. Any of the herbs and advice listed under 'Pruritis' may be helpful for atopic skin disorders.

PEP is the second most common of the dermatoses of pregnancy, occurring in around one in 160 pregnancies.[25] Itchy, urticarial papules develop, commonly in the same place as abdominal stretch marks, typically with periumbilical sparing. The eruption can spread quickly to the trunk and extremities, but rarely affects the face, palms, or soles of feet. It tends to affect primigravidae in their third trimester, is rarely seen immediately postpartum, and usually resolves completely over an average of four weeks, spontaneously or with delivery. There is no increased maternal or foetal risk. The exact aetiology is unknown but it has associations with multiple pregnancy, in vitro fertilisation, and increased maternal weight gain.

Pemphigoid gestationis (PG, formerly called herpes gestationis) is a rare autoimmune condition causing skin blistering in mid to late pregnancy, or immediately postpartum. The incidence has been variably estimated to be between 1:2000 to 1:60,000 pregnancies.[26]

Intrahepatic cholestasis of pregnancy (ICP or obstetric cholestasis) is considered the most common liver disease unique to pregnancy. Its reported incidence varies widely worldwide, ranging from less than one to over twenty seven percent. Aetiology is unclear although genetic, environmental, and hormonal factors are thought to be involved. It is characterised by itching which may be severe. Patients show abnormal liver function tests (LFTs) and/or raised serum bile acids, both of which resolve after delivery. The condition requires urgent medical attention, being associated with a range of problems for the foetus including premature birth, foetal distress, stillbirth, and postpartum haemorrhage. Itching tends to be worse at night, frequently affecting sleep, and often more noticeable on the palms of the hands and soles of the feet although it can be anywhere. Patients may have dark urine, pale stools, jaundice, fatigue, malaise, nausea, anorexia, and pain in the right upper quadrant. The condition may be linked with gall stones and/or dietary deficiencies. A nourishing vegan diet is recommended, avoiding fatty foods and sugar. Dandelion root (*Taraxacum officinalis* radix.) decoction can be taken to support the liver.

General topical applications for skin conditions of pregnancy (can be employed as creams, ointments, lotions, compresses, poultices):

Marigold (*Calendula* off.) to promote healing, treat/prevent infection, stop bleeding
Chamomile (*Chamomilla recutita*) for an allergic skin response, anti-inflammatory
Chickweed (*Stellaria media*) to cool and relieve itch
Comfrey (*Symphytum officinale*) to soothe, speed healing and reduce inflammation
Rose (*Rosa* spp.) petals to soothe and reduce inflammation
Witch Hazel (*Hamamelis virginiana*) for inflammation and dryness
Oak bark (*Quercus robur/petraea*), decoction or diluted tincture as a compress for weeping skin conditions
Nettle (*Urtica dioica*) tea as a cooling lotion for urticaria, allergic rashes, inflammation

Sleep disorders

See also 'Emotional and Stress-Related Conditions'.

Sleep disturbance is a common problem in pregnancy, especially in the first and third trimesters. This can be due to a variety of causes: difficulty in finding a comfortable position in bed, frequent nocturia, heartburn that worsens lying down, movements of the baby, anxiety, an over-active mind, excitement, or restlessness (see also 'Restless Legs'). It is also common to have vivid dreams especially in the third trimester.

Basic measures include using extra pillows to support the body and having a bucket to pee in by the bed. Breathing, relaxation exercises, and meditation can all be helpful (see Chapter 4), as well as taking regular daily exercise and not eating large amounts of food late at night.

Herbal treatment

Take a relaxing bath before bed, a footbath or preferably whole body bath, adding strong herbal infusions such as Chamomile (*Chamaemelum nobile, Chamomilla recutita*) Lavender (*Lavandula* spp.), Lemon Balm (*Melissa off.*), Limeflowers (*Tilia europaea*) or Rose (*Rosa* spp.) petals. Up to five drops of essential oils can be added to the bath (from 16 weeks), selecting from Lavender, Chamomile (Roman), Bergamot (*Citrus bergamia*), Geranium (*Pelargonium graveolens*), Ylang-ylang (*Cananga odorata*) or Rose otto. Blend 1–3 of the same oils to make a 1% dilution in carrier oil for a relaxing foot or body massage.

A herb pillow can aid restful sleep. This can be made by sewing a piece of muslin, or similar lightweight cotton cloth, to make a small bag about 6 inches square, leaving one side open. Fill with herbs, stitch closed and place inside a cotton pillowcase, between the pillow and the pillowcase. Suitable herbs include Hops (*Humulus lupulus*), especially for hyperactive states; Rose petals, particularly for grief and low self-worth; Lavender flowers for fear, hypersensitivity and those prone to headaches; Limeflowers to calm anxiety and tension (combine with Hawthorn (*Crataegus* spp.) flowers to soothe the heart). Add a pinch of Mugwort (*Artemesia vulgaris*) if excessive dreaming is causing a problem. Mugwort and Vervain (*Verbena off.*) flower essences are also helpful to calm disturbing dreams, taken as drops or made into a room spray for the bedroom. Many room sprays are helpful to create a calming atmosphere and promote restful sleep (see Chapter 16).

Internal treatments for insomnia include: Valerian (*Valeriana off.*), Passionflower (*Passiflora incarnata*), Chamomile, Skullcap (*Scutellaria lateriflora*), Limeflowers, Hops, Rose petals, Lemon Balm, and Lavender. These can be taken singly or combined as teas or tinctures. A cup of tea or 5–10ml of tincture can be taken 30 minutes before bed and if disturbed in the night. Passionflower is helpful for excitability and feelings of panic. Skullcap relieves nightmares and can be combined with Wood Betony (*Betonica off.*) for waking in the night in fear. If heartburn is a problem, take a cup of Slippery Elm (*Ulmus rubra*) before bed.

Stillbirth

See also Chapter 9 'Healing After Loss'.

Stillbirth is typically defined as foetal death at or after 20, 24, or 28 weeks of pregnancy, depending on the source. Diagnosis is usually made by ultrasound and results in a baby being delivered without any signs of life. This is a devastating experience often causing overwhelming feelings of shock, grief, and guilt in the mother. Causes of stillbirth include pregnancy complications, such as pre-eclampsia, birth complications, infections, and general poor health in the mother. In one third of cases the cause is unknown. Risk factors include maternal age over thirty five, smoking, drug use, first pregnancy, and use of assisted reproductive technology.

As well as bereavement support (see next chapter), it is important to ensure there is no physical infection or other post-partum complication. Look out for any offensive vaginal discharge; heavy vaginal bleeding (especially with clots); fever; persistent abdominal pain; pain, redness or swelling in the legs, particularly the calf area; chest pain or dyspnoea. See Chapter 13 Postpartum Care, Endometritis page 249.

Stretch marks

Striae gravidarum (SG or stretch marks) are tears in the dermal collagen that appear during pregnancy as linear purple-red lesions over the abdomen, thighs, breasts, buttocks, upper arms, lower back, and inguinal areas. They tend to lose their pigmentation postpartum, typically remaining as irregular, silvery-white bands. SG are considered the most common connective tissue change in pregnancy, affecting between 50% to 90% of pregnant women. They do not cause any significant medical problems but can lead to itching and discomfort during pregnancy. The aetiology is unclear but they are believed to arise from hormonal changes combined with rapid stretching. A woman's skin type and genetic history play a significant role in their development, with other risk factors including younger maternal age, high pregnancy weight gain, and concomitant use of topical steroids. Teenagers seem to be the group at most risk.

Zinc and vitamin E, as part of a healthy diet and included in a pregnancy supplement, can help their prevention (see page 36). Evening Primrose (*Oenothera biennis*) or Starflower (*Borago off.*) Oil, 1–2g daily, or Flax seed oil, one tablespoon daily, will also help to maintain skin health.

Herbal treatment

Daily massage with a nourishing herbal oil can prevent these entirely. I have seen excellent results with countless women by using a massage oil containing Lady's Mantle (*Alchemilla vulgaris*).

Preventative massage oil: Prepare a hot infused oil of fresh leaves of Lady's Mantle in almond oil (see page 63 for preparation instructions)

Combine infused oil of *Alchemilla vulgaris* 70ml, Wheatgerm oil 20ml, Avocado oil 10ml. This can be used as it is or add essential oils (from 16 weeks) 10–20 drops per 100ml, selecting from Lavender (*Lavandula* spp.), Lemon (*Citrus limonum*), Petitgrain (*Citrus aurantium*), Geranium (*Pelargonium graveolens*), Bergamot (*Citrus bergamia*) or Ylang-ylang (*Cananga odorata*).

Add one capsule vitamin E per 100ml (pierce with a pin and squeeze out contents).

Massage once daily into abdomen, breasts and thighs, preferably after a warm bath or shower. Lady's Mantle is specific and brings the added benefit of toning the breasts, but if unavailable it can be substituted by Marigold (*Calendula off.*) or Comfrey (*Symphytum off.*) infused oil.

If stretch marks have already developed, add vitamin E to cold-pressed Rosehip (*Rosa canina* fructus) oil (1 capsule to 25ml Rosehip oil) and 5 drops of Lavender essential oil (not in first trimester). Massage a small amount into stretch marks every night. Rosehip oil is superb for tissue regeneration.

Threatened Miscarriage see 'Miscarriage'

Urinary tract conditions

Increase in frequency

Urinary frequency is an early symptom of normal pregnancy, caused by hormone changes and increased blood volume leading to congestion around the bladder and increased urine production. This usually settles down in the second trimester as the uterus rises higher in the abdominal cavity and may recur later in pregnancy as the baby drops lower in the pelvis putting pressure on the bladder.

Urinary tract infection

Urinary tract infections (UTIs) are one of the most frequent complications of pregnancy. UTI is often classified as either involving the lower urinary tract (acute cystitis) or the upper urinary tract (acute pyelonephritis). A predisposing factor or precursor to UTI is bacteriuria, which occurs in 2% to 7% of all pregnancies. This is similar to the non-pregnant population but bacteriuria during pregnancy has a greater tendency to progress to ascending infection.

Several factors combine to make pregnant women more prone to UTIs than non-pregnant women. The enlarging uterus can lead to a slowing of the passage of urine and to vesicouteral reflux where urine refluxes back into the ureters. The weight of the uterus along with progesterone relaxing the smooth muscle of the ureters can lead to urinary retention. Further expansion of blood volume and increased load on the kidneys causes increased urine output in the face of decreased efficiency of the ureters. Finally, pregnant women tend to have higher levels of glucose in the urine than non-pregnant women.

If cystitis occurs, increased frequency may be accompanied by dysuria, suprapubic pain or aching, low grade fever, recurrent contractions, and haematuria. Some women with cystitis are symptom free and the condition may be picked up on routine urinalysis. Ideally, laboratory screening for asymptomatic bacteriuria should be performed at 12 to 16 weeks gestation for all women. Acute infection needs immediate attention since it is implicated in the onset of preterm labour and low birthweight babies. Also, a lower urinary tract infection can easily ascend to the kidneys (pyelonephritis) with fever, chills, malaise, loin pain, or costovertebral angle (CVA) tenderness, haematuria, nausea, and vomiting. Pyelonephritis may also develop independently of a

UTI, for example linked with a kidney problem, diabetes, or a weakened immune system. Most kidney infections come from existing bacteria in the vaginal or anal areas that spread upwards through the urinary system. Pyelonephritis usually needs quick treatment with antibiotics to prevent kidney damage and spread to the bloodstream.

General measures for cystitis

General measures include fresh air, exercise, and deep breathing. Acid urine is a common factor in cystitis. Avoid tea, coffee, alcohol, acid-producing foods such as sugars, red meat, refined carbohydrates, and processed foods. In acute conditions avoid fruit juices and instead take vegetable juices and barley water, which is soothing and anti-inflammatory to the urinary tract (recipe below). Drink plenty of water or herb teas. Empty bladder fully, wear loose cotton underwear, avoid wearing tights, no perfumed soaps, use herbal sitz baths or washes. Urinate after sex, wipe from front to back. Do pelvic floor exercises to improve muscle tone. Drinking cranberry powder in water can help by preventing bacteria from sticking to the walls to the urinary tract. Take vitamin C, up to 3g daily in acute infection (reduce if this causes diarrhoea or causes acid urine). Aim for urinary pH of 7 to 7.5. Check for Candida since cystitis may be linked to candidiasis and food allergies. In recurrent cystitis, it can be helpful to keep a food and symptom diary.

Barley water: Put 40g pearl barley in a pan with 200ml cold water, bring to boil and simmer covered for 30 mins, add a slice of lemon in last 10 mins, strain. Drink 3 cups daily.

Herbal treatment

The kidneys and urinary system have to work very hard during pregnancy and the load on the kidneys is greatly increased. Not only that, the urinary system is competing for space with the growing uterus. For me, it is frankly amazing that the body can function so well when organs are packed into such a small space! The entire urinary system needs particular support at this time and it is an area where herbal treatment excels. Herbs are extremely effective at promoting the health of the kidneys and urinary tract, helping to prevent infection, toning tissues, and providing nutrition. As stated in Chapter 2, herbs for kidney support are a relevant inclusion in prescriptions for many different conditions of pregnancy. Where there is a history of chronic urinary tract infection, supportive and prophylactic herbs can be given from the start of pregnancy. As always, assess the whole person, looking at underlying causes and tissue states. For instance, is the immune system under-functioning? Is there a need to address poor diet, exhaustion, anxiety, shock, depression, or chronic constipation?

Treatment for cystitis is ideally given in tea form, with additional tinctures if needed. For acute cystitis, I most commonly give Meadowsweet (*Filipendula ulmaria*) and Cornsilk (*Zea mays*), equal parts as a warm infusion, drunk frequently (1 heaped teasp. per cup, a cup every two hours). Meadowsweet is an astringent urinary antiseptic, alkalinises the urine and is analgesic. Cornsilk is demulcent and tonic for the urinary tract, diuretic, astringent and antiseptic. The two make an excellent combination.

Add Buchu (*Barosma betulina*; no more than 3g dried herb daily) for acute severe infection, along with ingesting raw Garlic (*Allium sativum*; 1 to 3 cloves daily; not 1st trimester) and Echinacea (*Echinacea* spp.) tincture (up to 10ml tds/qds).

Other useful dried herb additions include Couchgrass (*Agropyron repens*) as a soothing, demulcent, diuretic and Nettle (*Urtica dioica*) as a nutritive, astringent, that helps to counter inflammation. Add Plantain (*Plantago lanceolata*), Shepherd's Purse (*Capsella bursa-pastoris*) or White Deadnettle (*Lamium album*) if needed for haematuria, or Yarrow (*Achillea millefolium*) in case of fever (maximum seven days). In all cases, dosage is 1 heaped teasp of a mix of herbs, every two hours in acute infection, tds when symptoms subside. Wild Yam (*Dioscorea villosa*) or Cramp Bark (*Viburnum opulus*) tinctures can be included if there is severe spasm, 20gtt tds. Marshmallow (*Althaea off.*) root, infused for two to three hours in cold water, then heated, can be taken as an additional demulcent tea, one cup as required.

When treating cystitis, you will usually see good improvement within two days and the infection may take up to five days to clear. If symptoms are not responding, the woman should see her doctor.

For long term prophylactic support, give an infusion such as Meadowsweet, Cornsilk, Couchgrass, and Nettle combined, one heaped teaspoon per cup, one or two cups daily throughout pregnancy.

For kidney support, Pellitory-of-the-Wall (*Parietaria judaica*) and Goldenrod (*Solidago virgaurea*) can be recommended as kidney tonics. If kidney pain is present or there is a history of kidney infection, give a supportive prophylactic tea throughout pregnancy, such as a blend of Pellitory, Goldenrod, Meadowsweet, and Cornsilk, dosage as above. Pellitory-of-the-Wall should be avoided in individuals with a tendency to hypersensitivity reactions, since it is reported to have caused rhinitis, hay fever, and rarely asthma-like symptoms in susceptible people.

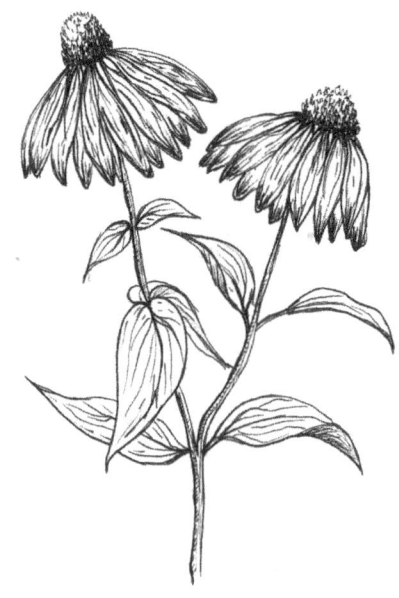

Stress incontinence

Relaxin relaxes muscles and ligaments during pregnancy. This includes the pelvic floor muscles and can cause urinary incontinence, especially from the second trimester onwards. This is the ideal time to start ongoing pelvic floor exercises (see Chapter 4 page 42), which are great preparation for delivery and postpartum recovery.

Vaginitis, Vaginal infections, bacterial vaginosis (BV)

Vaginitis is more frequent during pregnancy due to hormone levels, which change the normal balance of yeast and bacteria in the vagina and can cause the lining of the vagina to become inflamed. The hormone changes make it easier for pathogens, whether bacterial, fungal (see candidiasis), or parasitic (such as trichomonads) to establish themselves in the vagina and cause infection.

Bacterial vaginosis (BV) is a vaginal infection characterised by the presence of large numbers of organisms, such as *Gardnerella vaginalis* and other anaerobic bacteria, and by decreased numbers of the normal population of lactobacilli. BV may be present in between 10–41% of pregnant women.[27] It has been postulated as a cause of preterm birth but this has not been shown conclusively. Symptoms of BV include genital irritation, vaginal discharge (grey, white, watery, or foamy), inflammation of the labia and perineal area, dysuria, dyspareunia, and foul-smelling vaginal odour. Diagnosis is confirmed by vaginal swab.

For any case of vaginitis, employ the usual measures of avoiding soaps and shower gels, tea, coffee, alcohol, and refined sugar. Wear loose, cotton clothing. Take a daily probiotic and supplement vitamin C (at least 1g daily). Avoid intercourse in acute episodes, and bear in mind that partners may need concurrent treatment to avoid reinfection. Use a natural lubricant during intercourse, such as almond oil.

Herbal treatment

Topically, use Marigold (*Calendula off.*) tea as a genital wash, pat dry and apply Marigold or Chamomile (*Chamomilla recutita*) cream to affected areas. Take sitz baths with Marigold and Thyme (*Thymus vulgaris*), adding Lady's Mantle (*Alchemilla vulgaris*) if required to relieve vaginal itching.

Where infection is present, ingest raw garlic, at least a clove a day. Drink Marigold and Thyme tea, one cup, three times daily (1 teasp of each per 200ml cup). Take Echinacea (*Echinacea* spp.) 5ml tds or a tincture mix containing herbs such as Echinacea, Marigold, and Wild Indigo (*Baptisia tinctoria*).

Vaginal Thrush, Vaginal Candida see 'Candidiasis'

Varicose veins, haemorrhoids

Varicose veins are a common complaint of pregnancy, estimated to occur in between 20 to 50% of pregnant women. Varicosities most frequently occur in the legs and feet, the vulvovaginal area (vulvar varicosities), and the anus (haemorrhoids), generally becoming more pronounced as pregnancy advances. They usually regress after delivery and most are gone by six weeks postpartum, although they may recur in subsequent pregnancies.

Varicosities result from a combination of factors including pressure from the uterus on the inferior vena cava which reduces venous return from the legs and pelvis. High progesterone levels of pregnancy cause laxity of the venous system, and combined with the increased blood volume, can result in pooling of blood in the veins. Constipation will exacerbate. Varicosities may become visible as bulging, bluish veins, often tender and sensitive, sometimes aching without being particularly visible. In the legs, symptoms can start with feelings of heaviness or aching, especially at the end of the day, worse after prolonged standing.

Haemorrhoids often start with irritation and itching around the anus, they are exacerbated by straining, and can become prolapsed and protruding. Severe pain and fresh blood loss may ensue, especially on passing a bowel movement. Haemorrhoids frequently appear after delivery, due to the pressure of pushing.

With vulvar varicosities, some women will have visible varicose veins around the vulva, inner thighs and lower pelvis while others have no visible signs yet have a feeling of pressure, aching or pain around the pelvis and/or lower back. There may be vulvar swelling and discomfort, urinary frequency, and dyspareunia. The emotional aspect of vulvar varicosities can be a contributing factor in pre-natal anxiety and depression.

There is a strong inherited tendency to varicosities, but much can be done to prevent or reduce them through management of diet, lifestyle, and appropriate herbs. They do not harm the pregnancy, although they may increase the risk of deep vein thrombosis (DVT), which presents with a red, swollen, hot, or tender calf and needs immediate medical attention.

General measures for varicose veins

General measures include; avoiding standing for long periods or sitting with legs crossed, putting feet up as much as possible, avoiding tight underwear or jeans. Lie on back with legs up the wall for ten to fifteen minutes twice daily, or practice regular yoga (get help for full inverted postures). Sleep on the left side to take the pressure off large veins. Take regular exercise to improve blood flow, such as brisk walking, swimming, pelvic tilts, dancing, especially belly dancing. Use the shower for hydrotherapy to reduce varicosities by alternating hot and cold water directed at the legs, five minutes twice daily.

For vulvar varicosities, keep active and avoid being still for long periods of time, change positions when sitting or lying down. Practice pelvic floor exercises (see page 42) and avoid activities that cause straining, such as lifting, pushing, pulling, sneezing, or coughing (including uncontrollable laughter). When these activities cannot be avoided, use hands or a rolled towel to support the perineum.

Support stockings, compression shorts or leggings can provide gentle pain relief for varicose veins in legs and vulva, although they may be uncomfortable in hot weather. These are best put on before getting out of bed in the morning before gravity takes effect.

For haemorrhoids, avoid straining with bowel movements, and use a small footstool (or two piles of books) to enhance a squatting position and promote ease of passing. A range of squatting toilet stools are available online.[28]

Eat a healthy, wholefood diet, including plenty of green leafy vegetables and foods high in vitamins A, C, E, and B Complex (especially B6). Take foods high in the bioflavonoid rutin to strengthen the venous walls. High levels of rutin are found in buckwheat, unpeeled apples, figs, green tea, and Elderflower (*Sambucus nigra*) tea. Antioxidants in berries such as blueberries, blackberries, raspberries, and bilberries will all improve general blood vessel function. Include parsley and Nettles (*Urtica dioica*) in the diet to help elasticity of veins, and garlic and onion as circulatory tonics.

The above vitamins can also be taken as supplements (vitamin C is widely available together with bioflavonoids including rutin).

Herbal treatments

Local applications

Witch Hazel (*Hamamelis virginiana*) is a prime remedy for the external treatment of varicosities, being an astringent vasoconstrictor that is antiseptic, anti-inflammatory, antioxidant, and anti-haemorrhagic. The hydrosol, decoction and tincture are all effective in lotions, compresses, creams, and ointments. Witch Hazel combines well with Marigold (*Calendula off.*), which is antiseptic, anti-haemorrhagic, and promotes healing.

A simple and effective lotion can be made by combining equal parts of Marigold and Witch Hazel hydrosols, applied neat on cotton wool or as a cold compress, as often as required. Tinctures can be used instead of hydrosols, diluted in water twenty-five to fifty percent (or more in sensitive individuals). Always apply gently. Other herbs for a lotion or compress include Horsechestnut (*Aesculus hippocastanum*), Yarrow (*Achillea millefolium*), and Oak (*Quercus robur/patraea*) bark, tea, or diluted tincture.

Witch Hazel, Marigold, Horsechestnut, and Yarrow all make an effective cream or ointment. Comfrey (*Symphytum off.*) and Plantain (*Plantago lanceolata*) may also be used. Include Arnica if there is pain and itching. Avoid contact with broken skin with Arnica and Horsechestnut. A liniment can be prepared by adding tinctures to infused oil e.g. *Achillea millefolium* Tr 10, *Aesculus hippocastanum* Tr 10, Calendula oil 80. Add the contents of a vitamin E capsule as an antioxidant. Apply morning and night.

For topical applications, always work in the direction of the heart and never massage the varicose veins themselves since this could dislodge a clot and cause an embolism.

Support garments are helpful, apply a cold compress or cream to affected areas, then put on support socks or stockings.

For **vulvar varicosities,** apply an ice pack (or herbal ice cubes wrapped in cloth) or cold compress to relieve discomfort. Witch Hazel and Marigold hydrosols or cream can be applied topically to reduce inflammation and swelling, or saturate a thick sanitary pad with distilled Witch Hazel and wear it at night. Sitz baths, 15–20 minutes daily, can relieve pain and promote rapid shrinkage. Use dried or fresh Comfrey leaves, Plantain and Marigold, adding 10ml distilled Witch Hazel or Oak bark tincture to sitz bath for extra astringency. If varicosities occur inside the vagina, use pessaries of Witch Hazel and Marigold. Similar measures can be used for **haemorrhoids** as for vulvar varicosities. Apply cold compresses or lotion on cotton wool to rectal area to reduce pain and swelling. Marigold, Oak bark, or Witch Hazel are all indicated (hydrosol, strong infusion or decoction, cooled and refrigerated, or dilute tinctures). Add Yarrow or Shepherd's Purse (*Capsella bursa-pastoris*) to staunch bleeding, Dock (*Rumex crispus*) root if itch is severe. For internal haemorrhoids, Marigold and Witch Hazel suppositories.

Pilewort (*Ficaria verna*) cream is specific for haemorrhoids, it soothes inflammation, promotes rapid healing, and relieves itch. Alternatives include Comfrey, Marshmallow (*Althaea off.*), and Marigold.

Apply cream or ointment morning and night, after washing and after each bowel movement.

Internal medicine

If there is a history of varicosities, strengthen the venous system in advance as much as possible. Give venous tonics and decongestants such as a daily tea of Marigold, Yarrow, Limeflowers (*Tilia europaea*), and Hawthorn (*Crataegus monogyna/oxacanthoides*). Alternatively, a strong infusion of Nettle will tone blood vessels and gently stimulate the circulation, infuse 30g Nettles in 500ml boiling water for an hour, three cups daily (can be reheated).

Internal treatments include tinctures of *Urtica dioica, Achillea millefolium, Aesculus hippocastanum, Calendula officinalis, Crataegus monogyna/oxacanthoides, Allium sativum, Tilia europaea,* and *Vaccinium myrtillus*. Add Butternut (*Juglans cinerea*) for haemorrhoids with constipation and portal congestion.

Notes

1. The synonyms 'dilation' and 'dilatation' are frequently used when referring to the stretching out of the cervix in labour. Strictly speaking, 'dilatation' is etymologically more sound but this term is being gradually replaced by 'dilation', most likely driven by changes in the USA.
2. In the UK, *Ephedra sinica* is available for herbal practitioner use only. Ephedra cannot be prescribed in Republic of Ireland.

3. World Health Organization (WHO) Haemoglobin thresholds used to define anaemia www.who.int [last accessed 29/7/21]
4. Kaibara, M., Y. Marumoto, and T. Kobayashi. "Hemodilution and anemia in pregnancy and fetal development." *Nihon Sanka Fujinka Gakkai zasshi* 36, no. 10 (1984): 1893–1900.
5. Khan, Khalid S., Daniel Wojdyla, Lale Say, A. Metin Gülmezoglu, and Paul FA Van Look. "WHO analysis of causes of maternal death: a systematic review." *The lancet* 367, no. 9516 (2006): 1066–1074.
6. La Leche League International: www.llli.org [last accessed 27/7/21]; UK: www.Laleche.org.uk [last accessed 27/7/21]; Ireland: www.Lalecheleagueireland.com [last accessed 27/7/21]
7. A herbal simple describes the use of a single herb on its own.
8. Personal correspondence with Juliet Fishbourne, 2021.
9. Mor, Gil, and Ingrid Cardenas. "The immune system in pregnancy: a unique complexity." *American journal of reproductive immunology* 63, no. 6 (2010): 425–433.
10. Shah, Duru, and Nagadeepti Nagarajan. "Luteal insufficiency in first trimester." *Indian journal of endocrinology and metabolism* 17, no. 1 (2013): 44.
11. The IUCN (International Union for Conservation of Nature's Red List of Threatened Species) is the world's most comprehensive information source on the global extinction risk status of animal, fungus and plant species. This group is currently undertaking a global assessment of plant species. United Plant Savers www.unitedplantsavers.org/species-at-risk-list publish a list of endangered plants and initiate programs designed to preserve them.
12. Alberman, E. "The epidemiology of repeated abortion." In *Early Pregnancy Loss*, pp. 9–17. Springer, London, 1988.
13. Hyde, Kassie J., and Danny J. Schust. "Genetic considerations in recurrent pregnancy loss." *Cold Spring Harbor perspectives in medicine* 5, no. 3 (2015): a023119.
14. Thomas Bartram, Encyclopedia of Herbal Medicine, page 352. Grace Publishers 1995.
15. Hypertension is defined here as a blood pressure ≥140 mmHg systolic or ≥90 mmHg diastolic on two separate readings taken at least four to six hours apart after 20 weeks' gestation in an individual with previously normal blood pressure. In a woman with essential hypertension beginning before 20 weeks' gestational age, the diagnostic criteria are an increase in systolic blood pressure (SBP) of ≥30 mmHg or an increase in diastolic blood pressure (DBP) of ≥15 mmHg.
16. Al-Jameil, N. A brief overview of preeclampsia. *J. Clin. Med. Res.* 6, 1–7 (2013).
17. Davis, Jennifer A., and Gordon G. Gallup Jr. "Preeclampsia and other pregnancy complications as an adaptive response to unfamiliar semen." *Female infidelity and paternal uncertainty* (2006): 191–204.
18. Mustafa, Reem, Sana Ahmed, Anu Gupta, and Rocco C. Venuto. "A comprehensive review of hypertension in pregnancy." *Journal of pregnancy* 2012 (2012).
19. Carter, James P., Tami Furman, and H. Robert Hutcheson. "Preeclampsia and reproductive performance in a community of vegans." *Southern Medical Journal* 80, no. 6 (1987): 692–697.
20. Brewer, T. H. "Metabolic Toxemia of Late Pregnancy in a County Prenatal Nutrition Education Project: A Preliminary Report." *The Journal of reproductive medicine* 13, no. 5 (1974): 175–176.

21. https://www.who.int/news-room/fact-sheets/detail/preterm-birth Last accessed 25/1/22; https://www.tommys.org/pregnancy-information/premature-birth/premature-birth-statistics last accessed 25/1/22
22. The dermatoses of pregnancy are a diverse group of pruritic inflammatory dermatoses that occur exclusively during pregnancy and/or immediately postpartum. They include the following conditions: pemphigoid gestationis, polymorphic eruption of pregnancy (pruritic urticarial papules and plaques of pregnancy [PUPPP]), atopic eruption of pregnancy (eczema in pregnancy, prurigo of pregnancy, pruritic folliculitis of pregnancy), Intrahepatic cholestasis of pregnancy.
23. Trenkwalder, Claudia, Birgit Högl, and Juliane Winkelmann. "Recent advances in the diagnosis, genetics and treatment of restless legs syndrome." *Journal of neurology* 256, no. 4 (2009): 539–553.
24. Allen, Richard P. "Restless leg syndrome/Willis-Ekbom disease pathophysiology." *Sleep medicine clinics* 10, no. 3 (2015): 207–214.
25. Vaughan Jones SA, Black MM. Pregnancy dermatoses. *J Am Acad Dermatol.* 1999; 40:233–41.
26. Fong M, Gandhi GR, Gharbi A, et al. Pemphigoid Gestationis. [Updated 2021 Jul 21]. In: StatPearls [Internet]. Treasure Island (FL): StatPearls Publishing; 2022 Jan-. Available from: https://www.ncbi.nlm.nih.gov/books/NBK470287/
27. McGregor JA, French JI. Bacterial vaginosis in pregnancy. Obstet Gynecol Surv. 2000 May;55(5 Suppl 1):S1–19. doi: 10.1097/00006254-200005001-00001. PMID: 10804540.
28. Often known as the 'SquattyPotty'. Watch a light-hearted online video at https://www.youtube.com/watch?v=YbYWhdLO43Q [last accessed 27/7/21]

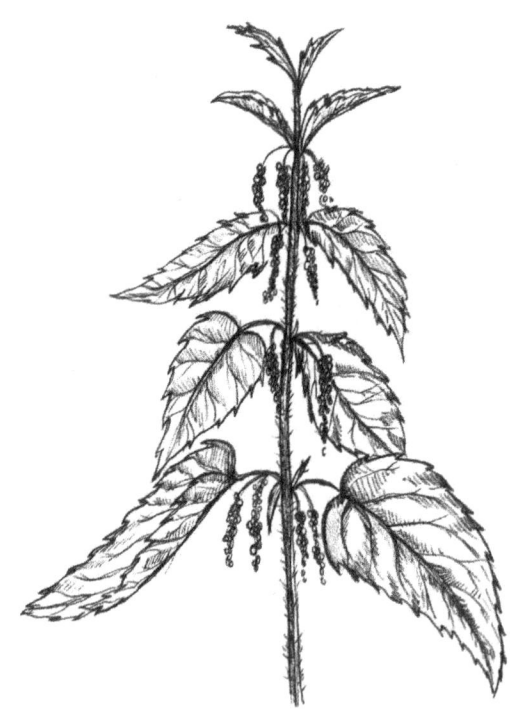

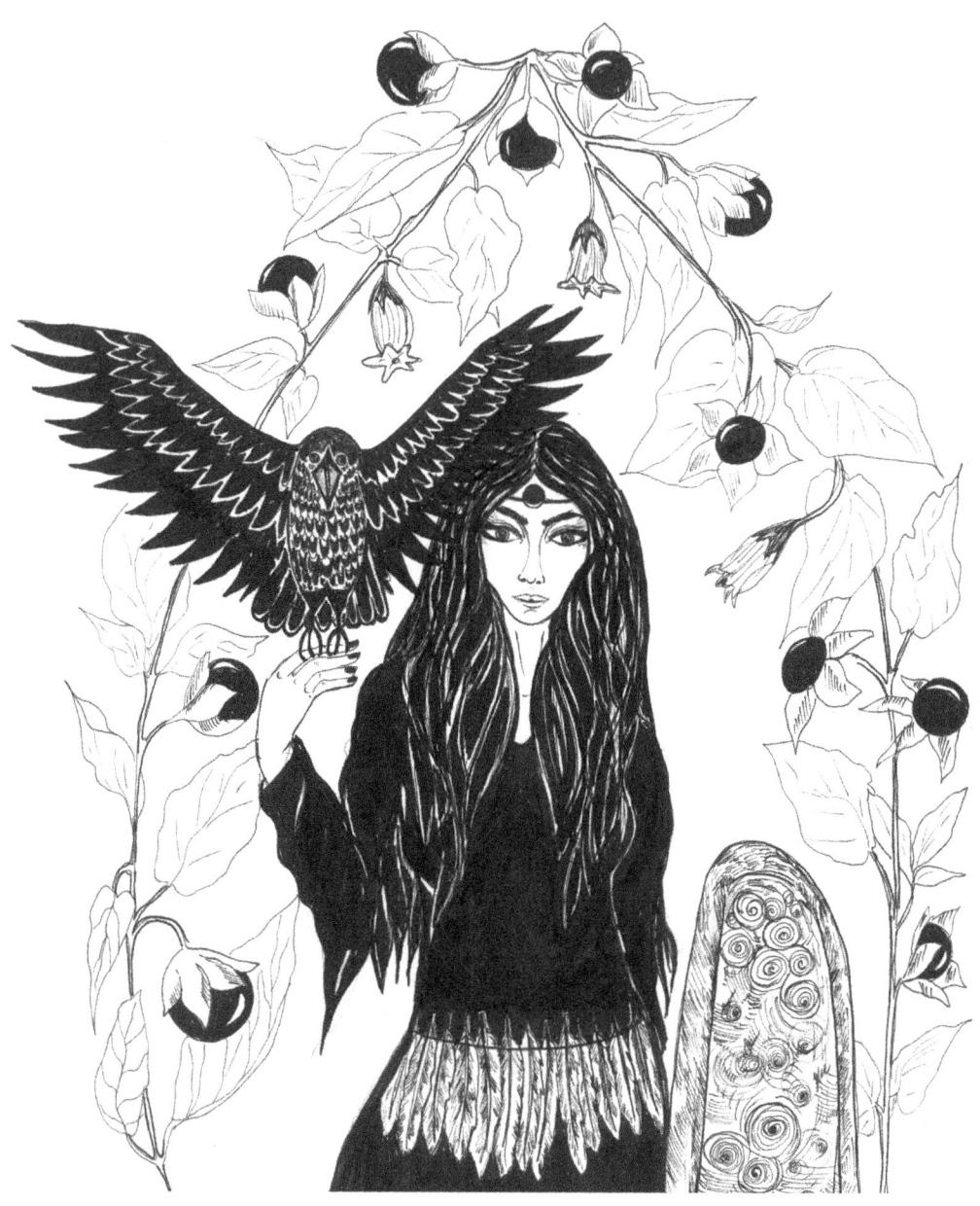

Morrigan. Goddess of birth, death, and sovereignty. Guardian of the dead. Transporter between life and death.
Deadly Nightshade (*Belladonna off*). Beautiful lady and guide in the underworld.

CHAPTER 9

Healing after loss

Many women experience devastating loss in pregnancy. Loss may stem from miscarriage, ectopic pregnancy, termination, or stillbirth. The previous chapter focused on physical recovery after the loss of a pregnancy. Here we look at mental and emotional recovery.

The pain of an early miscarriage or ectopic pregnancy is often underestimated but frequently causes severe mental suffering and anguish for the woman and her partner.

The loss of a pregnancy at any stage can lead to a host of difficult feelings including shock, grief, anxiety, fear, anger, confusion, guilt, shame, and blame. A woman may feel numb with a sense of unreality. If it is a first child, she may experience the loss of her self-concept as a mother and all expectations of self and family. Many women experience symptoms of post-traumatic stress disorder (PTSD) after a pregnancy loss, including flashbacks to the experience, nightmares, and the avoidance of places that remind them of the traumatic event. Recurrent loss can be particularly difficult, with each new pregnancy bringing both hope and anxiety, and each new loss feeling harder to bear, especially as women may feel that time is running out.

A termination can be equally devastating and the ensuing grief is often not validated by society or even the woman herself. Some women feel nothing but relief afterwards but many others are beset by feelings of sadness, guilt, and regret. In the case of an unplanned or unwanted pregnancy, women are often in crisis beforehand, feeling overwhelmed by emotions, and needing to make a life-changing decision in a short space of time. Many women report fears around sharing their feelings, fearing that others will judge them. Women commonly feel that they do not have the same right to grieve the loss because it was their choice or because of the judgement and stigma around termination. A termination carried out for medical reasons can be particularly traumatic, often leading to severe and complicated grieving, including pathological anxiety and depression.

When a baby is delivered after 24 weeks or more of pregnancy and is not alive, this is known as a stillbirth and it is one of the most devastating experiences that can happen. Many parents react with disbelief and it is common for them to think they hear their baby crying. It helps if parents can spend as much time as they need with their baby, holding the baby if they wish. Everyone needs time to grieve in their own way. If there are other children, letting them see the baby may help with the grieving process. Many parents like to choose a name for their baby and it can help to take photos or preserve the baby's memory in other ways such as by keeping a lock of hair. Most hospitals provide bereavement support and counselling, and many have midwives who specialise in supporting bereaved parents, helping them to make informed choices. The hospital may offer remembrance services for babies who die in pregnancy or soon after birth, or parents may like to organise their own funeral or alternative ceremony. Parents are usually offered tests to try and discover the cause of death, which can help with the grieving process and may give useful information for future pregnancies. In about one third of cases, cause of death is unknown.

Having a baby adopted is another major source of grief, sometimes unacknowledged until years after the event. Here in Ireland in past times, countless young women were forced to give up their babies for adoption leaving a legacy of sadness.

Grief affects everyone differently and takes its own time, often a slow and painful process that goes through various stages until the experience of loss is integrated into the pattern of a person's life.[1] If grief is not honoured it prevents full recovery and can impact future pregnancies. As herbalists, we can offer a listening ear and/or recommend other counselling support, a safe space where a woman can share her feelings, process emotions, and think through decisions. Herbs, vibrational essences, and sacred ritual or ceremony can be hugely supportive at times of loss, assisting the release of emotional trauma and facilitating healing.

Herbal Support for Grief and Loss

See also 'Emotional and Stress-Related Conditions' Chapter 8 page 120, and Chapter 13 page 248.

Rose (*Rosa* spp.) is my favourite plant for easing grief. It is calming and uplifting and has a special role in soothing the heart and helping people to overcome loss. Rose is the great comforter, gently lifting the spirits and restoring self-love and self-worth. Drink an infusion of Rose petals three times daily or take Rose tincture, 20gtt as often as required. Rose works well as a simple or combines beautifully with other herbs. The scent of Rose is a strong part of her healing gift, and Rose petals or essential oil make a lovely addition to baths, massage oils, or inhalations.

Other herbs for grief include:

Hawthorn (*Crataegus monognya/oxathoides*) blossoms as long-term support and strengthening for the heart.

Lady's Mantle (*Alchemilla vulgaris*) to soothe emotional heart pain and aid letting go and acceptance.

Lemon Balm (*Melissa off.*) for extreme low mood and tearfulness. Good as a simple, 20 drops of tincture as required.

Limeflowers (*Tilia europaea*) for anxiety and tension. A protective, comforting guide through grief.

Motherwort (*Leonorus cardiaca*) for emotional heart pain, palpitations, and tension. Feelings of emptiness.

Sage (*Sage off.*) to ease grief and release anger, blame, and shame. Restores emotional balance.

Skullcap (*Scutellaria lateriflora*) and Dandelion (*Taraxicum off.*) root are both helpful if there is a lot of anger.

Tulsi (*Ocinum tenuiflorum/sanctum*) for lifting mood and clearing the mind. Moves stagnant energy in the heart.

Wild Pansy (*Viola tricolor*) for soothing and healing the heart, especially good in infusion.

Willow (*Salix alba*) bark for comfort in bereavement.

Any of these can be taken, singly or combined, as **teas or tinctures**.
Dosage:
>Teas: one cup three times daily.
>Tinctures: up to 5ml tds

Baths: Select any of the herbs above. Combine for foot bath or full body bath.

Limeflower baths are traditional for grief, said to open gateways and help with feeling the presence of other dimensions. Combine Rose petals, Limeflowers, and Borage (*Borago off.*) flowers for a comforting and restorative bath to ease grief and lift the spirits.

An alternative option is Rose petals with Oatstraw (*Avena sativa*) to soothe the heart and strengthen the nervous system.

Heart Oil: Rose essential oil heals and unburdens the wounded heart, making a beautiful oil for emotional heart pain (which often manifests as physical pain in the heart area). Combine Rose essential oil 1% dilution in Almond oil. Apply a few drops over the heart area three times daily or as often as required to ease pain.

Other essential oils for grief include Violet leaf, (*Viola odorata*) Hyssop (*Hyssopus off.*), and Cypress (*Cupressus sempervirens*). For healing soul wounds, use Spikenard (*Nardostachys jatamansi*), which helps anxiety, or Yarrow (*Achillea millefolium*) which gives protection and is indicated for highly sensitive people. Geranium (*Pelargonium graveolens*) is uplifting and balancing, Lavender (*Lavandula spp.*) is calming and soothing. Sacred Basil (Tulsi) is helpful for reconnecting with Divine Life Force.

Massage Oil: It is usually best to invite the woman to choose the oils she is drawn to. One essential oil may be all that is required although you could blend up to three. Make a 1% dilution in Almond oil. Apply morning and night.

Vibrational essences See Chapter 16 'Vibrational Essences' for a full description.

I find essences an invaluable support for grief and loss. They can be made into room sprays or a few drops added to water, tea, or other herbal medicine for internal use.

A 'Rescue' spray is a general-purpose standby for any situation of shock and trauma, easy to spray into the environment without being intrusive. Borage, Motherwort, and Pink Heart Crystal are all indicated for grief, bringing comfort to the wounded heart. Valerian (*Valeriana off.*) eases emotional distress, and White Buffalo is particularly indicated for children affected by loss. Airmid restores hope, Oak (*Quercus robur/petraea*) assists recovery from exhaustion and despair. Lapis relieves anger and rage, Banishing Guilt helps eliminate feelings of guilt, and Elecampane relieves shame. Forgiveness clears blame, whether of oneself or others. Marshmarigold assists with letting go, Angelica and St John's Wort help with feeling safe and protected. Plantain helps ancestral or generational grief, Sacred Waters aids acceptance, and Lousewort helps with the expression of difficult feelings. Forget-me-not brings understanding of our spiritual connections with others.

Ritual and ceremony for bereaved parents

Funerals and remembrance services

As mentioned above, some hospitals offer remembrance services for babies who have died very young, or parents may choose to organize their own type of ceremony. For parents who choose to have a funeral, they may like to place something in the coffin with their baby. If there are other children, they may like to draw a picture to put in the coffin.

This is a time when plants have much to offer. Flowers can be uplifting at a funeral and certain plants are traditionally associated with helping with death. These can easily be incorporated into ceremony or planted in remembrance. Plants can be placed in the coffin and used to decorate the grave. In the West of Ireland there is a beautiful tradition of lining the grave with moss and appropriate plants prior to the burial. A herbal infusion or tincture can be made into a wash that is sprinkled on the earth or incorporated into a room spray together with essences. Equally, herbs can be burnt as incense, used decoratively or made into a posy or amulet (a small bag or bundle that can be placed in a coffin, buried in the earth, or carried by the bereaved).

Elder, Rosemary, and Yew are three prime plants to help with death:

Elder (*Sambucus nigra*), known as the 'Elder Mother', brings protection and is intimately connected with burial rituals. Elder is often planted in graveyards along with evergreens, which signify eternal life.

Rosemary (*Rosemarinus off.*), "for remembrance", is a rites of passage herb, carried in the hand during funerals and placed inside the coffin. Purifies and helps the dead to pass and helps the living to remember the dead. At funerals or memorials, it can be thrown onto the fire, burned as incense or drunk as a ceremonial drink while mourners recall memories of the dead. It can also be planted on graves.

Yew (*Taxus baccata*) is a symbol of death and regeneration, commonly planted in graveyards to protect the spirits of the dead. As an evergreen, it represents eternal life. Yew renews spiritual strength and helps us to see and understand the past (not to be taken internally).

Below is a selection of other helpful plants (these are not intended as internal medicines, as some are poisonous):

Blackberry's (*Rubus fructicosus*) five-petalled flowers are associated with the Goddess. The fruit that turns from green to red to black is seen to represent the three stages of the Goddess (maiden, mother, crone) and the completion of a cycle.

Cedar (*Cedrus spp.*) is a funeral herb, representing the continuation of the soul and the passage of spirit from this life to the next.

Forget-me-not (*Myosotis scorpioides*) helps the living to remember the dead and to understand their karmic connections with those who have passed.

Hawthorn (*Crataegus monogyna/oxacanthoides*) is associated with helping the dead to pass, and offers a doorway to the otherworld.

Hyacinth (*Hyacinthoides non-scripta*) is planted on graves as a token of grief.

Iris (*Iris spp.*) flowers are used at funerals to signify hope for the departed spirit.

Juniper (*Juniperus spp.*) to bless the dead.

Linden (*Tilia spp.*) helps the bereaved to feel the presence of other dimensions. Makes a good bath to comfort the grieving.

Lotus (*Nelumbo nucifera*) to encourage the dead to seek their highest possible incarnation.

Marjoram (*Oreganum majorana, Thymus mastichina*) to bring joy to the deceased and comfort to the bereaved.

Mugwort (*Artemisia vulg.*) is a herb of transitions, it clears energetic blocks, helps with letting go of the old and making way for change.

Myrrh (*Commiphora molmol*), widely used at funeral rites, burnt as an incense to raise vibrations and increase spiritual awareness.

Nettle (*Urtica dioica*), connected to the energies of life, death, and rebirth, helps us to see that our most difficult experiences are those that offer us the most growth. Used at funerals.

Oak (*Quercus spp.*) helps the dead to pass over. Boat burials were traditionally performed by casting the body to sea in a vessel (often made of Oak), or by placing a boat in the tomb.

Parsley (*Petroselinum spp.*) is sacred to Persephone, a herb of the Underworld, dedicated to the Death Goddess. Included in funeral wreaths and used to decorate graves to honour death.

Pasque Flower (*Anemone pulsatilla*) is planted on graves to ease grief. Said to have grown from the tears Venus shed for the dead Adonis.

Periwinkle's (*Vinca minor*) blue flowers and their five petals associate Periwinkle with the Goddess. It connects with the Mother and reminds us that we are all connected as children of the earth. The flowers are used in ceremonies after the death of a child, bringing gentleness, love, and spiritual connection.

Pine (*Pinus spp.*), an evergreen whose boughs are placed on graves to remind the living of everlasting life. Alternatively, the coffin is adorned with Pine branches and Pine-resin incense or essential oil are burned to bring harmony and healing to the bereaved.

Rowan (*Sorbus aucuparia*) honours death and brings protection for the living.

Rue (*Ruta graveolens*) brings protection and repels negativity. Strongly purifying.

Tansy (*Tanacetum vulg.*) branches are used to sprinkle sacred waters over a grave or ceremonial space.

Thyme (*Thymus spp.*) is used for purification and protection.

Violet (*Viola odorata*) is sacred to the Goddess of Love. It is associated with twilight and facilitating our passage to the next world. Used to decorate the graves and corpses of children.

Willow (*Salix spp.*) is seen as a guardian tree in graveyards, helpful to bless the dead and protect them from evil influences.

Burial ceremony for when there is no physical body

This ceremony uses a small "medicine bundle" to represent the lost baby, and can be especially helpful after a miscarriage, termination, or other loss where a funeral has not been possible. In advance of the burial, you will need to locate a suitable spot in nature for burying your bundle. This could be a spot in your garden, if you have one, or some wild place in nature.

Method:
Obtain a piece of cloth, large enough to make a pouch or bag. This can be any fabric you choose, felt can be a good option, being easy to cut and sew. Alternatively, you could cut a piece of cloth from a suitable garment that was intended for your baby. This bag, known as a "medicine bundle", will represent your departed child. It can be large or small. Many women find a bundle around 5–10 cm by 5–10 cm is suitable, but this is entirely your choice. Choose a colour that has meaning for you. Fold the cloth and sew up two sides, making a bag with an opening at the top. Do this mindfully, connecting to the memory of the one you have lost, and allowing yourself to feel your grief or whatever feelings arise.

Now choose items to fill the bundle. You might like to include items of baby clothing (or cut a small piece) if you have them, or any other reminders of your baby that feel appropriate. If you have no physical reminder, find a seed, flower, small stone, or piece of rose quartz, asking to be guided to one that is willing to stand for your lost baby. This can then be placed in the bundle to represent your child. You can also include plant material such a Rosemary or Hawthorn to help your loved one on their journey. Speak to the herbs as you add them, asking them to bring their blessings to the one who has departed. The filling of the bundle may be quick or it may take some time. Allow yourself all the time you need.

Once the bag is filled, sew up the top. Hold the bag in your hands, expressing your love and gratitude to this soul who came into your life for such a short while. Wrap the bundle in another piece of cloth and take it outside to your burial spot.

Prepare a hole in which to bury the bundle, placing a sprig of Rosemary in the bottom of the hole. Unwrap your medicine bundle and hold it in your hands, calling for blessings for the departed soul. Express your love and good wishes and anything else you would like to say, feeling the bundle infused with loving energy. Gently place the bundle in the hole, sprinkle on some rose petals to signify your unending love, say goodbye and fill in the hole with earth. Depending on practicalities and your own preference, you can either sprinkle the grave with more rose petals or plant something appropriate. If you so choose, another person or persons may be invited to participate in the burial.

Sacred rose bath to heal the wounded heart

This sacred bathing ceremony can be done at any stage to ease grief and bring healing to the heart.

Items needed:
One or two handfuls of red Rose petals (enough for a bath, plus two additional fresh petals if you have them), candle(s), bath or footbath, face cloth, room spray of appropriate essence (such as Pink Heart crystal) in a base of Rosewater, Rose massage oil.

Method:
This is best done at night before bed. Prepare the space by spraying the room spray. Prepare the bath or footbath, either adding the Rose petals directly to the water (can be lovely to be surrounded by floating petals), or if preferred, placing them in a muslin bag under the hot tap. Light the candle(s) and lie in the bath, feeling the energy of Rose infusing your body. Inhale the scent and imagine you are a sponge soaking up Rose into your cells. Rose is bringing love and comfort to every cell in your body. Feel your body relaxing as Rose dissolves tension and knots of pain. If you are in a full bath, soak the facecloth in the Rose filled water, and place it over your heart. Inhale, and as you do, visualize the energy of Rose entering, soothing, and healing your wounded heart. If you are in a footbath, visualize drawing the Rose energy up through the soles of your feet and feel it entering your heart to soothe and heal. Place the two additional Rose petals on your eyelids, a traditional way to soothe your tears. Speak to Rose, saying "gentle and sacred Rose, soothe my tears and heal my heart". Stay here, fully receiving the Rose energy, for twenty minutes or until the bath starts to get cold.

Dry yourself and massage your body (or feet, in the case of a footbath) with the Rose massage oil, knowing that you are sealing the loving energies of Rose into your body. Blow out the candle.

Herbal bath ceremony for letting go and healing the soul

The following is a sacred bathing ceremony for healing the soul after loss. This is ideal as a full body bath although a footbath will also work. You can either use the words suggested or your own words. Feel the words coming from your whole being: body, mind, and spirit.

Items needed:

Sacred Space room spray or smudge, candle, three healing herbs (see below), 5ml Mugwort (*Artemisia vulgaris*) infused oil (St John's Wort oil (*Hypericum perforatum*) can be substituted).

Prepare the space by using a room spray such as 'Sacred Space' to purify, protect, and bring blessings. Alternatively, burn smudge,[2] such as Sage (*Salvia off.*) or Mugwort if you are familiar with this method. Light your candle. Run the bath, adding:

Lady's Mantle (*Leonurus cardiaca*) or Raspberry leaf (*Rubus idaeus*) for healing the womb

Rose (*Rosa* spp.), Borage (*Borago off.*), or Hawthorn (*Crataegus monogna/oxacanthoides*) for healing the heart

Valerian (*Valeriana off.*), Skullcap (*Scutellaria lateriflora*), or Lemon Balm (*Melissa off.*) for healing the mind.

The herbs can be in the form of tinctures, dried or fresh herbs, all in separate bottles or bags. Use a handful of each fresh herb, a dessert spoon of dried or 20ml of tincture.

Call to each of the three herbs as you add it to the bath, asking for healing for your womb, heart, and mind, respectively, for example "beautiful and sacred Raspberry leaf, come into these waters and bring healing for my womb" and so on. After addressing all three herbs, say "sacred plants, help me in my grief".

Step into the bath, lie back and soak, imagining your body like a sponge, soaking up the potent healing waters and plant energies.

As you soak, put your hands over your womb area, saying "I open my womb to receive the healing blessings of [*name of womb herb*]". Feel the blessings entering your womb and be aware of healing taking place. Speak to your womb, speak of the one you have lost, honour your womb's journey. Allow yourself to feel whatever feelings arise, without judgment. Stay with this process as long as it takes.

When this feels complete, move your hands to your heart area, saying "I open my heart to receive the blessings of [*name of heart herb*]". Speak to your heart, honouring its grief and encouraging it to open. Feel the plant blessings entering your heart and be aware of healing taking place. Let yourself feel your feelings as fully as possible Again, take as long as you like.

Now, move your hands to your head, saying "I open my mind to receive the blessings of [*name of mind herb*]". Speak to your mind, honouring its struggles and reassuring it that all is well. Feel the blessings of peace entering your mind and be aware of the healing plant energies cleansing, calming and healing your mind. Allow yourself to feel whatever arises and take as long as needed.

Lie quietly, soaking in the waters, aware of the healing and renewal that is happening. When you feel finished (not before twenty minutes), or when the bath is getting cold, get out of the bath and dry yourself. Apply the Mugwort oil to your navel,[3] saying "I call to the cleansing powers of Mugwort. I let go all unhealthy attachments. I embrace a new beginning".

When you are finished, give thanks to the spirits of the plants for their assistance and blow out the candle. Go forward in life, knowing that this is a new beginning.

Saying goodbye to a loved one who has passed

Below are two different ways of saying goodbye to a loved one that can assist with letting go of a loved one. These can be tailored to individual requirements and preferences.

A. Write a letter to the departed soul, expressing how you feel and anything else you would like to say. Allow yourself to express all the feelings and all the words you were not able to share for whatever reason. Allow your tears to fall. The words may come quickly or this may be a process that takes several days. Take all the time you need. Have a special place to keep the letter while it is in process. When you feel it is completed, ritually burn it on a fire (in a safe place), offering it to the flames with your love and saying goodbye to your beloved.

B. Another way to say goodbye is to choose a cushion to represent your departed child. Sit with the cushion in front of you, reminding yourself that love never dies and is unending. Take the cushion in your arms and hold it to your heart. Talk to your child and express all the feelings and all the words you would like to share. Allow your tears to fall. Take all the time you need. When you feel complete, say goodbye to your beloved. Afterwards, burn some dried Sage (*Salvia spp.*) or Mugwort (*Artemisia vulgaris*) and "de-role" the cushion by holding it in the smoke to cleanse it, saying "this is just a cushion". Alternatively, you could use a cleansing essence spray to de-role the cushion in the mist of the spray.

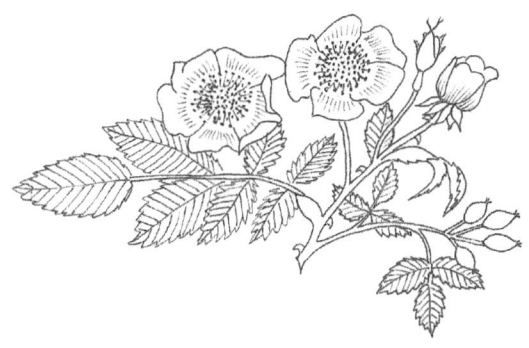

Spiritual perspectives on pregnancy loss

Some grieving parents find immense comfort in having an opportunity to talk about their loss from a spiritual perspective. For many parents this would be an entirely inappropriate conversation, but for others it can help them find meaning in their experience, and assist them in coming to terms with their grief and loss, even if long after the event. This is a delicate area where practitioner sensitivity, care, and compassion are critical.

In many cultures around the world, it is widely believed that the incoming soul chooses his or her parents in advance. Many believe that the soul chooses parents with whom it can best fulfil its spiritual goals, and who will provide life experiences in line with their own learning and karmic agenda. Ancient agreements are believed to be made between child and parents, for reasons that are usually forgotten during life, and events experienced at conception and birth are chosen in advance as part of this agenda. Children discover their own moment to arrive (coinciding with their personal astrological picture), and all is in perfect timing and divine order.

When a stillbirth occurs, although this can seem the most cruel of lessons, it can nonetheless be a learning experience that the parents may have signed up for, perhaps to learn the pain and grief of producing a dead baby, although there could be a host of different reasons. Similarly, with miscarriage and termination, there may be a pre-birth agreement, and it is believed that some souls make a contract to come for a very short time. Sometimes, when a woman is planning a termination, it can be helpful for her to dialogue in advance with her unborn child. By explaining her situation to the incoming soul, it can greatly ease the process. Also, it is possible that a soul returns to the same parent or parents at a later date. In the case of disability, some babies may abort during pregnancy, while others may be born with their disability because that is what offers the perfect learning experience for parents and child.

Sometimes one soul appears to enter in order to help another soul incarnate, for instance, in the case of twins, where one baby may be stillborn or die soon after birth. It may be that these souls have come with a joint purpose and the soul who leaves has completed its mission. The surviving twin may have feelings of loss or insecurity that are part of its learning journey in this lifetime.

Pre-birth experiences may be encountered in therapy, such as in hypnotherapy[4] and shamanic healing, and young children often recall previous lives.[5]

Practitioner self care

It is important to remember that working with loss can be intense and challenging work for practitioners, particularly if the practitioner is closely involved with a woman's pregnancy and an unexpected complication occurs. Witnessing another's grief may feel nearly unbearable and to be present at the death of a baby can be completely devastating for everyone involved. We are all human and grief is normal. As well as helping the bereaved, it is important to recognize our own grief, to know our own limitations, and be mindful of self-care. Counselling and peer supervision are frequently of benefit, if not essential.

Always call back all parts of yourself if you experience trauma as part of your work. Disassociation is one of our natural responses to an overwhelming experience, and from a shamanic perspective, at the time of a trauma, part of a person's soul may spontaneously leave the body as a survival strategy in order not to be totally devastated by the shock of the experience. This is known as "soul loss" and if not dealt with promptly, can cause problems later on. A full discussion of soul loss is outside the scope of this book, but even being aware that it is a possible consequence can be protective.[6] A rescue essence, such as Bach's Rescue Remedy or the Derrynagittah Rescue, is good to have on hand, and consciously using a vibrational essence spray, such as Rosemary, Tulsi, or Bugarach, can be a simple way to help gather oneself after experiencing trauma, useful for both practitioner and client. See Chapter 16 for more information on vibrational essences. Seek help if you are finding it difficult to recover after a traumatic event.

Below are some common-sense self-care points that all practitioners will be aware of, but sometimes may need reminding:

Drinking enough water, sufficient sleep, rest and relaxation, healthy nutrition, adequate exercise, plenty of play and laughter, loving personal relationships, walks in nature, or whatever works for you to give you a daily dose of sensual beauty.

Do you have a support network? Do you have regular self-care practices? These might include journaling, meditation, yoga, massage, or cleansing practices, such as washing hands, baths, or visualising standing under a shower or waterfall, all useful after working deeply with a patient. What helps you stay grounded? Regularly assess your own physical, emotional, mental, and spiritual state and find your own way to fulfil your personal needs. Make this a priority. Herbs and essences can help!

Notes

1. Classic stages of grieving include denial, bargaining, anger, depression, acceptance, and surrender (to a more expanded experience of life with grieving done). These do not necessarily proceed in a straight line. For a more detailed description, see *On Death and Dying* (New York: Scribner Book Co, 2014) and other books by Elizabeth Kübler Ross.
2. "Smudge" refers to herbs that are burnt to produce sacred smoke for cleansing and other purposes. This could be a bunch of herbs tied together in the form of a "smudge stick" or simple loose dried herbs in a heatproof bowl.
3. This ceremony incorporates an oil that is applied to the navel. As a student herbalist in the UK, a neighbour who was raised in Ghana taught me that many plant medicines are applied to the navel in that country. She told me that this area of the body is considered highly significant due to its early connection with the mother. I found this fascinating, and as it made a lot of sense to me, I began exploring this in my work with women. Some years later, when apprenticing with a Native American Medicine Woman, I learned that the navel is an important energy centre in the body and a place where many energetic "cords" are located. It is an area where we frequently hold energetic attachments to

186 THE HERBALIST'S GUIDE TO PREGNANCY, CHILDBIRTH AND BEYOND

others, often in an unhealthy way. Cleansing this area and releasing cords is a valuable aid to letting go.
4. See Robert Schwartz, *Your Soul's Gift, The Healing power of the Life you Planned before you were born* (London: Watkins, 2012).
5. See Wayne W. Dyer and Dee Garnes, *Memories of Heaven* (London: Hay House, 2015), which documents the words of young children from around the world who have spoken of pre-birth memories.
6. See Sandra Ingerman, *Soul Retrieval: Mending the fragmented self* (San Francisco: Harper Collins, 1991).

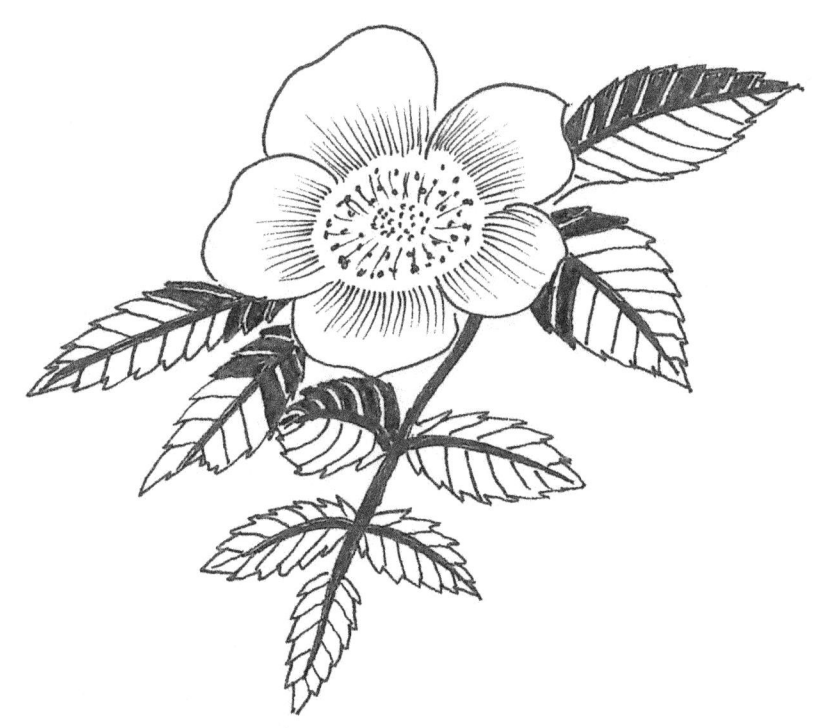

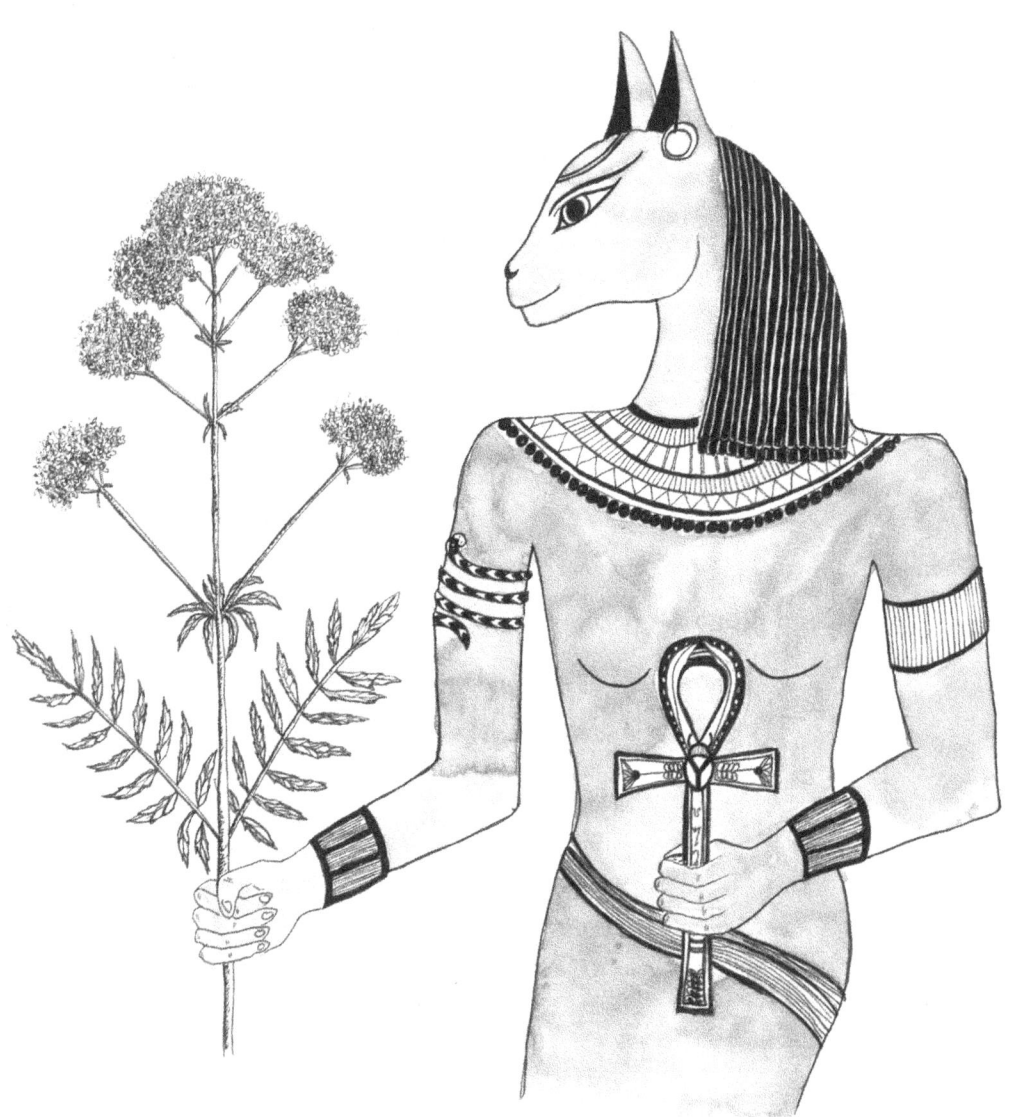

Bast. Joyful, playful cat Goddess. Protector of women in childbirth. Giver of life and abundance.
Valerian (*Valeriana off.*). Reliever of pain and anxiety, carrier of sensuality and relaxation.

CHAPTER 10

Preparation for labour and birth: week 36 onwards

The topics in this chapter are most applicable from week 36 onwards, although some issues, such as dealing with old trauma and fears, are usefully addressed much earlier in a woman's pregnancy.

Birthing options

Preparation for labour and birth involves making choices. For an expectant mother, these help bring clarity and peace of mind. Questions such as: Where do you want to give birth? Who do you want to be present at the birth? Do you want to use a birthing pool or stool? Do you want access to pain relief? If so, what kind? How do you feel about being induced? Do you want the birth to be filmed or photographed? Do you want your baby to be placed on the breast as soon as possible after giving birth? Who would you like to cut the baby's cord? Do you want to keep the placenta? Do you want a birthing partner to offer massage? What kind of herbal support would you like? (For herbal options for labour, see 'Birthing Pack' later in this chapter)

These answers can be used to formulate a birth plan or document that informs midwives, birth partners, and health care workers of a woman's preferences for labour and birth. For women planning a home birth, as well as a home birth check list, it is useful to have an alternative plan just in case they need to go to hospital.

Women's choices often change over the course of their pregnancy and it is helpful if they do not have rigid expectations of how a birth *should* be. Labour and birth are unpredictable and anything can happen. An overly fixed attitude can lead to unnecessary disappointment if things turn out differently, and in some cases, this contributes to postpartum depression. It is best to have clear intentions and then to surrender to the experience with flexibility and acceptance, viewing the process of birthing as an exciting adventure.

Conscious childbirth

In childbirth, the ordinary and routine becomes extraordinary. In this remarkable and commonplace event, a woman is blessed with an opportunity to enter into the mystery of life itself. She can directly experience the spiritual forces of the universe. Birth can just happen, in which case, it is likely to be the result of a woman's subconscious expectations and the expectations of those around her. On the other hand, birth can be prepared for in a conscious way, helping to unlock the potential of a transformative spiritual experience.

Preparing in a conscious way means having a strong intention as well as acceptance of whatever transpires. It involves being well-informed, trusting one's intuition, and making active choices. A woman's intuition and connection with her body during birthing are probably the most powerful and protective aids to a straightforward and empowered birth. Conscious birth also means aligning with one's soul purpose and not being driven by fear, accepting that life events cannot be completely controlled and at the same time making efforts to attain the results wished for. This could be defined as active hope.

As practitioners, we can encourage intentionality and fearlessness by providing information and herbal support, while facilitating safe ways for women to look at their subconscious fears and expectations. All these preparations empower women in childbirth and can help open them to an experience of higher consciousness.

Fear of childbirth

During the last weeks of pregnancy, women can feel eager and excited, overwhelmed and fearful, or a mixture of all of these. Fear is probably the single biggest cause of complications during childbirth. All sorts of fears may arise, including the fear of not being able to cope with labour, fear of something going wrong (especially after a previous difficult birth for oneself or a relative), fear of how to cope once the baby is born. Where practicable, we will have discussed and hopefully resolved fears earlier in the pregnancy; however, it can be common for fears to emerge in the final weeks. These need to be addressed as fully as possible, and vibrational essences can fulfil an enormously helpful role in this (see Chapter 16). Hypnobirthing is another valuable tool. Hypnobirthing teaching sessions include deep relaxation looking at any possible underlying fears and offering methods to resolve them pre-labour.

Also, as part of preparation for labour, guided visualisation can help a woman to gain experience of going within, connecting with her baby and being fully present in the moment (see "Connecting with one's baby' Chapter 4 page 46).

Regarding labour itself, there is often a fine line between fear and excitement. Practitioners can do their best to shift the emphasis to the latter, underlining the delight of finally meeting one's baby outside of the womb. Labour can be viewed as an exciting time of joyful anticipation, with mother and baby acting in partnership. The more a woman feels connected with her child and can surrender to the process of birth, the easier it is to feel empowered, rather than imagining oneself a victim of unwelcome forces. This connection with the baby facilitates mother-child bonding and can lead to a deeply spiritual birthing experience, with body, mind, and spirit united.

Pain in labour

Even though labour is usually described as painful, this *pain* is very different from our usual experiences. The pain of labour is part of a process where mother and baby are working together to bring forth the wonderful outcome of a new birth. As opposed to pain from injury, which sends a survival message of fight or flight, the sensations of labour and birth send a message of "surrender and relax your pelvic muscles". In Western culture, we are taught as girls and then women that labour involves pain and this can create an inbuilt fear that manifests as intensified pain in labour. American midwife, Ina May Gaskin, suggests that rather than "uterine contractions", they are thought of as "interesting sensations that require all of your attention".[1] Hypnobirthing mothers frequently report that they do not experience labour pain, describing the contractions as tightening and then release. Some women experience pleasurable feelings and orgasm while giving birth, and a whole range of simple factors can completely change the inner sensations of labour for a woman. These include the use of a simple breathing technique, changing one's physical position, a change of atmosphere or the arrival of a different midwife. Privacy and trusted female support are known to have a positive effect on childbirth.

For herbal pain relief see page 198, below, and Chapter 12 page 229. Alternative pain relief for labour is discussed in Chapter 11 page 217.

Vaginal delivery and self-doubt

Women, especially first-time mothers, may doubt their ability to give birth. Sadly, this is a tendency that can be propagated, covertly or otherwise, in our society and through the media, leading women to feel disempowered and even to choose a caesarean section (major surgery) rather than vaginal delivery. Elective caesareans are becoming more and more common in many developed countries, with the result that women are missing out on the amazingly beautiful and memorable experience that a vaginal birth can be. Giving birth is an experience of a lifetime, no matter how many babies a woman has delivered before. I consider giving birth to be one of the privileges of being female. Women have been birthing babies for thousands of years and our bodies have a primal instinct of what to do. Vaginal delivery offers numerous health benefits, such as a quicker recovery time and easier breastfeeding, as well as many benefits to the baby including receiving beneficial bacteria in the birth canal and a lowered incidence of breathing problems in the newborn. In practice, I do my very best to advocate for normal vaginal delivery wherever possible, aiming to help women believe in themselves and their bodies, and to ensure that they can make well-informed choices. My intention is to empower women by building confidence and self-assurance, in order that they have the most positive birthing experience possible.

Vaginal birth after caesarean (VBAC)

For women who have had previous births by caesarean section, if their pregnancy is straightforward, there is generally no medical reason why they cannot have a vaginal delivery, known as vaginal birth after caesarean (VBAC). The only exceptions are when:

- a woman has had three or more previous caesarean deliveries
- the uterus ruptured in a previous labour
- a woman has had a high uterine incision (classical caesarean)
- there are other pregnancy complications necessitating a caesarean delivery

In these cases, VBAC is not advisable and repeat caesarean is a safer choice.

Breech presentation

A breech presentation is when the foetus presents buttocks or feet first rather than head-first (a cephalic presentation). Around 3–4% of babies are in breech presentation at term (37–40 weeks), with a higher incidence in preterms.[2] In around 20% of cases, breech is not diagnosed until labour. The main implication of breech birth is on delivery, increasing the likelihood of needing suction (Ventouse), forceps or Caesarean section, primarily due to a lack of experienced medical practitioners in attendance. Possible complications include cord prolapse and intracranial haemorrhage from the rapid compression of the head during delivery. Experienced midwives and obstetricians can safely deliver breech babies but this skill is being lost due to the infrequency with which the procedure is performed.

Breech presentation is usually identified on palpation of the abdomen, where the hard round foetal head can be felt in the upper part of the uterus, and an irregular mass (foetal buttocks and legs) in the pelvis. Alternatively, the mother may feel the baby's head under her ribs, or she may have sudden urinary urgency by being kicked in the bladder.

If breech is discovered after 36 or 37 weeks of pregnancy, external cephalic version (ECV) is usually offered to manually turn the baby via the maternal abdomen to cephalic presentation. This is successful in around 50% of cases. In my own second pregnancy, the baby was breech at 36 weeks and my doctor turned him by ECV (this was a completely painless procedure with no medication or force). However, the baby clearly preferred the original position and turned back to breech that evening, only to turn himself to a cephalic presentation at 39 weeks. Babies do move around a lot and some have been known to turn at 40 weeks. If ECV is unsuccessful, contraindicated, or declined by the woman, she will generally be offered either an elective caesarean or vaginal breech birth, requiring an experienced midwife.

For women with breech presentations, it is helpful to visualise the baby lying head-down in the uterus in a perfect position for delivery. Do this every day for at least five minutes. Talk to the baby, explaining why you would like him or her to move. Swimming, or if possible, inverting head-down in a swimming pool, for as long and often as possible, will often effect a shift (although this may be a little extreme for most women!). Another option is to lie for at least twenty minutes daily with hips higher than head, for instance by kneeling on the floor with bottom in the air and head resting on arms on the floor. Pregnancy yoga, acupuncture, shiatzu, and homeopathy all have methods for turning a foetus (practitioners often like to start treatment by week 35).

Preparation for childbirth

Whatever the type of delivery, relaxation exercises, visualisation, and talking to the baby are invaluable preparation. There is inestimable value in being able to go within and be fully present in the moment with one's baby. Communicating with the foetus helps build a bonded relationship prior to the birth, making it easier for a woman to feel that she and her baby are operating as a team. Fathers/partners can also build this pre-birth bond with the baby by talking, singing and playing music to the unborn child. In addition, regardless of the presentation of the foetus, it is helpful for a mother to visualise the baby lying in the perfect position for a smooth and easy labour. Even if a woman knows she is having a caesarean, she can still intend for and visualise a smooth, easy, and joyful birthing. Many women find it helpful to envisage holding their newborn baby in their arms.

Guided visualisation: preparing for childbirth

Text can be tailored to suit the individual.

Lie down or sit comfortably with your feet on the floor…Take your attention to your breath as it comes in and out of your body.

Notice any areas of tension in your body and with each outbreath, let the tension release,

Allowing it to flow into the earth where it can be composted.

If other thoughts come into your mind, simply notice them and let them pass, returning your awareness to your breath.

With every in-breath, you are bringing light and oxygen into your own body cells and into the baby,

And with every out-breath you are letting go of stress and tension, becoming more and more relaxed…

> Take your awareness to your baby in your womb,
> Place your hands over your belly and feel your baby's body.
> Imagine you are inside in the safety of your womb with the baby.
> Greet the baby and feel your love for this wondrous being,
> This being who you will soon meet and hold in your arms.
> Send warm, loving thoughts through your hands,
> Enfolding the baby with your love,
> Knowing that he or she is held in safety and protection,
> And will soon make their journey outward.
> Visualise the baby lying in the perfect head-down position for a smooth and easy labour.
> If you have words you would like to speak to the baby, say them now.
> Take all the time you need, enjoying these precious moments together…
> You may like to envision holding your baby in your arms,
> Feeling your intense joy and love,
> Imagining the baby's warm body lying against your skin,
> Marvelling at his or her tiny, perfect features,
> Feeling the gentle movement as she or he breathes…
> When you are ready, again, send love to the baby in your womb.
> Bring your attention back to your breath.
> Prepare to return to your ordinary reality,
> Knowing that you are in constant communication with your baby
> And can speak to them at any time.
> Stretch your fingers and toes and gently open your eyes.
> Write down any experiences you would like to record.
> See also 'Connecting with One's Baby' in Chapter 4 Exercise and Lifestyle

Herbs to prepare for childbirth

Partus preparators or herbs to prepare for childbirth, have been used by women with excellent effect in cultures around the globe since ancient times. These herbs can improve uterine tone, assist the start of labour at the appropriate time, ease and shorten labour, reduce the incidence of complications, and expedite recovery.

Raspberry leaf (*Rubus idaeus*) is my favourite and probably the most well-known partus preparator. In an uncomplicated pregnancy, I routinely give Raspberry leaf tea for the last three months, one cup daily from week 28, increasing to three cups daily from week 36—see Chapter 2 page 21 for a typical antenatal care schedule. Dosage is one heaped teaspoon dried herb per cup (equivalent 1g). I nearly always give tea but if tincture is required, each cup of tea can be replaced by 5ml of tincture.

Raspberry leaf is a superb remedy that strengthens and tones the pelvic muscles, including the uterus, while softening and relaxing the tissues at the same time. It relieves excessive tension in the uterus and assists optimal function. Raspberry leaf does not make contractions stronger or more painful, but promotes effective contractions with a regular and co-ordinated rhythm. This can result in a shorter labour with reduced pain. Raspberry leaf is continued for one month after delivery, supplying valuable nutrients and helping to tone the pelvic musculature, including the uterus.

Contrary to some reports, I have never found Raspberry leaf to be over-stimulating at the dosages given, neither have I seen any contraindications in women with an athletic or muscular body type.[3] I cannot know how different a birth might have been without Raspberry leaves, but I have certainly seen countless cases of women who have had previous difficult births without Raspberry (sometimes several successive births) and their experience has been transformed after drinking this nourishing tea in the last three months of pregnancy. Raspberry leaves are said to soften the heart and allow for greater receptivity and intuition.

Partridge Berry (*Mitchella repens*) is a traditional and excellent partus preparator from the Native American tradition. A uterine tonic and astringent, it tones and strengthens uterine and pelvic muscles, preventing tension and spasm, and acting as a tonic to the nervous system. It primes the uterine muscle for contraction, relieves back ache and erratic pains, and assists quick dilation.

In cases of uterine atony and weakness, or if there is risk of haemorrhage, Partridge Berry can be combined in equal parts with Raspberry leaf from week 28 (dosage as for Raspberry leaf above), or add twenty drops to each cup of Raspberry leaf tea. Partridge Berry also combines well with Oatstraw (*Avena sativa*) for nervous exhaustion. It can be particularly indicated if a woman has low self-confidence.

Other helpful partus preparators include Black Haw (*Viburnum prunifolium*), Motherwort (*Leonurus cardiaca*), Lady's Mantle (*Alchemilla vulgaris*), Ashwagandha (*Withania somnifera*), and Black Cohosh (*Cimicifuga racemosa*). Any of these can be given as tinctures and may be combined with the above recommended dose of Raspberry leaf tea.

Black Haw relaxes the uterine muscle and is specific for uterine irritability. Motherwort tones the uterus and supports effective contractions. It has anti-anxiety effects and aids restful sleep. Lady's Mantle tones the uterus prior to birth and reduces the risk of haemorrhage. It is suited to soft, gentle women, and can help prevent postpartum depression. Ashwagandha, while not a classic partus preparator, can make a beneficial addition. It supports a healthy stress response, reduces fatigue, and assists general well-being. All the above can be given at a dosage of twenty drops of tincture per cup of Raspberry leaf tea. False Unicorn is excellent to strengthen the pelvic tissues and promote pelvic nutrition, especially helpful if there is lack of tone from previous pregnancies. Five drops can be added to tea.

Black Cohosh is sedative and helps relax excess spasm in the uterus. It is also anti-inflammatory and analgesic. At the present time, due to safety concerns, I only give Black Cohosh in the last two weeks of pregnancy, 5–10 drops three times daily. In past times I prescribed both Blue and Black Cohosh together for up to 6 weeks prior to delivery, with apparent benefit and no known ill-effects (see page 80 and Chapter 12). Black Cohosh can help if a woman feels cramped in her life, restricted by difficult circumstances or at the end of her tether.

If a woman is having an elective caesarian section, prophylactic Echinacea (*Echinacea* spp.) is recommended to prevent infection. Give 5ml tds for a week prior to surgery (see Endometritis page 249).

Preparation for after the birth

Preparing a woman for birth also includes discussion of the postpartum period, or what has begun to be termed the fourth trimester. This tends to be a neglected time for women, with attention being focused on pregnancy and labour, and a potential void after the birth. It is usual to prepare by having the physical items needed for the baby, but it is not so typical for a woman to consider and plan for her own postpartum care and recovery. In the same way that women frequently prepare a birth plan before labour, it is also beneficial to plan in advance for the postpartum period. The third trimester is an ideal time for a woman to assemble a support team and consider how she can create space in her life to rest, recover, and enjoy her baby after delivery. See Chapter 13 'Postpartum Care' page 237 for further details.

Perineal massage

Massaging the perineum from week 37 onwards encourages suppleness, elasticity, and perhaps even more importantly, a sense of trust and familiarity. It is good emotional preparation for birth, providing an opportunity to give some attention to this often neglected part of the body, and offering a chance to practice relaxing and opening the vaginal area. Massage also helps soften scar tissue. It is particularly important for women who may be left with discomfort, scarring, or associated painful memories from a previous experience affecting the perineum. Some practitioners recommend highly vigorous stretching of the perineum but a gentle approach can be just as effective. Avoid perineal massage in active vaginal infection.

Combine nourishing oils such as avocado or wheatgerm with almond oil to make a base. Marigold (*Calendula off.*), St John's Wort (*Hypericum perforatum*) or Chamomile (*Chamomilla recutita*) infused oils are also suitable. Add essential oils of Rose (*Rosa* spp.), Roman Chamomile (*Chamaemelum nobile*), Lavender (*Lavandula* spp.) or Geranium (*Pelargonium graveolens*) at 1% dilution, for instance:

Rx Almond oil 80, Avocado oil 20, E.O. Roman Chamomile 7gtt, E.O. Rose 1gtt, E.O. Geranium 12gtt. Apply daily to the perineal area from week 37.

PREPARATION FOR LABOUR AND BIRTH 197

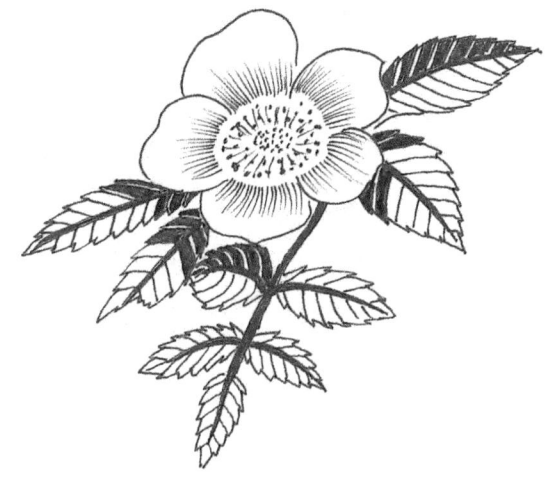

Birthing pack

Typically, around week 36, the expectant mother and I will discuss the various options available for herbal support for labour and birth. After discussing her wishes and my suggestions, she chooses whatever she would like to avail of. I then make up an individual *Birthing Pack* that the woman keeps at home in readiness for labour. It is important to give this pack well in advance, since even if I am due to be present at the birth, we cannot predict the timing. This gives her a basic kit that she can use herself whenever and wherever labour occurs, and also includes some remedies for immediately after the birth. If I am attending the birth myself, I will bring additional herbs at the time. These are described in Chapter 12 'Herbs for Labour and Delivery'. As part of the preparation, especially for first-time mothers, we might discuss signs of labour and coping mechanisms—these are also covered in the next chapter.

Birthing pack basics

1. Labour drops
These are general purpose drops to support labour and help keep it going effectively. A woman starts taking them as soon as true labour is established (see next chapter). Standard dosage is ten drops every half to one hour or as required. To restart a stuck labour or speed up a prolonged labour, the drops can be taken more frequently, such as every ten minutes for three doses (especially good combined with relaxation and visualisation). Alternatively, if labour proceeds very fast, a single dose may suffice.

Labour drops: Rx *Cimicifuga racemosa* 10, *Artemisia vulgaris* 10, *Trillium erectum* 7, *Zingiber officinalis* 3, Rescue remedy 2gtt = 30 sig 5–10gtt every 30–60 minutes or prn, starting at onset of labour.

I give a 30ml dropper bottle so there is no risk of overdosage. In many cases, only a few doses are needed.

2. Raspberry leaf tea (and ice cubes)

In normal circumstances, a woman will already be drinking daily Raspberry (*Rubus idaeus*) leaf tea. Some time in advance of her due date, she should make a strong infusion, strain and freeze in an ice cube tray, storing the ice cubes in a thermos flask ready for labour (this can be taken to hospital for a hospital delivery). Drink Raspberry leaf tea in early-stage labour and suck on ice cubes in later stages. Gives all the parturient benefits of Raspberry leaf as well as providing something to suck on and moisten the lips when in strong labour.

3. Ginseng 'energy sticks'

These are small pieces of Red Ginseng (*Panax ginseng*) dried root that can be chewed during labour to keep energy high and avoid exhaustion. If sticks are too hard to chew, they can be softened in a little hot water. Not to be taken in conjunction with caffeine or other stimulants, or where there is a history of hypertension.

4. Tinctures for relaxation and pain relief

When women feel supported, safe, and encouraged in labour, they often do not ask for pain relief. However, many women like to be prepared with a mix of tinctures, just in case. Herbs from the list below can be chosen to match the individual.

Motherwort (*Leonurus cardiaca*) combined with Black horehound (*Ballota nigra*) is a helpful mix for anxiety in early labour. The sedative action of Skullcap (*Scutellaria lateriflora*) can assist throughout, easing tension that may accompany and accumulate with pain. Valerian (*Valeriana off.*) relieves anxiety and tension. St John's Wort (*Hypericum perforatum*) soothes nerves and relieves erratic cramping and spasms. Lavender (*Lavandula* spp.) and Chamomile (*Chamomilla recutita*) are soothing and calming (be aware that some rare cases of anaphylactic shock have been reported with Chamomile). Pasque Flower (*Anemone pulsatilla*) is useful, especially in early labour, to ease pain, calm irritated nerves, and remove fear. All of the above can be taken as teas or tinctures, although tinctures are generally easier to administer in the later stages of labour.

Typical Pain Mix: Rx *Valeriana officinalis* 30, *Scutellaria lateriflora* 30, *Hypericum perforatum* 30, *Anemone pulsatilla* 10 x1 sig 5ml hourly for pain or anxiety.

5. Massage oils for pain relief, relaxation, or stimulation

Touch and massage can bring amazing relief when labour is painful. Relaxing massage oils are frequently given to reduce tension and ease pain, while stimulating oils can be helpful to encourage labour by energising and improving tone. For the Birthing Pack, some women like to have a small bottle of each. A woman may enjoy having her back, thighs, feet, hands, or any part of the body massaged during labour. Her likes and dislikes may alter rapidly and sometimes massage may be the last thing she wants! Essential oils can recreate scents associated with pleasure and relaxation during pregnancy. A woman's sense of smell is particularly acute during labour and small amounts of oils can have a powerful effect. You cannot predict how a woman will feel at the time, but many women love being massaged. It is best to ask a woman to choose the oils she is attracted to from an appropriate selection.

Suggested oils for relaxing massage during labour include Rose, Ylang-Ylang, Chamomile, Lavender, Geranium, and Bergamot, making a 1% dilution in carrier oil.

I consider Rose to be particularly suited to childbirth (avoid in first trimester). Energetically, it carries a vibration of love, has a sublime gentleness, and puts mother and baby into a warm and calm protective bubble. As a sedative and uterine tonic, Rose EO can relieve pain and will both relax and stimulate the uterus. It is highly recommended as part of a mix for labour, either singly or combined with other essential oils.

Sample relaxing massage oil: Rx Almond oil 70 Avocado oil 10 Wheatgerm oil 20 Geranium EO 10gtt Chamomile EO 5gtt Rose EO 5gtt apply prn.

For stimulation, Clary Sage and Jasmine are both appropriate.

Sample stimulating oil: Rx Almond Oil 70 Avocado oil 10 Wheatgerm oil 20 Jasmine EO 5gtt Clary sage EO 10gtt apply prn, especially around the sacrum. Clary Sage combines well with Roman Chamomile for back pain. Discontinue Clary Sage if woman has synthetic oxytocin. Frankincense is an alternative oil to enhance uterine tone and reduce anxiety.

6. Essential oils

As well as part of a massage oil, essential oils may be enjoyed in a burner/diffuser, inhaled or added to a bath during labour. These options can be discussed with the woman when preparing the Birthing Pack and additional oils supplied if desired. Clary Sage in a warm bath encourages smooth contractions and assists opening of the cervix. I have frequently seen this facilitate regular, effective contractions (usually within 30 minutes) where labour has been stalled or prolonged. Add 5 drops of Clary Sage to 20ml cider vinegar or a lotion base to act as a dispersant, shake well and add the full amount to a bath after running the water. A small pre-mixed bottle of essential oil plus dispersant can be included in the Birthing Pack for ease of use during labour. Alternative essential oils for the bath include Jasmine, Lavender, and Rose which can all promote effective contractions.

A blend of anti-infective oils can be placed in a burner or diffuser during childbirth to protect against infection, for instance Eucalyptus, Ginger, and Lemon, 3–5 drops. Alternatively, a woman might choose a relaxing, uplifting blend such as Bergamot, Geranium, and Lavender.

For inhalation during labour, Rose is particularly effective. Place 1–2 drops of Rose essential oil on a cotton pad or nasal inhaler tube and inhale as required. Other suitable oils include Lavender, Geranium, Bergamot, Jasmine, Mandarin, Neroli, Petitgrain, or Sweet Orange.

7. Room spray with vibrational essences

Women and babies are particularly sensitive to vibrational essences during labour. The use of a spray or spritzer is especially effective, combining a pleasurable scent with the subtle and energetic qualities of essences, hydrosols, and essential oils.

Ease of use is an added advantage, sprays being simple to administer, even in a hospital environment. General purpose sprays can be given or a personal spray specific to an individual woman's requirements (see Chapter 16 Vibrational Essences for details of sprays, including how to make your own). Sacred Birthing is a favourite generic spray, containing a mix of essences to assist labour, ease delivery, and welcome the new baby. Sacred Space is a useful space clearing spray to cleanse the atmosphere in the birthing room, clear negative energies, lift the spirits, and bring safety and protection. A Rescue spray is a general-purpose standby for any situation of shock and trauma. All sprays can continue to be used with benefit to mother and child postpartum.

8. Calendula lotion

A bottle of Marigold (*Calendula off.*) tincture is included in the Birthing Pack, an invaluable antiseptic lotion to heal the perineum and for general home use. Apply after delivery for tears, stitches or other wounds. Dilute in water to 25% alcohol strength and apply on cotton wool. Easiest for the woman if you give her a pre-diluted bottle that is ready to use. Add 20ml to bath to assist perineal healing and to treat or prevent infection. Calendula lotion is also applied on cotton wool to clean the baby's cord.

9. Postnatal tonic

In the Birthing Pack, I usually include 100ml of a general postnatal tonic that the mother can get started on straight away after delivery. Immediate post-partum herbal support makes a significant difference to long term recovery. As soon as possible after the birth, and depending on the woman's personal birthing experience, I dispense either more of the same or a personalised tonic to reflect individual needs (see Chapter 13 'Postpartum care' page 242).

Typical starter Postnatal Tonic:

Rx Vitex agnus castus 20 Verbena officinalis 20 Galega officinalis 20 Angelica sinensis 30 Astragalus membranaceus 15 Rescue essence 2gtt = 105 sig 5ml tds pc aq cal

Vitex balances hormones and is galactagogue. Verbena is galactagogue and restores the nervous system. Galega is galactagogue and balances blood sugar (which can be erratic after giving birth). Angelica sinensis is a woman's blood and energy tonic that combines well with Astragalus (two parts Angelica sinensis to one part Astragalus) to strengthen and restore after childbirth. The Rescue essence helps clear shock.

Dosage of chaste tree (*Vitex agnus castus*) in lactation

Recent studies suggest that low doses of Chaste Tree increase and higher doses inhibit prolactin. Current advice is to avoid doses greater than 250mg daily during lactation.[4] Readers may notice that the amount in the above prescription is higher: *20ml/week = 5g/week = 714mg daily.* I have been consistently giving this dosage to lactating mothers for 35 years and my personal clinical observations have all been highly favourable. To date, I have not seen any adverse effects on milk supply, quite the reverse. Is this because Chaste Tree only inhibits prolactin in certain circumstances? Is it due to the presence of other galactagogues over-riding any Chaste Tree inhibition? Is it a synergistic effect because I always prescribe a mix of herbs? Have I just been lucky? Or is it one of many other possible reasons? This is a question for further research and beyond the scope of this book. Practitioners must decide their own dosage.

NOTE: Women can take homeopathic Arnica (*Arnica montana*) 30 or 200 as an additional treatment for shock and bruising, starting as soon as practicable after delivery. Recommended dose is two tablets every 2 hours for 6 doses, followed by 2 three times daily for six days. If appropriate, this can be included in the Birthing Pack.

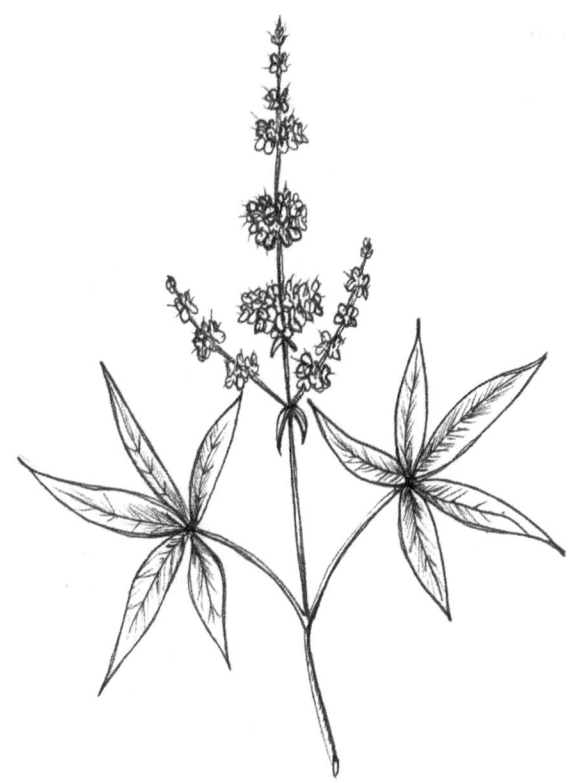

Induction of labour and post-term pregnancy

Post-term pregnancy is defined as pregnancy lasting 42 completed weeks or more. There are contradictory findings about the risks associated with post-term pregnancy and this has led to opposing views on the most effective form of medical care. Different policies exist depending on where a woman lives. These range from routine induction at or around 40 weeks, 41 weeks, or 42 weeks gestation, selective induction of labour based on abnormalities detected by antenatal foetal surveillance, to the intention to wait for spontaneous labour.

In most cases, it seems that post-term pregnancy is a variant of normal with a good outcome for mother and baby. However, in a minority of cases it is associated with increased perinatal mortality and early neonatal convulsions.

See Chapter 11 page 219 for details of medical induction.

As a herbal practitioner, I prefer not to interfere with nature's course, and unless there is good reason otherwise, I do not give herbs to induce labour. However, herbal induction is radically different from regular medical induction. The herbal approach does not force, but supports and encourages the body to go into labour by itself. It is well established that a spontaneous labour supports normal physiology, reduces the incidence of Caesareans, and prevents both iatrogenic prematurity and the cascade of interventions that commonly result from hospital induction.[5] There is no doubt that herbs can help to initiate and assist the progress of labour, and if hospital induction is imminent, herbs can offer a preferable alternative. Therefore, if there are no complications and a woman has been given a date for hospital induction, a herbal induction mix can be started in the preceding days. I usually start giving a mix three days prior to the induction date, starting at a low dose and increasing each day. In most cases, labour starts spontaneously in the days before the planned induction, often after only a few doses of herbs. In the unusual event that labour does not start before the hospital date, medical induction can proceed and having taken the herbs will only expedite the process.

If the cervix is already ripe, herbal induction is facilitated and labour usually starts promptly. During pregnancy, cervical ripening often begins prior to the onset of labour and is necessary for cervical dilation and the passage of the foetus. For women taking herbal partus preparators, it is common for the cervix to ripen and be partially effaced (thinned) for several days in advance of labour. If the cervix is unripe at term or beyond, ripening can be encouraged by having sexual intercourse. Human semen is a concentrated source of prostaglandins and pleasurable intercourse in the last weeks of pregnancy assists the woman's body to go into labour. Manual manipulation of the cervix can also stimulate the process. This can be done by vaginal self-examination[6] or during an internal examination by the midwife. Nipple stimulation also helps the process by encouraging the release of oxytocin and prolactin. This can be done by rolling the nipple between finger and thumb or by having someone suck constantly on the woman's nipples.

Herbal induction mix

Start this mix three days prior to induction (counting the induction date as Day 4)

Rx *Artemisia vulgaris* 35, *Cimicifuga racemosa* 35, *Cinnamomum zeylandicum/verum* 25, *Zingiber officinalis* 5 = 100

Dosage is 2.5ml qds on day 1, 2.5ml eight times daily on day 2, forty drops hourly on day 3, taking 15 doses over the day (30ml in total). In other words, day 1 10ml, day 2 20ml, day 3 30ml. Take the herbs in a little warm water.

Small frequent doses are recommended, but if this is difficult for compliance, the total for the day can be divided into fewer, slightly larger doses.

Alternative induction herbs include Golden Seal (*Hydrastis canadensis*), Fenugreek (*Trigonella foenum graecum*), and Garden Angelica (*Angelica archangelica*).

If desired, the herbal mix can be complemented by the use of a stimulating massage oil, as described in the Birthing Pack above, applied to the sacral area twice daily.

Vibrational essences for induction of labour

As well as a herbal induction mix, I may give vibrational essences to women facing hospital induction. These are by no means essential but dowsing for essences can reveal and treat subconscious issues for mother and baby that may be causing a block or some kind of resistance to labour and birth. This could be as simple as the mother not feeling that her home is ready for the new arrival, it could be a deeply held fear, it could even be that the baby is resistant to emerging into the world. All manner of unexpected issues can come to light and are remarkably accessible to treatment at this time. Essences may also be selected by other means as described in Chapter 16.

Adjuncts to herbal treatment

Craniosacral therapy can release compression in the pelvis resulting from previous difficulties giving birth. It also works on the sacral nerves to assist smooth dilation of the cervix. Hypnobirthing can also be a valuable therapy, to help release the effects of previous trauma, aid relaxation, reduce pain, and facilitate childbirth.

Notes

1. Ina May Gaskin, *Ina May's Guide to Childbirth* (London: Vermilion, 2003), 162.
2. Gray CJ, Shanahan MM. Breech Presentation. [Updated 2021 Aug 11]. In: StatPearls [Internet]. Treasure Island (FL): StatPearls Publishing; 2022 Jan-. Available from: https://www.ncbi.nlm.nih.gov/books/NBK448063/
3. Athletic refers to a body type described in the physique classification system developed by Ernst Kretschmer. In this system, an 'athletic' type is large boned and muscular, an 'asthenic' type is lean and narrowly built, the 'pyknic' type is small and rounded. A 'dysplastic' type has a unproportionate body. It has been suggested that Raspberry leaf (*Rubus idaeus*) can cause excess stimulation in women of athletic body type, but I have seen no evidence of this in practice.
4. Hananja Brice-Ytsma and Adrian McDermott, *Herbal Medicine in Treating Gynaecological Conditions*, (London: Aeon, 2020), 163.
5. Debby Amis, "Healthy birth practice #1: let labor begin on its own." *The Journal of perinatal education* vol. 23, 4(2014): 178–87.

6. Vaginal self-examination is a simple technique that women can safely perform in an uncomplicated pregnancy. Thoroughly wash hands and trim fingernails first. Find a comfortable position, lying with legs apart and knees bent, squatting or sitting on the toilet. Insert index and middle fingers into the vagina, pushing them up as far as needed until the cervix is felt (in pregnancy this feels like a pair of puckered lips). Use a gentle touch to feel the cervix, being aware that one finger may easily slip into the middle of the cervix if it is dilating. If this happens, the amniotic sac might be felt (may feel like a latex balloon filled with water). Dilation can be checked by using the two fingers to estimate the size of the opening in the cervix.

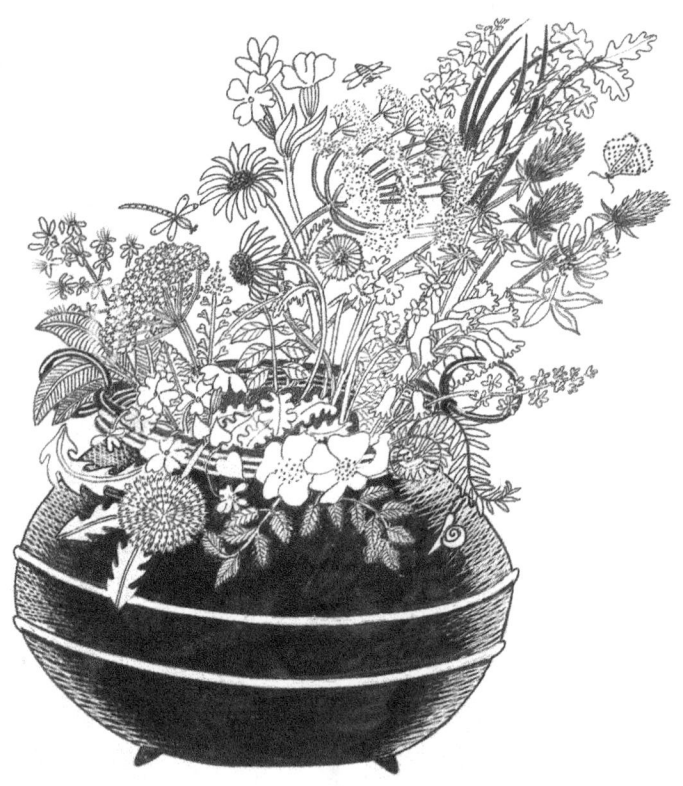

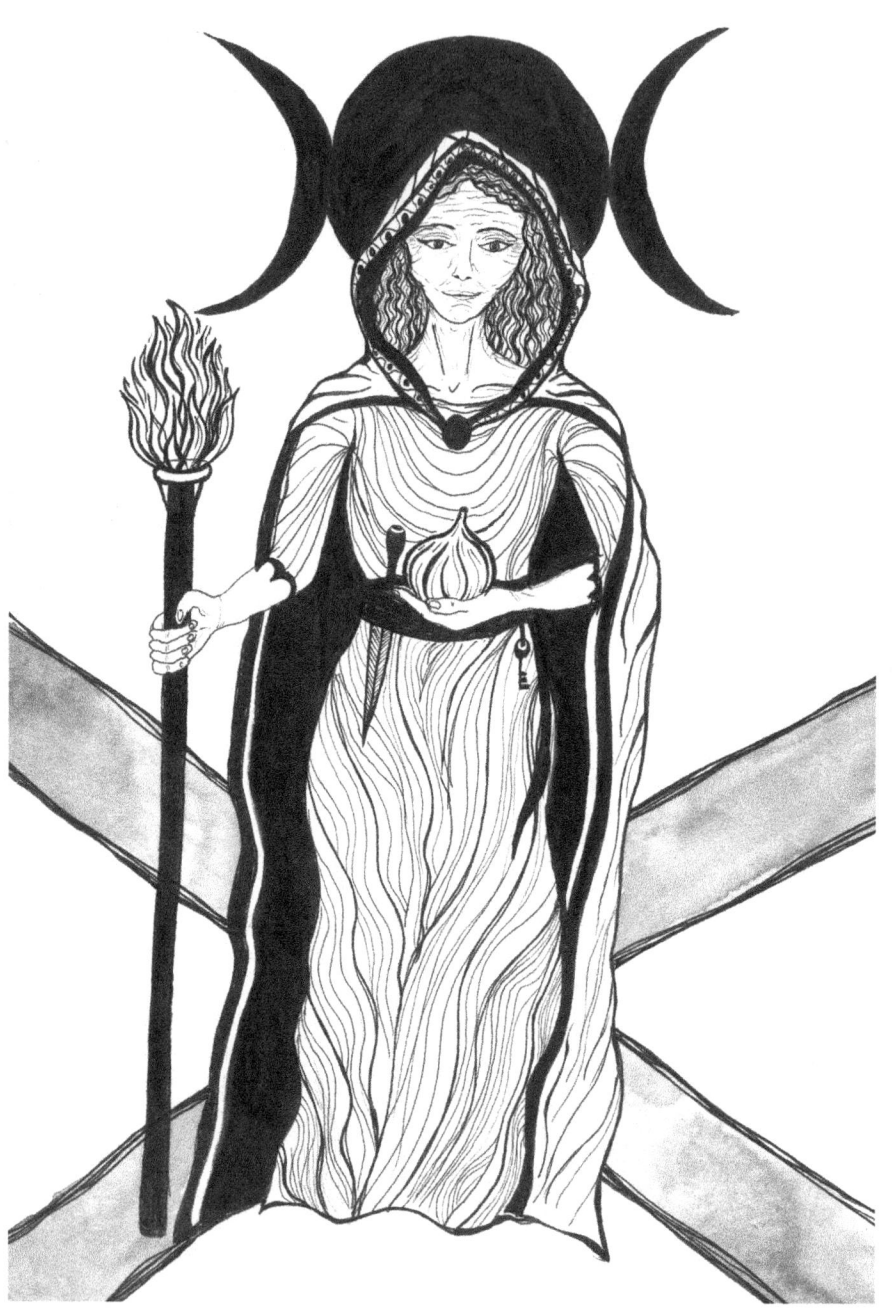

Hecate. Midwife and Wisdom Keeper. "She who cuts the cord with her sacred knife". Garlic (*Allium sativum*). The one who strengthens all, bringing purification and protection.

CHAPTER 11

The process of labour

The mystery of childbirth

Now is the time when a woman fully enters the mystery of childbirth. No matter how her birthing transpires, whether naturally or with numerous interventions, the experience reaches deep into her being and her identity, transforming her completely. A key teaching of this mystery is about surrender and letting go of the illusion of control. Only by letting go completely do we attain mastery. Childbirth is an opportunity to stand at a portal between worlds and experience the ultimate source of our creative power.

This can be seen as a sacred ceremony and may be dedicated to a safe and joyful incarnation for the baby. In addition, this is a rebirth for the mother, an initiation to a new state of Motherhood, whether with a first child or one of several. Like any initiation, we are asked to die to the old in order to embrace the new and enter a higher state of consciousness.

In childbirth, a doorway is opened between this world and the invisible world. Life and death are intimately connected, and birth itself is a kind of death, as the new soul chooses to leave the bliss and expanded consciousness of the interlife to enter the challenging world of human experience.

The Celtic tradition tells us that after the baby has travelled through the 'dark tunnel' of the cervix and the 'outer chamber' of the vagina, the new soul comes into the physical world and begins to ground itself. This is said to occur through the silver cord/spiritual umbilical *An Corda Geal*, which replaces the physical umbilical at birth, opening the central channel and bringing with it each of the body's energy spirals (chakras) that take up their place along the spine. The red spiral hooks into the child's anus and earths itself. This centre of fire energy is activated immediately, attracting and anchoring the newly arrived soul. The baby experiences the rainbow colours flooding in as the energy centres are established in the physical being. The silver cord settles at the crown of the head and does not stop pulsating until the spirals are in place which is usually complete around three months after the birth. This signifies that the baby's endocrine system is fully ready for activation.

In her book, *A Celtic Book of Dying*, Phyllida Anam-Aire describes how in the Celtic tradition a woman in labour was encouraged to "be in touch with the new life force with love and ease, showing it the beauty of nature through her eyes". The woman was massaged with oils and given herbs to ease the birth, while her partner sang to the new life force, encouraging it to the earth plane. When the waters released, they were known as "the flowing fountain", and a baby's first breath was considered an all-important bridge to a new life, welcomed with a chant by the attending family:

"Welcome, welcome, welcome
To the newborn child of grace,
We know the beauty of
The earth in the radiance of
Your face."[1]

Meditation for labour and birth[2]

You are reaching the sacred moment of the emergence of the beloved baby you have been preparing for. Your body knows what to do. Whatever happens will be exactly as you and your baby have planned. Between contractions, breathe and relax. Focus on your baby so that he or she can also relax. Re-align with your soul's purpose. Remind yourself of the awe of this event, you are delivering this beloved baby so that its soul can finally enter the world and fulfil its mission. Relax and allow love and light to pour into both of you. Be aware that there are a host of invisible helpers supporting you. Know that every contraction brings you closer to the moment of delivery.

As the wave of a contraction comes, ride it, surf it, knowing you are doing what women have done since time immemorial. Let your body take over. Ride the wave, feel your baby, and send him/her love and reassurance that all is well. Know that you are doing this together. Know that you are both held in safety and protection.

Hormone changes of labour

The exact physiological events leading to the onset of labour are not fully understood, but research suggests that the baby initiates labour by sending out particular proteins or hormones. This is thought to trigger a complex cascade of events including a rise in oxytocin and a drop in progesterone.[3] Oxytocin (often called the 'love hormone' as it triggers feelings of love and protection) causes regular contraction of the uterus and abdominal muscles, and together with oestrogen helps release prostaglandins, which assist in softening the cervix. Relaxin plays an important role in relaxing pelvic ligaments, softening the cervix, and promoting rupture of the membranes. Prolactin levels rise, and are needed to cause lactation to start. Together with endorphins and catecholamines, oxytocin and prolactin comprise four main birth hormones regulating labour and birth, breastfeeding, and mother-child bonding.

Foetal catecholamines increase a few days before the spontaneous start of labour. These play a crucial role in preparing the foetal lungs for air breathing immediately after birth. Babies born by scheduled caesarean or medical induction may lack this advantage and can be more at risk of respiratory problems at birth.

Pain-relieving endorphins are released by the mother's body as labour contractions intensify. These can induce feelings of elation and joy in the mother. Just before birth, her body releases large amounts of adrenaline and noradrenaline, causing a surge of energy and several very strong contractions, which can help deliver the baby. When the baby is born, oxytocin continues to contract the womb in order to restrict blood flow to the womb and reduce the risk of bleeding and to help detach the placenta, which is delivered shortly afterwards.

High levels of oxytocin and prolactin support bonding between mother and baby, and are further stimulated by skin-to-skin and mother-baby eye contact. The euphoria that many mothers describe just after labour is largely due to the effects of oxytocin, prolactin, and beta-endorphins.

Oxytocin is less available or effective under stress, and mothers who are fearful tend to secrete hormones that delay or inhibit birth. Mothers who are relaxed and without fear will secrete hormones to make birthing easier, less painful, and even pleasurable.

Stages of labour

In medical terms, labour usually means the full process of giving birth. It can be described in three phases: onset of contractions to full dilation of the cervix; delivery of the baby; and delivery of the placenta. First births may last on average fifteen to twenty hours, subsequent births averaging twelve hours, although herbal-assisted births tend to be quicker.

During most of pregnancy, the cervix holds the uterus tightly closed and is sealed with a plug of thick mucus. At the end of pregnancy, prostaglandins cause the cervix to soften and thin (effacement)[4] in preparation for labour. This is the 'ripening' of the cervix and usually happens in the last few days although gradual effacement can start much sooner or in some cases not at all. For most of pregnancy, the cervix feels something like the firm tip of a nose. Once it becomes ripe, it feels extremely soft and loses its neck-like shape. The mucus plug is usually expelled during the hours before the start of labour and is commonly blood-tinged caused by the membranes becoming detached from the uterine wall. If this is bright red and enough to soak a pad, the woman should call her midwife. The release of the plug is called having a 'show'.

Other possible signs of approaching labour include a sudden increase in the amount of vaginal discharge, a slowing down of the baby's movements in the last few days before birth, and an increased 'nesting' instinct where a woman may have an overwhelming desire to decorate or clean the house. I would encourage her not to go overboard and risk exhausting herself. There may be a feeling of increased pressure in the pelvis or the feeling that the baby is pushing down. Low back ache, nausea, loose stools, and the urge to pass frequent bowel movements can all be early signs of labour.

Rupture of membranes

It is common for the membranes to rupture during labour, but in 6–19% of all term births, the membranes rupture before labour starts (prelabour rupture). The membranes are the nearly transparent amniotic sac that hold the foetus and its umbilical cord in the uterus. Rupture of the membranes is referred to as the *waters breaking*. This may be followed by a gush or a trickle, the amniotic fluid leaking out gradually over a few days, bursting out explosively, or anything in between, depending on the size of the rupture and the baby's position in the pelvis. The salty fluid has a distinctive smell, which helps to distinguish it from urine.

If the amniotic fluid is stained with meconium from the baby's bowel (greenish, brownish, or black) or with fresh blood, the woman should be checked by her midwife. Fresh meconium is green and could indicate the baby being in distress. Thick meconium carries the worst prognosis.

If the waters break and baby is still high or not engaged, this should be reported to the midwife immediately since there is a slight risk of cord prolapse. If the cord is protruding, the woman should go to hospital immediately, lying face down with knees on ground and bottom raised in air. She should not touch the cord except to push it gently back into the vagina.

The rupture of membranes can trigger immediate contractions or labour may take several days to get started. 70% of women with term prelabour rupture of membranes (PROM) will give birth within twenty-four hours, and almost 90% will do so within forty-eight hours.

The main risk of PROM is maternal and neonatal infection entering through the vagina. The prognosis has changed considerably in the past few decades, no longer being associated with a high risk of maternal and perinatal mortality. Immediate induction was advocated in the past, but with current concerns about the possible increased risk of operative delivery after induction, it has become more popular to allow extra time. Policies vary, many midwives being content to wait for six days before considering induction, whereas some conventional obstetricians prefer babies to be delivered within twenty-four hours of spontaneous rupture—For rupture before 37 weeks, see 'Preterm Prelabour Rupture of Membranes' page 155. Sometimes antibiotics are prescribed, although their use is of questionable value in women without evidence of infection. Prophylactic Echinacea, up to 5ml tds, can be given in any case (concurrent with antibiotics if necessary), to help prevent intrauterine infection.

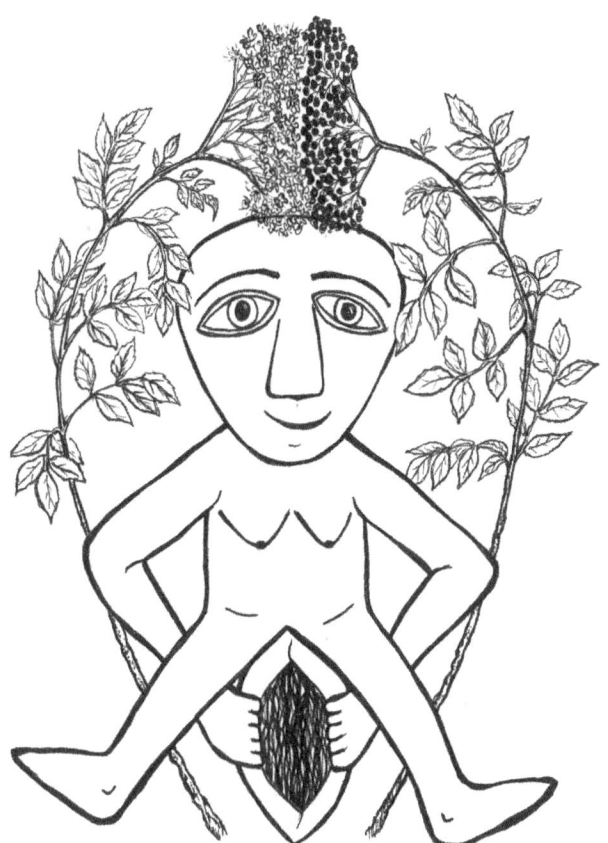

Sheela na Gig. Crone Goddess. The great opener who demonstrates the powers of the vagina[5]
Elder (*Sambucus nigra*). The Elder Mother who carries Earth magic, healing and protection, supporting women at all stages of life.

Eating raw garlic and taking 1g vitamin C daily are also recommended, as well as scrupulous hygiene, showers instead of baths, always wiping front to back after using the toilet, no sex, no vaginal examinations or anything put into the vagina. Induction herbs can be started three days prior to planned hospital induction, as outlined in Chapter 10 'Preparation for Birth' page 202.

PROM may also indicate an increased risk of the foetus being in an abnormal position or early detachment of the placenta (see 'Placental Abruption' page 152).

First stage of labour

The **first stage** of labour is when the cervix is opening, leading to full dilation of 10cm. This is usually the longest stage of labour, taking anywhere from minutes to days. It typically begins with the mother having occasional contractions, which happen increasingly often and last for longer as labour progresses. Contractions can be quite varied. Many women describe them as menstrual-like cramps, while others feel them mostly in their backs. During this stage the uterine fundus (upper uterus) stretches, causing the lower uterus and cervix to thin, with the cervix gradually becoming a thin sheet of tissue, eventually merging with the lower segment of the uterus.

Initially, there is a **latent phase**, which may last for hours or days before the woman is in established labour. During this time, contractions are likely to be irregular and may vary in intensity, becoming stronger and closer together. If this occurs at night, it is best for her to stay comfortable and relaxed, gathering energy, sleeping as much as possible, and allowing the cervix to dilate while she is resting. If labour starts during the day, it is wise to eat and drink, because energy will be needed later. Take light, easily digested foods, such as soup, avocado, omelette, fruit, seeds, or yogurt. Drink plenty of fluids and pass water every hour or so, which both avoid dehydration and also involves sitting on the toilet where there is likely to be a conditioned response to relax the pelvic muscles. Unless a woman is tired, it is helpful to stay upright and gently active in order to help the baby to move down and to speed up cervical dilation. Stay in a peaceful, calm, and unhurried atmosphere. Walking, dancing, singing, and playing music are all suitable pastimes, and now is the time to make any last-minute preparations, especially if having a home birth. This could include checking herbal medicines, lighting, flowers, music, candles, and camera. If tired, take a nap, a warm bath (if waters have not broken) or have a relaxing massage. Time the contractions, writing down the length and interval between the start of each one. Call the midwife or hospital when regular contractions have occurred every five minutes for an hour or are lasting for at least 60 seconds and coming every five minutes.

Established labour is when the cervix has dilated to about 4cm and regular contractions are opening the cervix. This is known as the **active phase** of labour and from a medical perspective is considered the start of labour. During this phase, the cervix dilates from 4 to 10cm, contractions have a more regular pattern, are closer together, and become more intense and longer lasting. There is a resting period between each contraction and it is important to take advantage of this time, relaxing as much as possible. It is also an opportunity to review affirmations made earlier. Midwife Ina May Gaskin has an interesting tip; she encourages women to arm wrestle between contractions, finding that this relaxes the pelvic floor muscles.

As labour progresses, the woman enters an altered state, with heightened senses and a changed sense of time. It helps to be in a warm, quiet, and dimly lit environment where she can feel relaxed, uninhibited, and free to go within to connect with her core essence. She becomes a vessel for a primeval force that is beyond our usual day to day experience. This highly sensitive state may easily be disrupted by other people's energies, changes in nursing staff, physical examinations, or even talking. Fear and anxiety stimulate a stress response that slows or stops the process of labour and disturbs the mother-baby relationship. Birth attendants need to be finely tuned to the mother in order to avoid disturbing her connection with the baby and her own inner knowing. Birthing is a natural animal instinct. Some women find they can more easily access their own wild nature if they imagine themselves as an animal giving birth. This is the moment the woman has been preparing for and her assistants are there to support and help empower her in her own unique process. It is crucial to be fully present with a woman, acknowledging and respecting her feelings, and providing whatever practical support is required. This could include helping her change position, giving herbs or massage, protecting her from unwelcome others, giving information, or simply keeping quiet. Laughter can be a great way to help the cervix open. Do not undermine her by either dismissing her pain or encouraging her to feel sorry for herself. She needs to feel strong and empowered rather than feeling like a victim.

As labour intensifies, or if a woman is distracted, she may find it helpful to realign with her core self in between contractions. Simple statements such as 'I align my intent with the intent of my soul' and 'My baby and I are aligned as one', or whatever wording fits for her, can quickly help a woman to return to her centre and stay present with the baby. She can send thoughts of love and welcome to the incoming soul, affirming that she is holding a place of safety and protection for this new being who chose her as the perfect mother for this lifetime. As a sacred ceremony, labour can be dedicated to a safe and joyful incarnation.

In the **late first stage**, as the cervix dilates to 8cm or more, regular contractions may increase to every two to three minutes, lasting sixty seconds or longer. The mother can be supported in adopting whatever position is comfortable, riding the waves of the contractions, like a surfer riding waves on the ocean and trusting that her body knows exactly what to do. She may find it helpful to focus on her partner's face or a curving shape in the room during a contraction.

Breath can be the key to a manageable and harmonious labour, helping to avoid resistance and pain. A good simple breathing technique can be learnt in advance and explained to the woman's birth partner who can remind the birthing woman to stay with her breath. For some women it helps if the birth partner keeps eye contact and breathes with her, saying 'I'm with you' or some other appropriate phrase.

At this stage the woman should call her midwife or go to hospital if she has not done so already.

As the cervix dilates to 10cm, there may be a build-up of pressure against the anus and rectum, or what can feel like a grapefruit behind the anus. Contractions may be as frequent as every one and a half to two minutes, being almost continuous as each one can last more than ninety seconds and some may have double peaks. The woman may experience a burning heat at the base of the uterus as the remaining tissues of the cervix are pulled up over the baby's head and the baby presses down through it.

Towards the end of the first stage, usually around 7–10cm dilation, many women experience a phase known as **transition**. This can last from a few minutes to a couple of hours (typically fifteen to sixty minutes) or may not be evident at all. The body is adjusting from the opening of the cervix to preparing to push. The woman can feel confused, irritable, fearful, hot and cold, drowsy, or completely exhausted. Her legs may shake, she may get cramp in her legs or buttocks, she may vomit or feel the desire to push, even though not fully dilated. There may be signs of an expulsive urge, such as hiccups, involuntarily held breath, grunting or groaning at the end of a contraction. She may forget she is having a baby or she might suddenly decide that she cannot cope and wants to give up the whole idea of childbirth. Encouragement and support are vital, using any rest periods for relaxation, and release of tension. If the woman wants to push but is not fully dilated, the midwife may ask her to pant through the contractions, since pushing too soon could exhaust the mother and cause damage to the cervix.

Second stage of labour

The **second stage** of labour begins once the cervix is fully dilated and lasts until the birth of the baby. This may coincide with an overwhelming desire to push (**active second stage**), or it may be that there is no desire and the body is in a **resting phase (passive second stage)**, during which contractions weaken or fade away for up to thirty minutes. If this latter scenario occurs, the woman should be encouraged to rest and enjoy these moments of peace.

The second stage becomes active when the woman has the desire to push. Powerful urges to bear down can occur in waves during each contraction. The anal pressure may feel enormous and she may pass small bowel movements when pushing.

She should be supported in choosing whatever position she is intuitively drawn to. Upright positions are ideal, including squatting, kneeling, all fours, and standing. For instance, she could be kneeling and leaning forward on a cushion, sitting on a birthing stool, lying on her side, or leaning against a table. Lying on her back makes contractions less effective and increases compression on the vena cava, which may precipitate reduced placental perfusion and put the foetus at risk of hypoxia.

There is no time limit for this stage, but on average a first baby will be delivered within three hours, and a multiparous woman will deliver within two. Longer than this used to be considered dangerous to mother and baby but it is now recognised that this view was based on out-dated evidence and health professionals are advised to consider a woman's individual circumstances and wishes when dealing with extended second stage of labour.

Using a mantra or positive affirmation

The mother can use positive words or affirmations to assist labour and help her to trust her feelings and her body. Affirmations can be repeated in the mind and are best designed to suit the individual. For instance, in the earlier stages of labour, a woman could repeat "My body is strong and knows exactly what to do" or "I open to the wondrous creation of life". Throughout the time of pushing, she might use "out, out, out" or "open, open, open" as an effective mantra.

Delivery involves synchronisation of the mother's uterine contractions, pressure from her abdominal muscles, and the baby's shifts in position in order for the baby to fit into the birth canal and travel along it to the outside world. In an uncomplicated cephalic delivery, the baby turns towards the mother's spine so that the widest part of the baby's skull is aligned with the widest part of the mother's pelvis and the skull temporarily moulds itself to pass easily through the mother's pelvic bones. The baby tucks in its chin and starts moving out of the uterus and into the vagina, which stretches to make room for the baby's head.

An upright maternal position reduces the risk of perineal tearing and if the birth is progressing too fast, getting onto hands and knees will help to slow it down. As the baby descends through the birth canal, the top of the head appears for the first time, known as 'crowning'. At this point the woman can put her hands down to feel the top of her baby's head in her vagina and know that birth is likely to be imminent. The baby has usually turned to face the mother's anus in order to negotiate the bend in the fully stretched vagina.

As the baby's head emerges from the mother's body, the mother's strong contractions will continue to push the baby out. The midwife can help the baby's head to emerge slowly and gently, helping to avoid perineal tears. The midwife will check that the umbilical cord is not wrapped around the baby's neck, and if necessary, mucus will be cleared from the baby's nose and mouth to facilitate breathing. The baby turns again so that the shoulders can slip out easily, one shoulder quickly followed by the other. As soon as possible, the baby can be placed directly on the mother's chest, covered in a blanket. Both mother and baby receive massive benefit from having uninterrupted skin-to-skin contact in the vulnerable period directly after birth. If, for some reason, she is not able to receive the baby straight away, the woman's partner, if present, can hold the baby next to their skin.

The umbilical cord should be allowed to stop pulsating before being cut and clamped.

Practices vary depending on where a mother is giving birth, but early cord clamping results in fewer red blood cells in the newborn and can predispose to retained placenta, postpartum haemorrhage, foetomaternal transfusion, and a range of possible unwanted effects in the baby, respiratory distress in particular. Delayed cord clamping results in a helpful placental transfusion to the baby and is of particular benefit for premature babies.

Third stage of labour

The **third stage** lasts from after the birth of the baby until the delivery of the placenta. The uterus resumes mild contractions soon after the baby is born, helping to seal shut any blood vessels that are still bleeding. The mother is encouraged to cuddle and suckle her baby with skin-to-skin contact, which increases the release of oxytocin, stimulating uterine contractions, encouraging placental separation, and reducing postpartum haemorrhage. This is a sublime period of deep bonding between mother and baby, an awesome time of joy and connection that will stay with mother and child for the rest of their lives. Skin-to-skin contact is essential at this time.

Typically, around five to fifteen minutes after delivery (although it could take up to an hour), the placenta detaches from the uterine lining and the mother becomes aware of a feeling of pelvic pressure. With a few gentle pushes, the placenta is usually delivered. Gentle massage of the lower abdomen can assist if desired. If a mother is lying down with her baby and the placenta has separated but not been expelled, she may be helped into an upright position to facilitate delivery. Nipple stimulation also helps. Depending on prevailing midwifery practices, the cord may be clamped and cut as soon as it stops pulsating, or this can be left until after the placenta is delivered.

The above is known as **physiological third stage** and is recognised as the appropriate care when labour is normal. Women may also be offered an **active third stage** where the cord is clamped and cut almost immediately after birth and an injection of oxytocin is given to the mother in order to stimulate contractions and cause placental separation. Usually after ten to fifteen minutes the midwife checks for signs of separation and if it is ready, she will apply traction to the cord and pull out the placenta while pressing on the lower abdomen. An active third stage might be suggested if a woman has had a very long labour, if she has low iron levels, or if she has had other medical interventions that can interfere with the natural processes of the body. If necessary, if a woman chooses to deliver the placenta naturally, she can change her mind and have an oxytocin injection at any time.

Possible complications of the third stage include postpartum haemorrhage (PPH) and retained placenta. PPH is the leading cause of maternal death worldwide. The World Health Organization (WHO) defines primary PPH to be all blood losses over 500ml occurring within twenty-four hours of delivery. It has been suggested that an estimated loss of more than 1,000ml is an appropriate cut-off point to define major PPH requiring emergency measures. A loss of more than 2,000ml is considered severe PPH.[6]

The most common cause of PPH is uterine atony, where the uterus fails to adequately contract following delivery. Contraction of the uterine muscles during labour compresses the blood vessels and slows blood flow, helping prevent haemorrhage and facilitating coagulation. Therefore, if the uterine muscles do not contract sufficiently, it can lead to an acute haemorrhage. This can happen for various reasons, such as when the muscles are overtired from an extended labour, or if the muscles are overstretched from the distension of a multiple pregnancy, or if the uterine muscles are over-relaxed from pharmaceutical medications given during labour. Uterine atony is also a common cause of retained placenta where part, or all, of the placenta remains in the body. Inversion of the uterus is a rare but life-threatening complication of third stage.

After delivery, the placenta is carefully examined by the midwife to check if it is healthy and complete. Afterwards, many parents choose to keep their placenta and it can easily be frozen to preserve for later. This is a nourishing and spectacular organ! Some women choose to eat it, making soup, adding it to smoothies or having it encapsulated.[7] Many women choose to bury it, often planting a special tree or shrub over it, and honouring it as sacred.

Phyllida Anam-Aire says that in the Celtic tradition the midwife helped expel the placenta by means of oils, massage, and sound, and the baby was wrapped warmly and placed on the mother's breast. Later the mother ate the placenta herself or put it in the earth. The eating of it ensured that no disease would come to the mother and subsequently to the child. The place where the placenta was buried was called the "place of treasure" and if ever the child needed a reminder of his or her value, they could go to the place of treasure to be reminded.

Medical pain relief in labour

See next chapter for herbal pain relief.

Inhalation analgesia, gas and air (entonox)

This is a mixture of oxygen and nitrous oxide gas. It is inhaled through a mask or mouthpiece as a contraction begins. It is fast-acting and easy to use, the mother stays awake and uterine activity is not affected. It takes the edge off the pain, can be used at any time during labour, does not affect the baby and can be used with other forms of pain relief. Disadvantages can be a dry mouth, nausea, and lightheadedness. The effects quickly dissipate once it is discontinued. Its use has declined in recent years, partly because it does not provide complete pain relief and partly due to concerns about the effects of exposure to inhalation agents on medical staff.

Opioid pain relief

Pethidine, diamorphine, and other opioids may be given by intra-muscular injection. Each one works slightly differently and has different unwanted side effects. They may help lessen pain, especially if used alongside other methods. They can cause drowsiness, orthostatic hypotension, nausea, vomiting, and dizziness in the mother. They also delay stomach emptying, which can be an issue if a general anaesthetic is required for delivery. They cross the placenta and can cause respiratory distress in the baby, or cause drowsiness.

Epidural analgesia

The epidural route is one of the most commonly used methods of providing pain relief during labour and delivery. Anaesthesic or analgesic agents are delivered via a needle into the space between the vertebrae and the spinal column in the lumbar region. This affects the nerve fibres that detect contraction pains and can be used for analgesia, with or without total motor blockade. A catheter is passed through a fine needle and inserted into the epidural space. This is left in place, allowing drugs to be topped up throughout labour. Sometimes a lower-dose variant is used, known as a mobile or walking epidural, which reduces pain without removing sensation, allowing women to move around during labour.

Epidurals are associated with a longer second stage of labour and an increased likelihood of assisted birth. With an epidural, mother and baby need to be monitored more closely and there can be unwanted side effects, including hypotension, loss of bladder control, pruritis, nausea, headaches, infection, and nerve damage.

Alternative pain relief and assistance for labour

All the methods below are complementary to herbal treatment (see next chapter).

A transcutaneous electrical neurostimulation (TENS) machine delivers small electrical pulses to specific nerves, thought to block pain signals to the brain and stimulate the release of endorphins. Two electrodes are attached to the skin and connected to a hand-held device. Women experience a tingling sensation around the site of the electrodes. TENS seems to give the most effective pain relief if women start using it at the beginning of labour. It needs at least an hour for the body to build up endorphins in response to the stimulation. TENS helps women feel in control of their pain and feel less anxious. Apart from some possible local skin irritation to the areas where the electrodes are applied, TENS does not appear to have any adverse effects on women or their babies, it can be used as long as a woman wants and then be removed.

Hypnobirthing involves using relaxation and self-hypnosis techniques to promote relaxation and reduce pain in labour and birth. It aims to help a woman deal with any fear or anxiety she may have around childbirth, helping to boost the release of endorphins and assist pain management. During hypnobirthing classes, the physiology of the process of labour is clearly explained, empowering the woman and her partner. Self-hypnosis techniques, taught and practised in advance, allow the woman to enter a deep trance state, totally focused on the birthing process and her own innate abilities and power.

Music therapy is used to decrease anxiety and increase pain tolerance in labour. Music can aid relaxation and can also be part of using hypnosis. Like scent, sounds associated with pleasure and relaxation can be recreated during labour to have a calming effect on the woman.

Birthing balls are inflatable, burst-resistant balls that can be gently bounced upon or rocked on while in labour, to aid relaxation and ease pain. These are available in varying sizes to suit different sized women, and can be useful to support different positions in labour.

Water births, in an uncomplicated pregnancy, involve immersion in water for labour and/or birth and results in excellent outcomes for women and babies. Many women find that being in water helps them cope better with pain and feel more relaxed. Sometimes being in water will slow down a fast labour. A birthing pool is larger and deeper than a bath so there is space to move around, supported by the water. Birthing pools can be hired, borrowed, or purchased for home use or they are available at some hospitals or birth centres. For a home birth, it is worth doing a trial run of filling the pool in advance in order to find out how long it takes to fill with hot water and to reveal any potential problems ahead of time. This is particularly important if a woman suspects a quick birth since she may not have time to use the pool. Avoid using essential oils in the water in order to protect the baby's eyes from contact.

When labour is not straightforward

Monitoring

The well-being of mother and foetus must be carefully monitored during any labour but does not necessarily need any special equipment.

Foetal monitoring

Monitoring the baby can be done with a stethoscope or by hand-held Doppler ultrasound monitor. If a delivery is not proceeding as expected, electronic foetal monitoring (EFM or cardiotocography) may be used. EFM can be done externally with two devices strapped to the mother's abdomen, or internally with an electrode clipped to the baby's head and attached to the electronic foetal monitor. The baby's heart rate can now be monitored remotely, so it is possible for the mother to remain mobile during labour.

Medical induction

Induction may be advised for sound medical reasons or simply because of hospital policy. The approach varies widely between midwives and obstetricians and in different hospitals in different countries. For instance, in Ireland currently, if a woman's membranes rupture, one Dublin hospital will wait twenty-four hours before induction, another will wait only eighteen hours, and a home-birth midwife may wait up to six days. Similarly, if a woman in in hospital in active labour, varying opinions and policies exist as to what constitutes 'failure to progress' or a delay needing medical intervention. For a woman with an uncomplicated pregnancy who is planning a hospital birth, it is generally wise to stay at home as long as possible.

Medical induction includes the following measures:

- A sweep of membranes (digital separation of the foetal membranes from the lower wall of the uterus), aimed at stimulating intrauterine prostaglandin synthesis, softening the cervix and avoiding a formal induction of labour. This technique can only be done if the cervix is ripe. It can often initiate labour but there are no clear benefits reported on substantive outcomes, such as reduction in caesarean section.[8] In some cases of sweeping of membranes, women have reported associated discomfort, bleeding and irregular contractions. Other mechanical induction methods have also been developed, such as the use of small balloon catheters that are placed in the cervix.

- Prostaglandin pessary. This is a pessary containing synthetic prostaglandins, typically administered to the cervix as a gel to ripen the cervix and initiate labour. It is often given the night before a full induction and may initiate spontaneous labour.
- Artificial rupture of membranes (amniotomy). The midwife inserts a plastic hook called an amnihook into the vagina and uses the point of the hook to 'nic' the membranes and create a hole so that the amniotic fluid leaks out. This can be very painful if the cervix is not ripe. It can start or accelerate labour, often triggering sudden, strong, and painful contractions.
- Oxytocin. Synthetic oxytocin, given by intravenous infusion, usually only after the membranes have ruptured. This usually starts contractions and makes them stronger. These artificially stimulated contractions tend to be much harder to cope with than natural contractions. This is associated with more frequent use of epidural analgesia and of internal foetal heart-rate monitoring. It carries a slightly increased risk of operative delivery or Caesarean section.
- Unlike natural oxytocin, the synthetic form does not support mother-child bonding.[9] If this method fails the woman will be offered a Caesarean section.

See previous and next chapters for herbal alternatives to induction.

Posterior presentation

Also known as the occiput-posterior position (OP, 'face to pubes' or 'sunny side up'), a posterior presentation is when the baby's back is against the mother's back, so the baby's occipital bone is against the back of the pelvis. Most babies turn during labour, but if not, it can lead to a longer and more painful labour that may result in an assisted delivery. Visualisation and talking to the baby can help, and midwives can advise on various positions to use during labour.

Assisted birth

An assisted birth (also known as an **instrumental delivery**) is when forceps or a ventouse suction cup are used to help deliver the baby. Assisted birth is less common in women who have had a previous spontaneous vaginal birth, and in women who have a support partner (as well as a midwife) present during labour, particularly if the support comes from someone the woman knows. It also helps to use upright positions in labour and not to have an epidural.

Episiotomy

An episiotomy is a deliberate cut made in the perineum in order to enlarge the outlet for the baby. This has become one of the most commonly performed surgical procedures in the world but it is now recognised that it should only be used to relieve foetal or maternal distress, or to achieve adequate progress when the perineum is responsible for lack of progress.[10]

An episiotomy can cause pain that lasts for weeks or months and can dominate the experience of early motherhood. It increases blood loss, may become infected and can cause serious tears because it makes the perineum less resistant to laceration. In some cases, an episiotomy may result in significant disability for months or years. Episiotomies can be either 'midline' or 'mediolateral', the latter being more common in the UK and Europe, while the former is more common in the United States.

Midline episiotomy is a major cause of third- and fourth-degree laceration to the anal sphincter, often resulting in anal incontinence postpartum. The most important step in preventing anal sphincter laceration in vaginal delivery is restricting the use of midline episiotomy. Prior to delivery, it can be helpful for a woman to have an open discussion with her midwife or doctor about how often episiotomy is used, particularly midline episiotomy.

A spontaneous tear may happen during delivery, but this tends to heal more quickly and easily because it follows the natural stress line instead of having a cut through muscle. A skilled midwife will often be able to avoid a cut or tear occurring. It helps if a woman only pushes when the urge arises, and slows down her pushing when the baby's head is about to come out.

Caesarean section (C-section)

In a caesarean section the baby is delivered through incisions made in the abdominal wall and uterus. This may be scheduled in advance or it may be performed as an emergency. An 'elective' C-section may be booked for a variety of reasons including, placenta praevia, uncontrolled hypertension, active herpes infection, or if the baby presents in a difficult breech or transverse position—the latter often occurring with multiple births. Other complications such as heart disease in the mother can also necessitate a caesarean. If a woman has had a previous C-section it does not automatically mean she needs another (see 'Vaginal birth after C-Section' page 192). Emergency C-sections may occur due to conditions such as premature labour, placental abruption, cord prolapse, or foetal distress. They are frequently the end result of an induced birth or a failed assisted birth.

If a woman is having a C-section and has the choice, it is generally preferable to have epidural anaesthesia where she avoids the risks associated with a general anaesthetic, can be awake for the delivery and have immediate contact with her baby. Either way, a caesarean entails recovery from major surgery for the mother, and the baby has a sudden transition to life, missing out on the benefits of coming down the birth canal and receiving the oxytocin and endorphins released by the mother in a natural birth. Babies are often delivered with anaesthetic in their bloodstream and bonding is more difficult. Mothers have an increased likelihood of postpartum depression.

Women who deliver by C-section are at high risk (27%) of contracting postpartum endometritis (see Chapter 13 Postpartum Care page 249). It can be prudent to prescribe prophylactic Echinacea (*Echinacea* spp.) at up to 5ml tds for a week prior to an elective C-section.

Since a C-section is major surgery, scarring and adhesions may occur afterwards. Adhesions can attach to bladder, intestines, bowel, sacrum, or other areas of the pelvic floor, causing pain, urinary or bowel dysfunction, fertility challenges, and other subsequent disorders in the pelvic floor and lower abdomen (see 'Scar Tissue' page 259).

A woman may feel particularly upset after an unplanned C-section, especially if she had a fixed and very different idea of how her birthing would or should be. It is easy to feel guilty, or cheated, or like a failure. Many women feel a deep sense of loss by not experiencing a vaginal delivery. For practitioners, it is important to raise a woman's self-esteem and gently help her come to a state of acceptance, so that she can go forward joyfully. For some women, it may be appropriate to offer the view that greater forces are at work here and everything is in divine order. The soul paths of mother and baby are intertwined—she and the baby may have made a pre-birth agreement to be here at this time and place, and the choice of caesarean could be part of that pre-birth plan. Life is mysterious.

Notes

1. Phyllida Anam-Aire. *A Celtic Book of Dying* (Forres, Scotland: Findhorn Press 2005), 50.
2. Adapted from Brenda Davies, *Journey of the Soul* (London: Hodder and Stoughton, 2002).
3. Condon J. C, Jeyasuria P, Faust J. M, Mendelson C. R. Surfactant protein secreted by the maturing mouse fetal lung acts as a hormone that signals the initiation of parturition. Proceedings of the National Academy of Sciences of the United States of America. 2004; 101(14): 4978–4983.
4. Effacement describes the shortening and thinning of the uterine cervix in labour. It is generally expressed as a percentage. Prior to effacement, the cervix is like a long bottleneck, about three to four centimetres in length. When it is 50% effaced, it is about 2cm long. When it is 100% effaced, it is "paper-thin".
5. Ina May Gaskin, in *Ina May's Guide to Childbirth* (London: Vermilion, 2003), states her view that sheela-na-gigs depict the act of giving birth and can reassure women about the capabilities of their bodies in birth. She suggests having a 'large rendition of a sheela-na-gig as part of the décor of birth rooms in maternity units'.
6. HSE home birth policies. https://www.hse.ie/eng/services/list/3/maternity/new-home-birth-policies-and-procedures/hb010-pph-guideline-hse-home-birth-service.pdf [Last accessed 15/5/21]
7. In Ireland, UK and US there are many companies offering a professional placenta encapsulation service e.g. Placentatlc in Cork, Ireland https://placentatlc.ie [Last accessed 17/7/21]. It is recommended that women who test positive for group B streptococcus should only consume their placenta after it has been heated above 70°C e.g. take steamed, dehydrated capsules rather than raw smoothies.

THE PROCESS OF LABOUR   223

8. Murray Enkin et al., *A guide to effective care in pregnancy and childbirth*, (Oxford: Oxford University Press 2000), 384.
9. Synthetic oxytocin "tends to disrupt the maternal-infant connection, interrupting natural rhythms that provide resourcing pauses, and instead causing unbearably painful, strong contractions." Franklyn Sills. *Foundations of Craniosacral Biodynamics*. (Berkeley: North Atlantic Books, 2012), 64.
10. Murray Enkin et al., *A guide to effective care in pregnancy and childbirth*, (Oxford: Oxford University Press, 2000), 295–6.

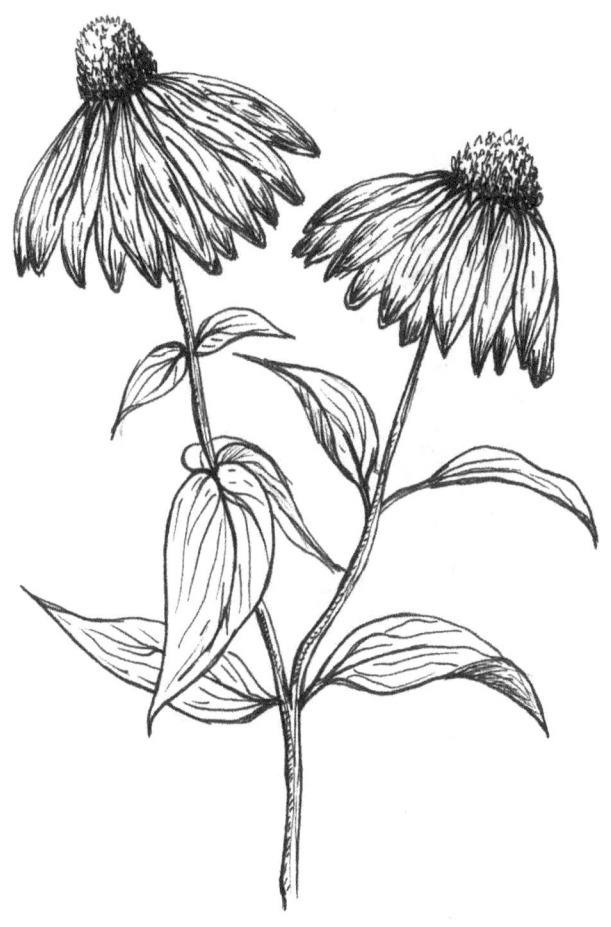

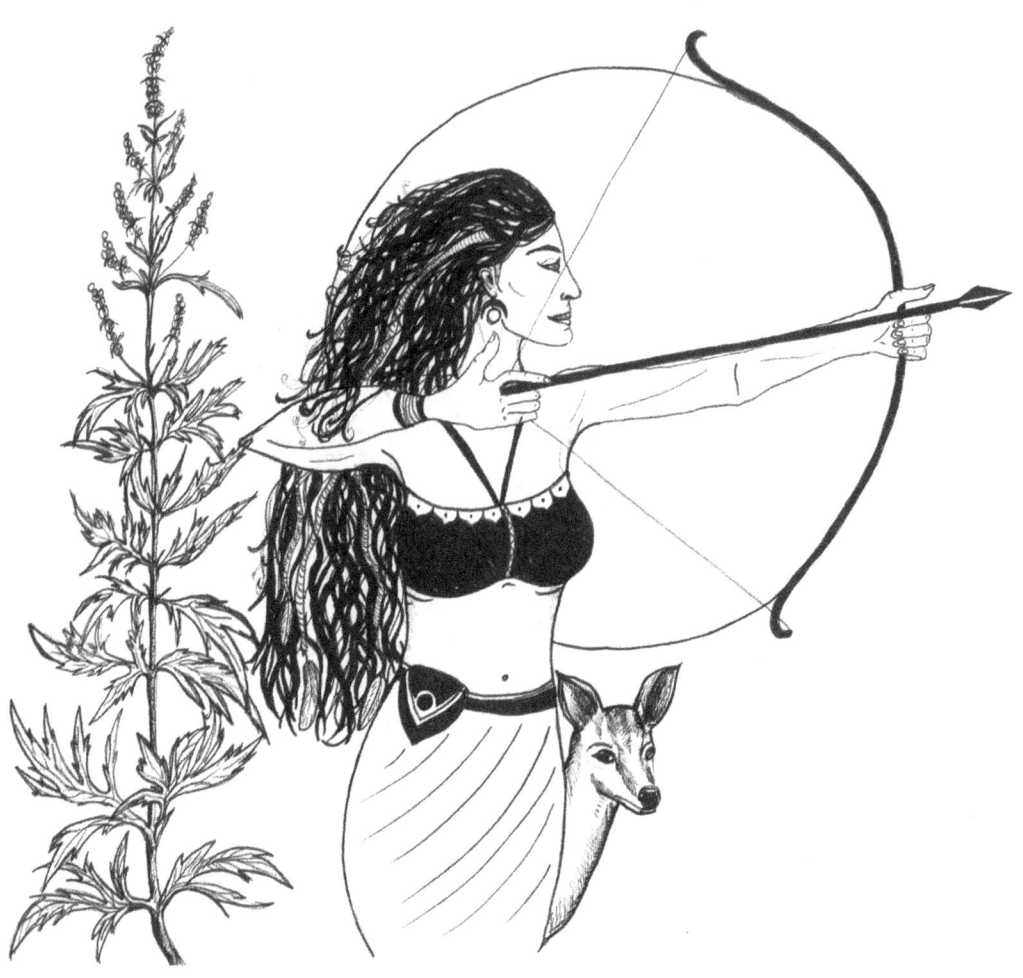

Artemis, Patron of women and Goddess of the wild and free. Protector of women and children in childbirth.
Mugwort (*Artemisia vulgaris*). Magical visionary, guardian of transitions.

CHAPTER 12

Herbs for labour and delivery

Herbs to bring to a delivery

The **Birthing Pack** page 197, contains the key items needed to support mother and baby during labour and birth. These items easily cover most common eventualities, and are suitable for the woman or her birthing partner to administer.

If you are attending a delivery as a practitioner, you may like to bring some extras that will enable you to tailor prescriptions to mother and baby as events unfold. While exact requirements cannot be predicted in advance, your knowledge of the mother and her pregnancy will help guide you in deciding what to bring. Below is a list of conditions you may encounter with additional medicines that can be helpful.

Many items in the regular Birthing Pack are useful (or can be quickly adapted) for a variety of situations, so you do not necessarily need anything extra. For instance, a relaxing massage oil can ease anxiety, relieve pain, aid contractions, and assist opening of the cervix. That said, if you are planning to attend births regularly, it is worth making up your own **Practitioner Birthing Kit** with a range of extra items that can easily be added to for individual women. At the end of this chapter is a suggested generalised practitioner kit that can be adjusted to your own requirements and preferences.

Herbs for first stage

An uncomplicated 1st stage

When labour commences, drink Raspberry (*Rubus idaeus*) leaf tea freely and take labour drops as directed on page 197. If contractions are strong, labour drops may not be needed.

Anxiety and fear

Fear and anxiety can slow contractions or stop them altogether, they represent a major underlying cause of complications during labour (see also 'Contractions'). Effective treatments include the following:

Tinctures: Skullcap (*Scutellaria lateriflora*), Motherwort (*Leonurus cardiaca*), Valerian (*Valeriana off.*), St John's Wort (*Hypericum perforatum*), Chamomile (*Chamomilla recutita*), Lavender (*Lavandula* spp.), or Black Horehound (*Ballota nigra*), 2–5ml hourly of one or a mix for up to 10 hours. See Birthing Pack for details.

Footbath: a generous handful of Rose (*Rosa* spp.) petals

Essential Oils: 1–2 drops of essential oil Lavender, Rose, Lemon, Mandarin, or Sweet Orange for inhalation on cotton pad or nasal inhaler tube.[1] Any of the same oils applied to pulse points from a rollerball or 5gtt in an oil burner or diffuser.

Essences and Sprays: 2–3 drops Chamomile or St John's Wort essence under the tongue or added to tea and sipped regularly, or made into in a spray to use around the body. If major anxiety exists, individual prescribing is the preferred option (see Chapter 16 'Vibrational Essences').

Contractions—To increase their effectiveness

Sometimes contractions are ineffective, making labour excessively long, painful, or exhausting. Herbs can support the body to increase the effectiveness of contractions, making for a shorter and less painful labour, and reducing the risk of medical intervention.

Herbal treatment is tailored to the individual and we need to be aware that contractions may be ineffective for a number of reasons, including maternal fear or foetal position, both of which can have considerable impact. In order to enhance contractions, it is helpful to assess pelvic tone in each individual. Some women have naturally high or low tone. A **hypertonic** state can lead to short, sharp, painful, and ineffective contractions, and is frequently linked with fear and anxiety causing unhelpful muscle tension. A **hypotonic** state may lead to weak, waning, irregular, and ineffective contractions, often occurring in second stage labour due to a long first stage, pharmacological sedation or uterine distension from a multiple pregnancy. Multiparous women often find that birthing becomes easier with subsequent pregnancies, however, in some cases, the more children a woman has had, the less tone and the more relaxation exists in the uterus and pelvis resulting in a hypotonic state. Both hypo- and hyper-tonic conditions can result in slow cervical dilation, a prolonged labour, exhausted mother, and an increased risk of assisted birth.

The length and ease of labour are also related to circulatory efficiency, and circulatory tonics may be indicated, as well as attention to breathing and physical movement. The woman's energy levels and vital force are naturally of significance too.

Raspberry leaves are invaluable, being a great balancer for both hypo- and hypertonic states. The tea can be drunk freely throughout labour. In late first stage and second stage, Raspberry leaf ice cubes can be sucked between contractions.

Tinctures: The **Labour Drops** (page 197) also help both hyper- and hypo-tonic conditions. Black Cohosh (*Cimicifuga racemosa*) and Mugwort (*Artemisia vulgaris*) work as a team to balance tone and promote effective labour.[2] Black Cohosh reduces excess tone and normalises contractions, dissipating those that are short, sharp, and ineffective. It assists dilation of the cervix and helps allay fear, tension, and erratic pains, as well as helping prevent post-partum haemorrhage.

Mugwort is a stimulating tonic with an affinity for the uterus. It helps sustain the uterine circulation, increases the power of contractions, eases pain, and aids delivery of the placenta.

Beth Root (*Trillium erectum*) is parturient, a uterine stimulant, anti-haemorrhagic, and oxytocic, supporting Black Cohosh and Mugwort in facilitating natural hormone release, promoting effective contractions, and decreasing risk of haemorrhage. Ginger (*Zingiber off.*) energises the pelvic area, improves circulatory efficiency, enhances stamina, and reduces mental resistance to the birthing process. Rescue essence treats the effects of any shock that may arise for mother and baby.

In most cases the Labour drops dosage of 5–10 drops every 30–60 minutes is sufficient. However, if needed, for instance if labour is stalled, 10–20 drops can be taken every 10 minutes, until strong, regular contractions are established. For stalled labour, one drop Cayenne Pepper (*Capsicum minimum*) can be added to each dose, up to 5 doses. (CAUTION: avoid Cayenne in second stage labour). Vervain (*Verbena off.*) also has a reputation for restarting labour, although I have not used it this way.

If necessary, additional herbs can be taken with the labour drops:

For severe **hypertonic** states, Cramp Bark (*Viburnum opulus*) or Black Haw (*Viburnum prunifolium*), or Wild Yam (*Dioscorea villosa*), 2–5ml hourly for up to 10 hours. Motherwort and Partridge Berry (*Mitchella repens*) are also suitable. Relaxing, antispasmodic nervines and sedatives may be included in this dosage if appropriate (see 'Anxiety and fear' above).

For severe **hypotonic** states, Golden Seal (*Hydrastis canadensis*), 5 drops every 20 mins for up to 10 hours. This is oxytocic, promoting and sustaining vigorous contractions (discontinue if woman is given synthetic oxytocin). Alternatively, Feverfew (*Tanacetum parthenium*) 20gtt hourly for up to 4 hours, to increase the circulation to the uterus and support regular effective contractions.

Lady's Mantle (*Alchemilla vulgaris*), Myrrh (*Commiphora molmol*), and Cinnamon (*Cinnamonum zeylandicum/verum*) combined with a small amount of Lavender (*Lavandula augustifolia*), will improve tone, stimulate effective contractions, and relieve pain, especially where a woman feels the need for gentle protection Rx *Alchemilla vulgaris* 25 *Cinnamonum zeylandicum/verum* 10 *Commiphora molmol* 10 *Lavandula augustifolia* 5 = 50 sig 5ml hourly.

Compress: A Ginger compress or poultice, from tincture or grated fresh Ginger, can be applied over the belly to stimulate circulation and strengthen weak, irregular contractions. A poultice over the navel is particularly indicated for a long first stage.

Massage oils: Combine suitable oils for a relaxing or stimulating massage oil as outlined in the Birthing Pack page 198.

Baths with essential oils: See Birthing Pack page 199
Inhalations with essential oils: See Birthing Pack page 199.

In her book *Women's Health Aromatherapy*, Pam Conrad, nurse and clinical aromatherapist, describes a visualisation exercise with Rose essential oil to enhance contractions: Apply 2 drops Rose oil to a cotton pad, close eyes, inhale, and visualize a Rose bud slowly opening to full bloom.

Room sprays: See Birthing Pack page 199.

Essences: Specific essences to promote effective labour include Motherwort, Derrynagittah Lily, Nurturing Mother, Skullcap. For stalled labour, Primrose. Any of these can be taken 2–3 drops under the tongue, added to tea, bath, room spray, or applied directly to skin.

Depression, low mood

Essential oils: Jasmine, Rose, Lavender, Bergamot, or Geranium (blend of 1–3) for inhalation, 1–2 drops on cotton pad or inhalant tube, or added to spray or diffuser.

If there is a risk of postpartum depression, these can be continued postpartum (see page 255 'Postpartum Depression').

Essences: Borage 2–3gtt under the tongue, added to tea, bath, room spray, or applied directly to skin. 2gtt Borage essence added to 30ml Lemon Balm tincture, 20gtt prn for a severe drop in mood.

Exhaustion

Exhaustion in the mother is a common cause of complications in labour. Women should be encouraged to rest completely between contractions and to follow their natural rhythms in eating and drinking.

Chew Ginseng (*Panax ginseng*) 'energy sticks' (see Birthing Pack) throughout labour to sustain energy. If these are unavailable, take tincture *Panax ginseng* 20gtt hourly for up to 10 hours (not with hypertension).

Ginger (*Zingiber off.*), infusions of fresh root, alone or combined with Raspberry (*Rubus idaeus*) leaf, can be sipped freely in first stage of labour with a little honey to enhance stamina and mental focus. Alternatively, add 10 drops Ginger tincture to Raspberry leaf tea.

Essential oils: Geranium and Lemon in a diffuser, oil burner, or spray to freshen room and raise energy.

Room spray: Ginger or Geranium Hydrosol 50ml Grapefruit EO 5gtt Essences of Lady's Smock and Comfrey aa 3gtt to lift the spirits and restore energy for mother and baby.

Grief

If stillbirth or other profound trauma has occurred, the mother, with or without her partner, can be encouraged to use an essence spray around herself to establish a sacred space and bring comfort. The spray can also be used around the baby wrapped in his or her blanket. The Sacred Space spray (see Chapter 16 page 305) is appropriate for this or a heart soothing Rose spray with Rose hydrosol, Rose essential oil and essences of Rescue, Borage, and Motherwort.

Headache

For headache during labour, *Scutellaria lateriflora* tincture, 5–10gtt in water or Skullcap essence, 2–3gtt under the tongue. Massage with Lavender EO, 2% in carrier oil, applied to temples, forehead, back of neck, and temporomandibular joint.

Hypertension

Combine tinctures of *Scutellaria lateriflora*, *Valeriana officinalis*, and *Viburnum opulus*, 5ml every hour for up to 10 hours.

Leg cramps

Ensure the woman is not dehydrated. Massage lower legs with Chamomile and Lavender EO 2% dilution in carrier oil.

Nausea

Sip Peppermint or Chamomile tea. Inhale 2% Lemon EO on cotton pad or inhalant tube.

Pain

Herbal treatment for pain cannot be compared to the power of pharmaceutical analgesia, but herbs can relax the mind, ease tension in the body, soothe the spirit, and take the edge off physical pain. These actions have a significant impact on how pain is perceived by a woman in labour, and how much is bearable. Perhaps even more importantly, herbs can increase the effectiveness of contractions, thereby shortening the duration of labour and reducing pain in the first place (see 'Contractions' above).

Herbal infusions tend to be more suitable in the early stages. As labour progresses, especially if in a hospital environment, it is generally both easier to administer and easier for a woman to take small amounts of tincture. All the herbs listed as tinctures can be taken as teas if preferred.

Tinctures: see Birthing Pack for suggested tinctures for pain relief. The labour drops are essential and *Scutellaria lateriflora* and *Valeriana officinalis* may be particularly helpful in addition.

Massage and essential oils: see Birthing Pack

Essences: Emotional or psychological issues may easily interfere with childbirth and result in a painful labour. Essences to ease labour pain include Motherwort and

Lady's Smock, either as stock essence or in spray form. Useful combination sprays include Sacred Birthing, Sacred Space, and Rescue.

Panic

Use any of the remedies for anxiety and fear.
>**Tea:** Cinnamon tea with 2gtt Rescue essence, sipped frequently.
>**Tincture:** Valerian with 2gtt Rescue essence 5–10gtt every ten minutes.
>**Inhalation:** Frankincense EO 2gtt on cotton pad or nasal tube. Slow, deep breaths.
>**Essence:** Rescue essence in water, sipped frequently. Rescue spray.

Rigid Os

The os is the opening in the centre of the cervix. This needs to soften and dilate in preparation for childbirth. If the os is tense and rigid, relaxation may be aided by a warm bath, relaxing music or other distraction. Laughter is good!

>**Tinctures:** Labour drops, 10–20 drops taken every 10 minutes, are usually sufficient. If additional help is needed, an effective remedy for a rigid os[3] is Yellow Jasmine (*Gelsemium sempervirens*) ☘ combined with Pasque Flower (*Anemone pulsatilla*), equal parts given as a single dose of 10gtt to relax the cervix. Yellow Jasmine relaxes pelvic nerves, allays pain, and rectifies ineffective contractions. Alternatively, 5gtt Yellow Jasmine can be mixed into 5ml Evening Primrose (*Oenothera biennis*) oil and applied directly to the rigid lip of the cervix, rubbing gently around and into the os with fingertips. The same oil can be massaged into a rigid perineum to soften and assist opening. If Yellow Jasmine is unavailable, Myrrh (*Commiphora molmol*) 10gtt can be taken as a single oral dose in water, or Lobelia (*Lobelia inflata*) ☘ 10gtt.

>See 'Contractions' above for other suggestions to relax the uterine area. If sedative nervines are needed, Black Cohosh (*Cimicifuga racemosa*) and Skullcap (*Scutellaria lateriflora*) are indicated, singly or combined, 10gtt every 30 minutes.

>**Pessaries:** If this is something that appeals to the mother, a pessary can be quickly made by soaking a tampon in an strong infusion of Feverfew (*Tanacetum parthenium*).

>**Essences and sprays:** Sacred Birthing Spray. Essences of Primrose, Skullcap, or Nurturing Mother, 2gtt taken neat or in water to moisten mother's lips.

Herbs for second stage

Perineal care

A compress or massage oil can be used to reduce the risk of perineal damage as the second stage advances. Massage the perineal area with Rose EO 1% dilution in carrier oil, or use a warm/hot compress of Rose or Lavender hydrosol to facilitate stretching of the perineal tissues (if these are not available, substitute with diluted Marigold (*Calendula officininalis*) tincture from Birthing Pack). Alternatively, essential oils or hydrosols can be used in a perineal spray.

Vulvar varicosities

These may not become noticed until labour. A warm compress of Witch Hazel (*Hamamelis virginiana*) or Marigold hydrosol, infusion, or diluted tincture can be applied to distended veins to help prevent trauma. Gentle pushing is required for delivery.

Herbs for third stage

Mother child bonding

Essences and sprays: To assist mother child bonding after delivery, take Motherwort essence, 2–3gtt under the tongue, added to tea, water, room spray, or applied directly to skin. Sacred Birthing spray.

Postpartum haemorrhage

Tinctures: Herbs to arrest haemorrhage include Shepherd's Purse (*Capsella bursa-pastoris*), White Deadnettle (*Lamium album*), and Lady's Mantle (*Alchemilla vulgaris*), all of which are powerful astringent haemostatics with an affinity for the uterus. Give 20–40gtt of fresh plant tincture under the tongue every 2 minutes or as often as required to stop bleeding (up to a maximum of 10ml). All three are effective uterine tonics. Shepherd's Purse is probably my favourite: it is a vasoconstrictor and promotes contractions, stimulating the uterus to clamp down rapidly. White Deadnettle is mildly sedative and Lady's Mantle gently uplifting. Witch Hazel (*Hamamelis virginiana*) can also be used.

Where heavy blood loss has been sustained, give a tea of White Deadnettle or Lady's Mantle, combined with Raspberry (*Rubus idaeus*) leaf and Nettle (*Urtica dioica*), 3 cups daily for 3–4 days following delivery. Continue infusions of Raspberry leaf and Nettle for a further six weeks.

American herbalist Susun Weed, in the *Wise Woman Herbal for the Childbearing Year* recommends a single dose of Motherwort 10gtt immediately after delivery of the baby in order to prevent postpartum haemorrhage.

Essences and sprays: Comfrey, Motherwort, or Skullcap essence, 2–3gtt under the tongue, added to tea, water, room spray, or applied directly to skin. Sacred Birthing spray.

Retained placenta

Tinctures: Herbs to help expel a retained placenta include Tansy (*Tanacetum parthenium*), Black Cohosh (*Cimicifuga racemosa*), Mugwort (*Artemisia vulgaris*), Raspberry leaf (*Rubus idaeus*), Partridge Berry (*Mitchella repens*), Rose (*Rosa spp.*), Vervain (*Verbena off.*), Beth root (*Trillium erectum*), Angelica (*Angelica archangelica*), and Golden Seal (*Hydrastis canadensis*).

These can be combined as appropriate, for instance, equal parts of Black Cohosh (*Cimicifuga racemosa*), Raspberry leaf (*Rubus idaeus*), and Vervain (*Verbena off.*) or Rose (*Rosa spp.*) 40gtt neat or in water, repeating after 5 minutes if required.

Essences and sprays: as for Postpartum haemorrhage.

Shock, clinical

If clinical shock occurs, for instance as a result of haemorrhage, this is life threatening and needs urgent medical attention. A woman may develop a dangerously low blood pressure, cold and clammy skin, rapid or weak pulse, lightheadedness, nausea, anxiety, hypoglycaemia, thirst, weakness, or restlessness. She may lose consciousness.

The woman needs to be kept warm and still, awake and talking. Remedies listed above for 'Panic' can all assist.

Immediate after-care

Care of the baby's cord stump

Calendula tincture from the Birthing Pack is applied on cotton wool as a healing antiseptic to the baby's cord stump. NOTE: there is no evidence to warrant the use of routine prophylactic antibiotic powders or creams to prevent infection of the umbilical cord.

Tears, cuts, episiotomy

Tincture: Bathe wounds with Marigold (*Calendula off.*) tincture (from the Birthing Pack), or use the tincture in a spray.
Herb powder: If the perineal area is very sore and inflamed, mix Comfrey (*Symphytum off.*) or Slippery Elm (*Ulmus rubra*) powder to a firm paste with water or diluted Marigold tincture. Apply as a poultice between two layers of muslin and keep in place with a maternity pad, renewing the poultice whenever the pad is changed.

10ml Marigold tincture can be added to baths after delivery as a healing and soothing antiseptic.
Essence: Comfrey essence, 2gtt under the tongue or in a drink to promote healing and restoration.

See also 'Perineal healing' page 253, Chapter 13 'Postpartum Care'.

Vulvar varicosities and haemorrhoids

Existing varicosities often become enlarged at the birth, or new ones appear, due to the mother's pushing. These may persist postpartum, occasionally causing bleeding or haematoma.

Apply Yarrow (*Achillea millefolium*), Marigold (*Calendula officinalis*), or Witch Hazel (*Hamamelis virginiana*) diluted tincture, infusion or hydrosol on cotton wool.

See also 'Varicose Veins' page 168 Chapter 8 'Conditions of Pregnancy'.

Herbal practitioner birthing kit

Adjust as appropriate for an individual woman and according to your preferences.

A complete **Birthing Pack** (see page 197)

Dried herbs:
Raspberry leaf (*Rubus idaeus*) tea
Rose (*Rosa spp.*) petals – to add to a bath or footbath
Comfrey (*Symphytum off.*) or Slippery Elm (*Ulmus rubra*) powder

Tinctures (mainly 30ml bottles):
Labour Drops (bring an extra bottle)
Yarrow (*Achillea millefolium*)
Pasque flower (*Anemone pulsatilla*) (5ml) (omit if not bringing Gelsemium)
Mugwort (*Artemisia vulgaris*)
Shepherd's purse (*Capsella bursa pastoris*) (from fresh plant)
Cayenne (*Capsicum minimum*)
Black cohosh (*Cimicifuga racemosa*)
Yellow Jasmine (*Gelsemium sempervirens*) ☘ (10ml) or Myrrh (*Commiphora molmol*) or Lobelia (*Lobelia inflata*) ☘
Golden Seal (*Hydrastis canadensis*) (10ml)
Motherwort (*Leonurus cardiaca*)
Raspberry leaf (*Rubus idaeus*)
Skullcap (*Scutellaria lateriflora*)
Valerian (*Valeriana off.*)
Black Haw (*Viburnum prunifolium*) or Cramp Bark (*Viburnum opulus*)

Hydrosol: Witch Hazel

Essential oils: Clary Sage, Rose, Lavender, Lemon

Essences: Rescue, Borage, Chamomile, Comfrey, Lady's Smock, Motherwort, Nurturing Mother, Primrose, Skullcap, St John's Wort

Room sprays: Sacred Space, Sacred Birthing, Rescue

Almond oil or olive oil to use as a base oil for massage

Evening Primrose (*Oenothera biennis*) **oil** 10ml

Miscellaneous items such as cotton wool, cotton pads, surgical gloves, empty dropper bottles and inhalant tubes, medicine measures, muslin, scissors, pendulum if you use one.

A flask of hot water to dilute or prepare medicines or simply to make a cup of tea.

Anything else pre-prepared and specifically indicated for a particular woman.

Notes

1. Nasal inhaler tubes are readily available online. These are small, capped tubes containing a wick that essential oils or blends can be dropped onto. The cap can be removed for easy inhalation and replaced to preserve freshness. The smells are long-lasting and the tubes easily fit in a purse, pocket or bag.
2. For many years I regularly prescribed a combination of Black Cohosh (*Cimicifuga rasemosa*) and Blue Cohosh (*Caulophyllum thalictroides*) both during and in the weeks preceding labour. This seemed to be highly beneficial and had no observable ill-effects. Blue Cohosh is no longer available for use by herbalists in the Republic of Ireland. I have therefore been using Mugwort (*Artemisia vulgaris*), in combination with other herbs, with increased frequency for labour and have found it to be equally effective. In my own pregnancies, as well as regular Raspberry (*Rubus idaeus*) leaf tea, I took a mix of Blue Cohosh and Black Cohosh at 5ml bd for the last six weeks of pregnancy and was blessed to have two very easy and straightforward births. The labour drops I previously prescribed were Rx *Caulophyllum thalictroides* 9, *Cimicifuga racemosa* 9, *Trillium erectum* 9, *Zingiber officinalis* 3, Rescue rem 2gtt = 30 sig 10gtt every ½ hour or prn.

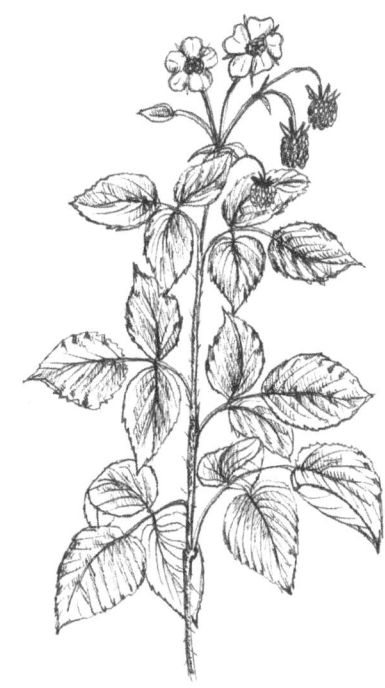

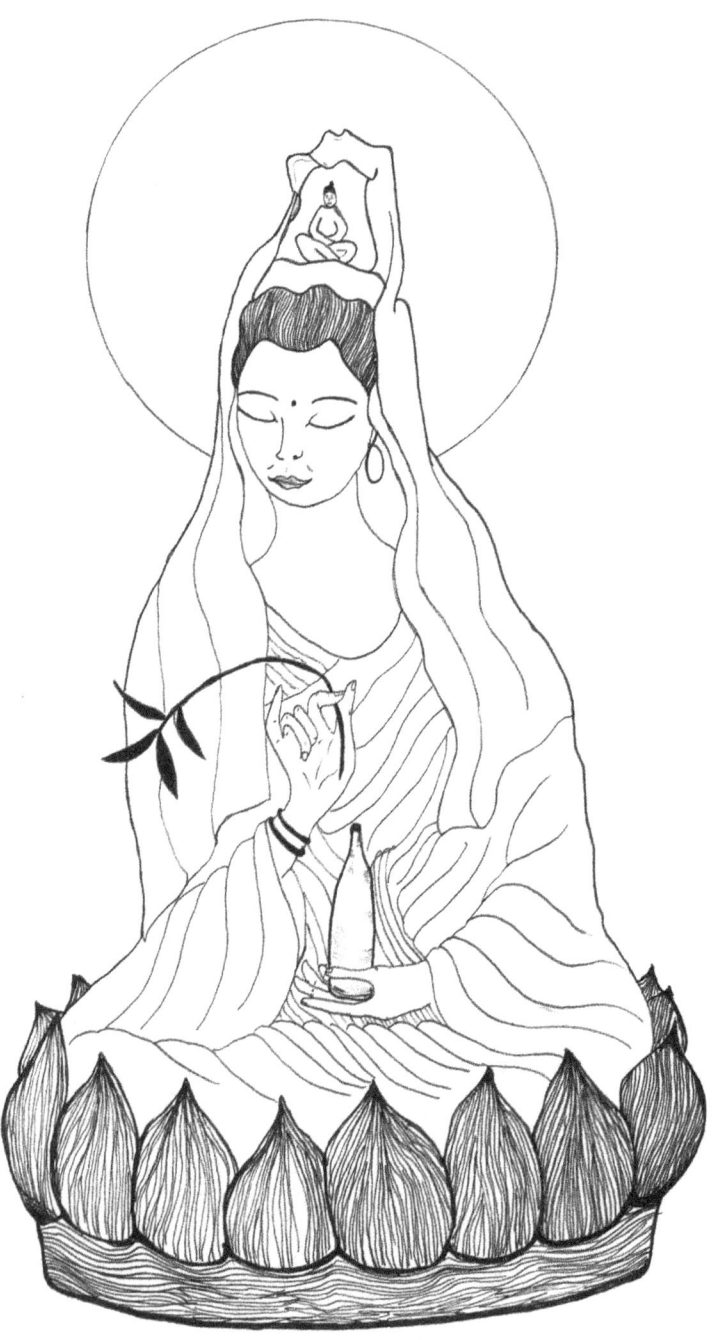

Kwan Yin. Goddess of infinite mercy and compassion. Healer who protects women and children. "She who hears the cries of the World"
Lotus Blossom (*Nelumbo nucifera*). Spiritual elixir and consciousness raiser.
Willow (*Salix* spp.). Brings flow and emotional release. Soothes pain.

CHAPTER 13

Postpartum care

Caring for women in the fourth trimester

The fourth trimester describes the first 12 weeks after the birth, a time that can be both exciting and overwhelming for a new mother. Pregnancy and birth are only one aspect of the initiation to motherhood, and care during the fourth trimester is equally important as care during pregnancy. Specific attention is needed in the days and weeks immediately following the birth to heal and restore a woman physically, emotionally, mentally, and spiritually as she embarks on the sacred journey of motherhood.

Hormonal changes after the birth

Most women experience a hormone-fueled period of euphoria that can last for 24 hours after giving birth. However, depending on circumstances, women may feel utterly exhausted, completely overwhelmed, or find themselves wishing they were still pregnant. Either way, women are likely to be wide awake and unable to sleep in the immediate postpartum period. This wakefulness is normal and seems to provide a crucial time to ponder recent events and start to make sense of the massive life changes that have just occurred.

With the release of the placenta, the hormones it was producing are gone too, including oestrogen, progesterone, relaxin, hCG, and human placental lactogen (hPL). Oestrogen and progesterone may fall to the lowest levels they will ever be until a woman enters menopause.

While oestrogen and progesterone are plummeting, there is a simultaneous surge in prolactin encouraging breast milk production, and oxytocin—which promotes a state of calm and enhances feelings of affection between mother and child. Oxytocin has been called the 'love hormone', reducing stress levels, promoting a sense of wellbeing, and strengthening bonding. High levels of oxytocin encourage the baby to seek out and latch onto the nipple.

When the baby suckles, oxytocin and prolactin are released from the pituitary, and pass through the mother's blood to the breast, where prolactin stimulates milk production and oxytocin stimulates the ejection or letdown reflex. Levels of cortisol, insulin, and thyroxine also play a part. Usually, between 50–73 hours (two or three days) postpartum, most women experience swelling of the breasts along with copious milk production (known as when the milk 'comes in'). In primiparous women, this stage is slightly delayed, and early milk volume is lower. The first milk a suckling baby receives after delivery is colostrum, the yellow nutrient-rich fluid that helps in the development of immunity. See Chapter 14 'Lactation' for details.

Oxytocin release is further triggered by skin-to-skin contact with the baby and increases in response to physical touch. Oxytocin also stimulates uterine contractions, helping the uterus and vagina to shrink back to their normal size and position in the body, and responsible for the cramps know as 'afterpains' that women may experience during breastfeeding for a few weeks postpartum. See 'Afterpains' below.

By three or four days after the birth, the rapidly changing hormone levels can cause widely fluctuating emotions, ranging from feeling sad and tearful to elated and joyful. Feelings of sadness may be exacerbated by sleep deprivation, which can contribute to decreased levels of melatonin (and, as a result, serotonin) and a rise in cortisol levels. These 'baby blues' are normal and usually last less than two weeks.

See 'Postpartum Depression' for a discussion of persistent unhappiness after childbirth.

Supporting the new mother

This is a time of great transition. Most new mothers need both emotional support and practical help in the days following childbirth. The first six weeks postpartum are a particularly important time—a woman's hormones are rapidly shifting, and she may be dealing with a host of physical discomforts, such as bruising, sleep deprivation, exhaustion, incontinence, haemorrhoids, engorged breasts, and recovery from stitches or caesarean. She also may be struggling with her changed role, new responsibilities, mood swings, and feelings of insecurity. The baby may sometimes be inconsolable, and a mother may have moments of feeling guilty, overwhelmed, and unable to cope or enjoy her new baby. Stress and worry can affect milk production.

Understandably, the baby usually becomes the focus of attention at this time and the mother's needs can easily be overlooked. In fact, it is critical that the mother's care is also made a priority. Her vital force will be depleted by childbirth and experienced herbalists will be well aware of the number of women's health conditions having their roots in the postpartum period. As part of a new mother's care, I consider it of the utmost importance to give strengthening restorative tonics after delivery, tailoring them to a woman's needs and continuing for as long as required (see below for more details).

Resting and 'lying in'

A new mother needs time to rest, recover, and be with her baby. She may also need help to develop the skills and self-confidence to care for herself and her newborn infant. The right kind of help is crucial. Some mothers are swamped by an exhausting number of visitors and need to be shielded from too many guests, over-long visits, and from looking after visitors if they do come.

Many traditional cultures have a 'lying in' period after childbirth where a woman is encouraged to stay in bed with her baby, bonding, resting, healing, establishing breastfeeding, and simply getting to know the new little person. In some traditions, a new mother is given a period of forty days to recover from childbirth and bond with her new baby. Traditional postpartum support usually lasts between twenty-one and forty days, during which the mother is prohibited from performing her usual household chores. This is commonly viewed as a way to value and protect the mother's future capacity for mothering and avoid ill health in later years. The mother is fed and taken care of by others so that she can rest, get to know her baby, and adjust to her new state of being. Forty days might be considered extreme in Western society; however, taking a period of time to rest and be with the baby is a wise decision and of massive benefit to mother and child. It is a circumscribed period of 'mothering' for the woman herself. If she is fortunate enough to have a supportive partner or other care-giver, it is realistic to suggest at least a week (preferably longer) of lying in. Some midwives advocate "five days in the bed, five days on the bed, and five days around the bed". In some countries a postpartum doula can be hired to give support during the postpartum period. These doulas offer non-medical physical and emotional support and household assistance, and can be worth their weight in gold. Receiving good postpartum care has countless benefits, enabling a woman to enjoy this precious time with her baby, and significantly reducing the risk of postnatal depression and other health issues.

Even a week of not 'doing' or caring for others can be a challenging thought for some women in Western culture, but it is well worth planting this idea as a seed in a woman's mind and may help a mother to give herself permission to be pampered.

When a woman is lying in, she and her baby will be together nearly all the time. Someone else is there to mind the baby while the mother showers, goes to the bathroom, or takes a bath. They can entertain older children while the mother rests, or if the baby is fretful, they can walk with the baby to calm him or her before the mother breastfeeds. Not only is this a time for rest and healing, but breastfeeding gets established much more easily if mother and baby are able to focus on each other. Women benefit from unrestricted access to their babies, allowing space and time for spontaneous interactions between mother and baby. Many women find it helpful to enjoy the presence and spiritual companionship of another woman (the classic 'wise woman'). A new mother can prepare for this time in advance by assembling a support team and, if necessary, by stocking the freezer and pantry to ensure she has the health-giving food she requires. Even better if kind members of her community support her by preparing and supplying nourishing food. In many cultures, bodywork such as gentle massage is an integral part of the lying-in period.

The next few weeks should be taken slowly, staying home as much as possible and with minimal demands on the new mother apart from eating well and enjoying the baby. This is the integration phase of her rite of passage. It involves an ego-death, letting go of one's previous self and one's previous life. As well as the physical replenishment, this is an immensely valuable time offering the mother an opportunity to reflect upon her experience of pregnancy, to honour what she has left behind and to consider what she may be holding onto. Who is the new self that is emerging? What has she learned through this process?

In numerous cultures, this profound transition is marked by sacred ceremony to bless and protect the mother. Many women in Western culture are rediscovering the beauty and power of marking their passage into motherhood in a ceremonial way. A blessing ceremony can be designed in whatever way a woman chooses and incorporated into the fourth trimester. Traditionally, this is women's business, the domain of the feminine. The ceremony could be with one trusted person, a few close companions, or a group, according to the mother's preferences. The intention is to help the mother feel loved, nurtured, and celebrated, offering blessings and honouring the process she has travelled through. This will empower and protect her, enabling her to step into her new role knowing that she is supported and surrounded by positivity.

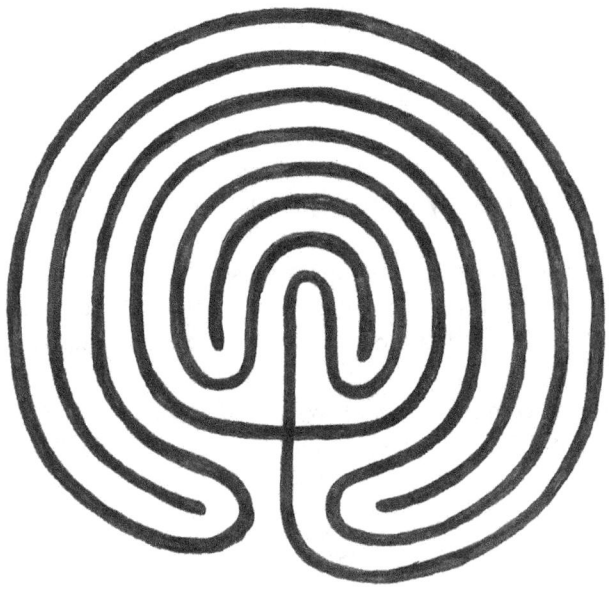

Seven-circuit labyrinth.

Simple Blessing Ceremony for a new mother

If you are performing a Blessing Ceremony for a new mother, you might begin by preparing the space with a space clearing spray, lighting candles, and filling the area with her favourite flowers. Make her a pot of a well-loved herb tea and run her a luxurious floral bath with fresh flowers and essential oils. Rose makes a lavish choice, but be guided by the woman's tastes and your own intuition. Add flower essences of choice. Mind the baby while the mother soaks in the bath and offer a listening ear if she would like to recount a story from her pregnancy or birth. Make a pampering massage oil, such as Lavender EO 4 drops and Rose EO 2 drops in 30ml Almond oil. After her bath, offer massage according to her preference: full body, feet, hands, or neck and shoulders. Play relaxing music while she takes time to rest. Feed her a delicious and nourishing lunch. If you are so called, bring a deck of beautiful Oracle cards and suggest she select one to help support and guide her at this time. Print or draw a simple seven circuit labyrinth as shown below (I use a sewn labyrinth cloth but you can easily use one that is drawn or printed on paper).

Invite her to finger-walk the labyrinth,[1] setting an intent to pass through the gateway of motherhood and be initiated into this new phase of her life. Explain that as she (finger)walks to the centre, she is letting go the residues of her previous life, including the pregnancy and birth (while retaining all happy memories). The centre of the labyrinth is a place of transformation and she should let her finger rest there awhile, being aware that transformation is taking place. When she feels complete in the centre, she (finger)walks the circuit back to the entrance, receiving blessings as she walks, and aware that she has moved to a whole new level, leaving transformed. Finally, she gives thanks for the miracle that she has accomplished and for all the blessings that she has received.

Have ready an anointing oil made with a drop of Rose EO in 5ml Rosehip oil. Anoint her head, heart and womb with the oil, offering blessings and sweet words as you anoint her into this new phase of motherhood.

Spray an appropriate essence spray around her, putting blessings into her auric field and surrounding her with love.

Shower her with Rose petals.

Blessed Be

Postpartum wraps

Postpartum wraps, also called rebozos, can heal and stabilise the body in the early weeks after childbirth. Postpartum binding has been a tradition in cultures all over the world, including Western culture, only falling out of favour in recent times.[2] A new mother is very open, physically, emotionally, and spiritually, and wrapping the hips and lower abdomen provides energetic protection, as well as giving nurturing support to help bring a woman back to her centre. Physically, it offers comfort and warmth, and supports unstable joints and muscles, helping to heal a diastasis recti (separation of the abdominal walls/rectus abdominis muscles that can occur during pregnancy), and helping the pelvic ligaments to gel back together. Wraps are warming, improve posture, and have been shown to reduce both pain and bleeding after caesarean-section.[3] They can also fulfil a woman's need for caring touch at this time (gentle massage is another option). Women tend to find wraps particularly helpful in the first week or two after birth. A strong, wide scarf can be used or special wraps can be purchased online.

Diet and exercise

Now is a time for a woman to really look after herself. She needs a nourishing and well-balanced diet with plenty of protein, fresh fruit and vegetables, unrefined carbohydrates, essential fatty acids, and adequate iron. Warming foods are indicated, for instance having stewed fruit instead of raw and generally avoiding cold, raw foods. Drink warm teas rather than cold drinks, and include warming herb teas, such as Ginger, Cinnamon, and Cardamom. Essential fats and vitamin A are depleted after pregnancy and it can take three months to a year to replenish iron and zinc stores. See Chapter 14 'Lactation' for dietary advice while breastfeeding.

Pelvic floor exercises should be started as soon as possible (see 'Pelvic Floor' below). When a woman feels strong enough, taking walks in nature with the baby is recommended as an ideal low-impact exercise.

Herbal treatment

As stated earlier, a woman's life force needs to be restored and strengthened after delivery. This is a vulnerable period for a mother. Chronic ill-health can be associated with a wide variety of postpartum issues, including the effects of injury and trauma, exhaustion, poor healing, hormone imbalance, and inadequate nutrition. What happens now can set the tone for months or years to come and may make a significant difference to the rest of a mother's life as well as her child's.

A new mother needs to be warmed, nourished, and given plenty of fluids. It is important that she stays in a warm environment, avoiding drafts, and well wrapped up with blankets, socks, and scarves if necessary. She should avoid heavy lifting, limit screen time on electronic devices, and be encouraged to stay as calm as possible.

Postpartum tonics

In my practice, postpartum tonics are a crucial part of a new mother's care, being both restorative and prophylactic. Typically, 100ml of a generalised tonic is included in a woman's Birthing Pack so she can start taking it as soon as possible after giving birth (usually the next day), for instance:

Rx *Vitex agnus castus* 20, *Verbena officinalis* 20, *Galega officinalis* 20, *Angelica sinensis* 30, *Astragalus membranaceus* 15, Rescue essence 2gtt = 105 sig 5ml tds pc aq cal.

Chaste Tree (*Vitex agnus castus*) and Goat's Rue (*Galega off.*) combine synergistically as supremely nourishing balancers after childbirth. Vitex is a hormonal adaptogenic, restoring female hormone balance, while Goat's Rue balances blood sugar and reduces the risk of insulin resistance. Chinese Angelica (*Angelica sinensis*) and Milk Vetch (*Astragalus membranaceous*) make a second powerful pairing, specifically indicated after birthing, Angelica as a warming blood and energy tonic, and Milk Vetch bringing its gifts as an immunostimulant tonic, strengthening the uterine energy. Vervain (*Verbena off.*) draws the whole mix together, combining with Chaste Tree and Goat's Rue as galactagogues, encouraging the secretion and flow of milk and thereby helping the establishment of breastfeeding. As a restorative nervine, Vervain raises energy and combats fatigue after a long labour, lifts mood, and supports the digestive process and kidneys. A few drops of rescue essence are included to help clear any residual shock and trauma. This synergistic blend restores a woman's depleted life force, warms, balances, and nourishes deficiency. If appropriate, a little Ginger (*Zingiber off.*) can be added to bring extra heat.

This prescription is reviewed after delivery and either repeated or adjusted as appropriate for the individual. In an uncomplicated pregnancy and birth, the standard mix might remain unchanged and be repeated for six to twelve weeks or longer. In other circumstances, adjustments are made; for instance, giving extra to restore energy, support hormone balance, promote healing, relieve pain, or calm anxiety. It is not unheard of for women to feel so well while taking their tonic, that at some point they forget to take it and almost invariably notice a decline in their sense of well-being in a short space of time. They rarely forget again. The wonders of preventative medicine!

Endocrine balance

The endocrine system undergoes profound changes during pregnancy and postpartum. The pituitary gland enlarges by approximately 136% during a normal pregnancy and the maternal hypothalamic-pituitary-adrenal (HPA) axis undergoes major changes, causing the adrenal cortex to secrete increased amounts of cortisol into the maternal bloodstream and leading to a threefold rise in maternal cortisol levels by the third trimester.[4] Normal thyroid activity also undergoes significant changes in pregnancy, with metabolic, haemodynamic, and immunological changes to the thyroid, enlargement of the mother's thyroid gland, and changes in thyroid hormone levels.

The postpartum period is a time of rapid change and readjustment, which for some women results in the exacerbation of a pre-existing hormonal imbalance, or the development of a new one.

For any woman with a history of hormonal imbalance (which could have manifested in pre-pregnancy conditions such as menstrual disorders, fertility issues, polycystic ovary syndrome, or thyroid disorders, to name but a few), it is especially important to pay attention to hormones and support the endocrine system. Careful questioning may reveal adrenal, pituitary/hypothalamus, thyroid, or blood sugar imbalances, which can appear after giving birth—often subtle and not necessarily detectable by medical testing. Herbal medicine can nip these in the bud, establish balance and prevent the development of a more serious condition. Chaste Tree and

Goat's Rue are invaluable here, with additional herbs as appropriate, and may need to be prescribed for several months or even years. Women who have had assisted fertility treatments such as IVF will need particular support in this area.

See also 'Thyroiditis' below.

Sitz baths and vaginal steaming—See also 'Perineal Healing' and 'Birth Trauma'

Vaginal steaming and sitz baths can speed up healing, relieve pain, and release trauma.

Unless bleeding is excessive, sitz baths can be started the day after delivery, or as soon as blood loss is manageable, soaking for twenty minutes, once or twice daily for as long as needed. Soak only once daily if sutures are in place. The new mother can enjoy a cup of Raspberry (*Rubus idaeus*) leaf tea while she soaks, and take the opportunity to practice her pelvic floor exercises, drawing up some of the bath fluid into her vagina. A combination of Marigold (*Calendula off.*) and Comfrey (*Symphytum off.*) is particularly healing and soothing for wounds, bruising, and inflammation. NOTE: use Comfrey once daily only, for a maximum of 5 days. Other suitable herbs, depending on the mother's condition, include Lavender (*Lavandula* spp.), Chamomile (*Chamomilla recutita*), Marshmallow root (*Althaea off.*), Plantain (*Plantago lanceolata/major*), Raspberry leaf (*Rubus idaeus*), fresh Shepherd's Purse (*Capsella bursa-pastoris*), Witch Hazel (*Hamamelis virginiana*) and Yarrow (*Achemilla millefolium*). Lavender EO 2% in grapeseed oil can be added to the warm sitz bath, to speed healing and encourage growth of new skin, and a handful of sea salt can be added for extra cleansing and soothing.

In an uncomplicated birth, vaginal steaming can be started once blood loss has ceased, and if the woman has no vaginal wounds, sores or inflammation. Steaming can be done as a one-off or repeated on a daily basis for up to a month, in order to cleanse and restore the uterine membrane and the pelvic area. Suitable herbs include all those listed for sitz baths, plus Motherwort (*Leonorus cardiaca*), Thyme (*Thymus vulgaris*), Partridge Berry (*Mitchella repens*), and Lemon Balm (*Melissa off.*). For caesarean deliveries, steaming can usually be started at six weeks postpartum.

Cease steaming if there is renewed fresh vaginal bleeding.

A–Z of postpartum conditions

Below is a list of common conditions encountered in the postpartum period, with suggested treatments.

Afterpains

These are uterine contractions that happen during the process of involution, as the uterus shrinks back down to its pre-pregnancy size. Involution begins during the third stage of labour, accelerates after expulsion of the placenta, and continues over the next five to six weeks. The contractions are not usually painful after a first baby but become increasingly painful after each subsequent birth, and are also likely to be painful after a multiple birth. Pain can range in intensity from mild cramps to the pain of labour, usually subsiding by 5–7 days after delivery. Breastfeeding and skin-to-skin contact trigger oxytocin release, which causes the uterus to contract, and afterpains tend to be strongest when breastfeeding.

Motherwort (*Leonurus cardiaca*) 10–20 drops before feeds is recommended to relieve uterine spasms.

Other suitable herbs include Black Haw (*Viburnum prunifolium*), Wild Yam (*Dioscorea villosa*), and Ginger (*Zingiber off.*), singly or combined. Catnip (*Nepeta cataria*) infusions can be drunk three or four times daily. A hot water bottle or hot Chamomile (*Chamomilla recutita*) compress over the abdomen will assist.

If tension and anxiety are contributing factors, relaxing teas are indicated such as Chamomile, Lemon Balm (*Melissa off.*), Skullcap (*Scutellaria lateriflora*), Lavender (*Lavandula* spp.), Valerian (*Valeriana off.*) and Vervain (*Verbena off.*), singly or combined, three or four cups daily. Any of these herbs can also be combined with Raspberry (*Rubus idaeus*) leaf tea, which assists the process of involution and is routinely recommended for a month following delivery.

Mugwort (*Artemisia vulgaris*) 10gtt tds is an alternative to assist involution.

Rose EO strengthens the uterine muscle and helps the uterus return to normal after delivery. Use a massage oil with 1% Rose EO for daily abdominal massage.

Anaemia

The prevalence of postpartum anaemia (PPA) among women in developed countries ranges from 10% to 30%, mainly due to bleeding and the amount of iron lost during childbirth. PPA is associated with fatigue, palpitations, increased maternal infection, reduced cognitive ability, emotional instability, and postpartum depression. The chronic tiredness of anaemia can also be a reason for new mothers to abandon breastfeeding. If a woman has lost an excessive amount of blood, for instance from a tear or episiotomy, follow advice on 'Herbs and dietary advice' for anaemia in pregnancy, Chapter 8 page 106.

Anal Incontinence see 'Incontinence'

Back pain

Back pain commonly persists postpartum, estimated to affect around a third of women. Pain may be considerable and last for several months or longer. A reliable chiropractor, osteopath, or craniosacral practitioner may be recommended. See 'Conditions of Pregnancy' for herbal treatment of back and pelvic pain.

Birth trauma

Medically speaking, birth trauma generally describes physical injury to the neonate. In this section I am describing trauma experienced by the mother during the birth, whether physical, emotional, mental, or spiritual. It is estimated that around 9% of women experience postpartum post-traumatic stress disorder (PTSD) following childbirth, and I suspect it is a much higher percentage of women who feel they have experienced birth trauma.

The definition of trauma is entirely personal and determined by a woman's own experience. She may feel traumatised by her birthing even if it appears smooth and easy to an observer. Her perception will be influenced by a number of factors, including personal or family history, fears, expectations, sense of control, feeling supported, or feeling disrespected. There may be an aspect of the birth that keeps coming back to her or that she wishes had been different. Her experience may trigger old memories of previous abuse. Whatever a woman's experience, she may require help in coming to terms with it and moving on. This can involve dealing with deep feelings of shock, grief, overwhelm, fear, sadness, guilt, or anger. My aim as a practitioner is to support women by being fully present with them, sensitively asking questions and listening without judgement, enabling them to feel safe enough to tell their stories. I am not necessarily there to 'fix' something, simply to bear compassionate witness, which of itself can be tremendously healing.

One method that can contribute to healing birth trauma is for a woman to write her story in a journal, describing the chain of events on one page and her feelings about it on the opposite page. For many women this helps them to process the experience, integrate, and release their painful feelings. However, another woman might find revisiting the memory only increases their anxiety, and as ever, we have to find the best methods to suit each individual. These could include professional counselling, body work, or other non-verbal expressions such as painting.

Vibrational essences can be invaluable, for instance; Rescue for shock, Borage for grief, Banishing Guilt for guilt, Blackthorn or Lapis for anger, Dog Rose for feeling alone.

The memory of trauma may be held in the physical body and prevent full recovery (this is especially the case with scar tissue—see 'Scar Tissue' below). Water is an excellent medium for facilitating the release of traumatic tissue memory, with baths, sitz baths, or vaginal steaming being particularly suited to the relief of birth trauma (see 'Sitz baths and vaginal steaming' above). Specific herbs for this purpose include Lavender (*Lavandula* spp.), Lemon Balm (*Melissa off.*), Limeflowers (*Tilia europaea*), Chamomile (*Chamomilla recutita, Chamaemelum nobile*), Comfrey (*Symphytum off.*), Marigold (*Calendula off.*), Motherwort (*Leonorus cardiaca*), Valerian (*Valeriana off.*), Marshmallow root (*Althaea officinalis* radix.), and Rose (*Rosa* spp.). Vibrational essences can be included in the water and the woman encouraged to ritually bathe or steam, with the intention of honouring her womb and pelvic tissues, dissolving the effects of trauma, and allowing the therapeutic properties of the herbs and essences to strengthen her and ease emotional, mental, spiritual, and physical pain.

Drinking teas or tinctures of Lavender, Chamomile, Motherwort, Valerian, Lemon Balm, and Limeflowers may also be indicated.

If a woman is suffering from grief and sadness, 'The Sacred Rose Bath to Heal the Wounded Heart' on page 181 can ease grief and speed recovery. Alternatively, you could design your own simple ritual for the woman to honour herself and her womb/vagina/perineum, releasing trauma and receiving blessings.

For physical injury to the perineal area, see 'Perineal Healing'.

Other physical trauma, such as injuries to the pelvic bones, may benefit from treatment from an osteopath, chiropractor or craniosacral practitioner. Some doulas and other healers are trained to perform a ceremony called 'Closing the Bones',[5] which physically restores a woman including guiding the pelvic bones back into place, as well as assisting in bringing her spirit back into the body after pregnancy and birth.

Bleeding (Lochia)

For the first 2–6 weeks following birth, a woman will experience some vaginal discharge, mainly originating from the area of the uterus where the placenta was attached. This discharge is known as lochia. For the first 2–4 days after the birth, bleeding is bright red and heavy and may contain clots or small pieces of tissue. As long as clots are no larger than a plum, this is normal. Women should use maternity pads rather than tampons since tampons increase the risk of infection and delay healing. Change the pad each time of visiting the toilet, and wash hands thoroughly before and after changing a pad.

Bleeding gradually diminishes over the next few weeks, slowly turning browny pink and eventually yellow/creamy brown/clear. Heavy bleeding or renewed bright red bleeding after the flow has tapered off is usually a sign that a woman is doing too much and needs to rest. If bleeding is excessive, it can signal a secondary postpartum haemorrhage and the woman should contact her midwife, public health nurse, or doctor. Secondary postpartum haemorrhage is defined as abnormal or heavy bleeding between 24 hours and 12 weeks after giving birth. This is usually caused by infection (see 'Endometritis'). Other signs of infection include an offensive smelling discharge, fever, and pelvic pain.

A woman's period may start again within the first six weeks, although if she is fully breastfeeding this is likely to be delayed. For most breastfeeding mothers, menstruation does not resume for at least six months after the birth and some find that their periods do not return until they have stopped breastfeeding. Mothers who do not exclusively breastfeed will usually start menstruating within two months.

Caesarean section

A caesarean section (C-section) is major abdominal surgery, requiring several days in hospital and plenty of rest afterwards. Women need to be especially gentle with themselves, avoiding heavy lifting, over-stretching, or driving for at least six weeks. Wear loose cotton clothing that does not press on the wound. Vitamin C, zinc, and essential fats all promote healing.

Caesarean section wound care

The wound can be cleaned with Marigold (*Calendula off.*) tincture from the Birthing Pack. Comfrey ointment is then applied liberally and gently to soothe and repair damaged tissue, relieve pain and inflammation, and accelerate healing.

Comfrey (*Symphytum off.*) also reduces scar tissue formation. A poultice of powdered Marshmallow root (*Althaea officinalis* radix) can be applied on top of the Comfrey ointment as an additional healing demulcent to relieve itching. Add Marigold (tincture, tea or powder) to prevent infection and further promote healing.

The area around the incision is often numb after surgery due to nerve damage. If numbness persists, apply St John's Wort (*Hypericum perforatum*) oil or ointment, or combine St John's Wort with Comfrey as oil or ointment.

Post-operative pain and healing

For post-operative pain, combine equal parts *Hypericum perforatum* tincture with *Valeriana officinalis* or *Chamomilla recutita* tincture, taking 5ml every three hours. Lavender EO inhalations also provide pain relief, inhale 10% Lavender EO for five minutes every four hours after delivery.

To assist recovery from surgery and promote rapid healing without the formation of scar tissue, Gotu Cola (*Centella asiatica*) 20 drops tds. For scarring, see 'Scar Tissue'.

Constipation

Constipation is particularly common after an episiotomy or stitches, due to anxiety about the wound breaking open or the amount of pain that may be experienced. After perineal suturing, it is normal not to pass a bowel movement until at least day three. When sitting (or squatting) on the toilet, some women find it helpful to put a clean pad over their stitches to hold them in place. Follow the advice for constipation, page 118 Chapter 8 'Conditions of Pregnancy'. Be cautious with Butternut Bark (*Juglans cinerea*), which could be passed through breastmilk and might cause diarrhoea in a sensitive newborn.

Dyspareunia see 'Sexual Dysfunction'

Emotional and stress-related conditions

See 'Emotional and Stress-Related Conditions' of Pregnancy Chapter 8 page 120, since any of the treatments suggested in that section are also helpful in the postpartum period.

Some of my favourite herbs for postpartum conditions include:

For fear, anxiety, stress, tension

Passionflower (*Passiflora incarnata*), St John's Wort (*Hypericulm perforatum*), Valerian (*Valeriana off.*), Skullcap (*Scutellaria lateriflora*), Chamomile (*Chamomilla recutita*), Vervain (*Verbena off.*), Lavender (*Lavandula* spp.), Cramp Bark (*Viburnum opulus*).

Sedative and pain relieving

Lavender, Valerian, Chamomile, St John's Wort, Skullcap, Limeflowers (*Tilia europaea*).

For mood and emotional well-being

See also 'Postpartum Depression' below.

St John's Wort, Oatstraw (*Avena sativa*), Skullcap, Lemon Balm (*Melissa off.*), Rose (*Rosa* spp.), Vervain.

Recommended essential oils can be used at 1–2% dilution postpartum. I find Rose, Lavender, and Ylang-Ylang to be particularly beneficial for postpartum emotional and stress-related conditions, whether for massage (foot, hand, or full body), inhalation, spray, diffusion, or use in an oil burner.

Endometritis (uterine infection)

Postpartum endometritis is infection of the endometrium or upper genital tract after childbirth. It occurs following 1–3% of vaginal births and up to 27% of caesarean sections. Most infections manifest more than 24 hours after delivery and are diagnosed within the first ten days after giving birth. However, postpartum endometritis may develop anytime in the first six weeks. It is typically caused by bacteria migrating into the endometrium during the labour and delivery process and grows into a full-blown infection in the following days or weeks. There is usually a mix of 2–3 organisms involved, some of which are found in normal vaginal flora. It is often a mixed aerobic and anaerobic infection.

Symptoms vary markedly from patient to patient but usually include fever, chills, malaise, abdominal or pelvic pain, offensive-smelling lochia, abnormal vaginal bleeding or discharge, dysuria, and dyspareunia. Along with a raised temperature, there may be tachycardia and uterine tenderness, possibly radiating to the adnexae. Diagnosis is clinical and rarely aided by culture.

Caesarean section delivery is the single biggest risk factor. This is further increased if the woman is HIV positive. Other predisposing factors include; long labour with multiple examinations, prolonged rupture of membranes, internal foetal monitoring, obstetrical manoeuvres, prolonged surgery, severe meconium staining in amniotic fluid, postpartum haemorrhage, retained products of conception, manual removal of placenta, maternal anaemia, diabetes or impaired glucose tolerance, pre-existing infection, history of pelvic infection, presence of bacterial vaginosis, or group B streptococcal infection, low socio-economic status, poor nutritional status, primiparity, obesity.

Herbal treatment

Home treatment is possible in early endometritis. It is vital that this is quick and effective since complications of infection include sepsis, peritonitis, pelvic abscess, and septic pelvic thrombophlebitis/septic pulmonary emboli, all requiring urgent hospital care.

At the first signs of infection, give Echinacea (*Echinacea purpurea*) 5–10ml every two hours, plus raw garlic one clove crushed into food or honey, three times daily. You will usually see significant improvement within 24 hours. Refer if no response by 48 hours or sooner if there is deterioration. Dosage of Echinacea can be gradually reduced as symptoms clear, going down to 5ml qds and continuing for at least a week. Drinking Marigold (*Calendula off.*) tea will help as an anti-infective cleanser.

In addition, if there is heavy bleeding, give astringent and antiseptic uterine tonics such as Yarrow (*Achillea millefollium*), Shepherd's Purse (*Capsella bursa-pastoris*), and Marigold. The tinctures can be combined, taking 20gtt hourly until bleeding subsides. If retained products of conception are suspected, give Mugwort (*Artemisia vulgaris*) tea, three or four cups daily. Alternatives to Mugwort include Vervain (*Verbena off.*), Feverfew (*Tanacetum parthenium*), Garden Angelica (*Angelica archangelica*), Motherwort (*Leonurus cardiaca*), and Rose (*Rosa* spp.), preferably 2 or 3 combined, as tea or tincture. Sitz baths may also be of benefit with the same herbs as above.

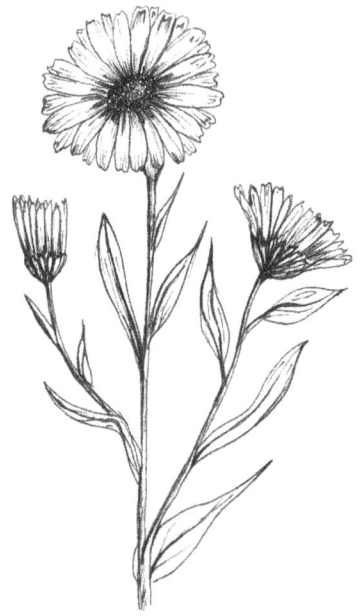

Fatigue

Tiredness is perhaps the most common postpartum complaint. It is estimated that most mothers lose between 400–600 hours of sleep in the first year of a baby's life, and that is without taking into account the extra demands of a toddler or other children.

As well as lack of sleep and normal initial depletion after childbirth, breast feeding requires significant energy, while physical healing, stress, and worry may all contribute to fatigue. Sufficient hydration and a nutritious diet remain crucial, avoiding stimulants such as caffeine and sugar. A specially formulated vitamin and mineral supplement for new or breastfeeding mothers can be recommended, as well as additional essential fatty acids. B complex vitamins are particularly helpful. This is not a time for weight loss diets.

Women should be encouraged to be gentle on themselves and to rest or nap while their baby sleeps. If this is difficult due to tension or agitation, breathing exercises or visualisations can help with relaxation (see pages 44–45). See also 'Sleep Disorders' Chapter 8 page 161 for herbs to assist. After the first six weeks, taking gentle exercise may help to boost energy.

As discussed above, herbal postpartum tonics play a significant role in restoring energy, treating, and preventing exhaustion. If a woman is very depleted, the regular tonic can be supplemented by a dedicated energy tonic. Oatstraw (*Avena sativa*) makes a valuable addition as a nutritive trophorestorative for the central nervous system, promoting energy, and calming irritated nerves. This can be taken as tea, tincture, or fresh plant juice (available commercially from Salus). Oats combine well with St John's Wort (*Hypericum perforatum*) if energy is affected by nervous disorders or low mood. Vervain (*Verbena off.*) and Skullcap (*Scutellaria lateriflora*) combine beautifully with Oats as relaxing tonic nervines. Siberian Ginseng (*Eleutherococcus senticosus*) may be helpful as a relaxing adaptogenic energy tonic (15ml mane for up to six weeks), although I tend to avoid it in the first six weeks postpartum since observing dizziness and transient visual disturbance occur in breastfeeding mothers taking the tincture. These may have been co-incidental or idiosyncratic reactions, or too high a dosage, but I have avoided re-trialing. In appropriate cases, Ginseng (*Panax ginseng*) can be prescribed as an adaptogenic stimulating tonic for lactating mothers (5ml mane for up to 12 weeks).

For a stimulating energy tea that does not cause a subsequent drop in energy, combine Ginger (*Zingiber off.*), Cinnamon (*Cinnamomum zeylandicum/verum*), and Cardamom (*Elletaria cardamomum*) and take a 20-minute decoction three times daily, or drink an infusion of Rosemary (*Rosemarinus off.*) in the morning.

Essential oils of Lavender or Sweet Orange can be used to combat fatigue as inhalations, in a diffuser, oil burner, or spray.

Haemorrhoids See Chapter 8, 'Conditions of Pregnancy' 'Varicose Veins, Haemorrhoids' page 168 for treatment.

Hair loss, telogen effluvium

Postpartum hair loss is known as postpartum telogen effluvium (PPTE), thought to be due to the rapid change in hormone levels after the birth. During pregnancy, hormone levels can cause more of a woman's hair to stay in the growth phase, often resulting in a thick, luxuriant head of hair. With falling oestrogen levels after delivery, the hair moves from the growth phase to the shedding phase (telogen). This usually begins one to six months after the birth and can last as long as eighteen months, although it usually resolves after three to six months. For normal postpartum hair loss, the best approach is to nourish, restore, and rebalance the body, having the usual herbal tonics and healthy diet. Be alert to other possible causes of hair loss, such as thyroid problems or anaemia. Combine Nettles (*Urtica dioica*) with Rosemary (*Rosmarinus off.*) for a scalp rub to help promote new growth.

Incontinence, stress incontinence

See 'Prolapse' below and 'Pelvic Floor Exercises' Chapter 4 page 42.

Incontinence of urine, faeces, or flatus is common in the days or months after delivery. Incidence and prevalence figures vary considerably, and are likely to be misleading since incontinence frequently goes unreported.

Urinary incontinence

This usually takes the form of stress incontinence, with involuntary leakage of urine that occurs on coughing, laughing, sneezing, or exertion such as picking up the baby. Urge incontinence (or 'overactive bladder') is also common, where the muscles of the bladder contract too early, causing an immediate urge to urinate and an unstoppable stream.

Vaginal delivery seems to be the biggest risk factor, and women who experienced bladder leakage during pregnancy are more likely to have stress incontinence postpartum. Other risk factors include delivery of a large baby, prolonged second stage labour, pre-pregnancy obesity, smoking, and excessive weight gain during pregnancy. Decreased pelvic floor muscle strength due to stretching of muscles during delivery is a contributory factor, as well as pelvic organ prolapse (see 'Prolapse') and postpartum uterine involution causing compressions on the bladder.

Pelvic floor exercises are an essential part of treatment (see Chapter 4 page 42) usually yielding effective results when practiced consistently. If symptoms persist or are severe, it may require the help of a physiotherapist or other specialist bodyworker.

Additional treatments include practicing timed voidings, voiding every 2–3 hours while awake to avoid the bladder getting over full. Avoid constipation and bladder irritants such as caffeine, carbonated beverages, tobacco, and very acidic or spicy foods which can all increase urgency.

Herbal treatment

Herbal treatment of incontinence may include Agrimony (*Agrimonia eupatoria*) and Horsetail (*Equisetum arvense*), taken three times daily to tone bladder muscles. St John's Wort (*Hypericum perforatum*), Cornsilk (*Zea mays*), Couchgrass (*Agropyron repens*), and Marshmallow (*Althaea off.*) calm hypersensitivity of the nerves supplying the bladder and reduce irritation.

Anal incontinence and urgency

Anal incontinence and urgency, of either stool or flatus, is associated with forceps or vacuum delivery, and anal sphincter damage such as third- or fourth-degree laceration.

It is particularly common in the first few months after delivery, and may also be associated with dyspareunia, lower back, and pelvic pain. Most women regain control of their bowels within a few months of giving birth, some may have chronic problems or go on to develop anal incontinence in later life. Postpartum anal incontinence has similar risk factors to urinary incontinence, and similarly benefits from pelvic floor exercises. Specific anal sphincter squeezes can be done to help control the release of wind and faecal urgency. Local treatment of scar tissue may also be indicated (see 'Scar Tissue').

Libido, Loss of see 'Sexual Dysfunction'
Lochia see 'Bleeding'
Mastitis see Chapter 14 'Lactation'

Pelvic floor exercises

See also 'Prolapse', 'Incontinence'.

Pelvic floor exercises, sometimes known as kegels, should be started as soon as possible after the birth, ideally during pregnancy. Following delivery, they improve muscle tone, promote healing, and aid drainage of the lochia. They do not put strain on sutures, and will start to be effective even if initially a woman cannot feel the muscles working. Strengthening the pelvic floor can help urinary and anal incontinence, treat pelvic organ prolapse, and improve a woman's sex life, giving increased sensitivity and stronger orgasms. See page 42 for details of pelvic floor exercises.

Perineal healing

It is estimated that 85% of women who have a vaginal delivery will have some degree of perineal trauma.[6] The perineum is likely to be sore and swollen, and is often bruised, torn, or may have been cut and repaired. This can cause a considerable amount of pain, as well as resulting in urinary retention and incontinence, usually taking the form of stress incontinence (see 'Incontinence'). Vulvar varicosities may have become enlarged during labour (see Chapter 8 'Conditions of Pregnancy', Varicose Veins page 168 for treatment, avoiding steaming until lochia is minimal). Perineal trauma can also contribute to constipation (see 'Constipation') and sexual dysfunction (see 'Sexual Dysfunction').

It helps to drink plenty of fluids to keep the urine dilute and reduce perineal stinging.

Some women prefer to sit on a rubber ring to take the pressure off the perineum.

Herbal treatment

For vulval bruising, swelling, soreness, wounds, tears, or varicosities, apply Marigold (*Calendula off.*) or Witch Hazel (*Hamamelis virginiana*), diluted tincture, tea or hydrosol, as a compress on a cotton pad or lotion on cotton wool. Add Yarrow (*Achillea millefolium*), if there is excessive perineal bleeding.

Alternatively, if the area is initially too painful to touch, the same lotion can be used in a spray bottle, spraying the tender area every time the woman goes to the toilet. Most women can tolerate the 25% alcohol strength Marigold provided in the Birthing Pack, but some may need it to be more dilute in the first day or two after birth e.g. diluted 1:10 in water. If necessary, try a high dilution first and work backwards. Tea or hydrosol can be a gentle option, although tea is less easy in hospital and hydrosol not generally as effective as tincture.

Homeopathic Arnica (*Arnica montana*) 30 tablets can be recommended as an additional treatment for shock and bruising, starting as soon as possible after delivery. Dose is two tablets every two hours for six doses, followed by two tablets three times daily for six days.

As well as using a compress or lotion, a healing ointment can be applied liberally to the perineum. Marigold has pride of place as a healing antiseptic while Comfrey (*Symphytum off.*) is ideal to accelerate healing, soothe inflammation, ease bruising, and prevent scarring. They can be used singly or combined with excellent effect. For instance, make an ointment of Marigold and Comfrey, adding a small amount of Rosehip (*Rosa canina* fructus) oil to further promote healing and reduce the risk of scar formation. A few drops of a Rescue essence can be included to help release the effects of trauma. Apply several times daily.

Regular use of a healing ointment will strengthen and restore the perineal area and also helps prevent irritation from menstrual pads which may otherwise sometimes occur when pads are required for a number of weeks postpartum.

For infected wounds, use Marigold lotion and ointment as above, or apply a poultice of Slippery Elm (*Ulmus rubra*) powder mixed with Echinacea (*Echinacea* spp.) or Golden Seal (*Hydrastis canadensis*) powders and Marigold tea. Reapply whenever pads are changed.

Sitz baths are particularly beneficial for healing the perineum and relieving pain. See 'Sitz baths' page 244 for details and suitable herbs. If pain is severe, take a sitz bath, and afterwards apply a soothing poultice of Marshmallow root (*Althaea officinalis* radix.) powder combined with Aloe Vera gel (*Aloe barbadensis*). If additional analgesia is required, combine equal parts of Valerian (*Valeriana off.*) and Hypericum (*Hypericum perforatum*) tinctures, taking 5 ml every three hours. Chamomile (*Chamomilla recutita*) tea or tincture is also helpful, or inhale 10% Lavender EO for five minutes every four hours after delivery.

For scarring, see 'Scar Tissue'.

Postpartum depression

Postpartum (postnatal) depression is a common and serious problem in new mothers, estimated to affect much higher numbers than the 10 to 15% widely reported.[7] It can also affect fathers and partners. Postnatal depression may start any time in the first year, although a danger point does seem to occur around 6–12 weeks after the birth.

Unhappiness after childbirth is closely related to a lack of social and psychological support at what is a time of profound change and transformation in a person's life. It often takes time to adapt to becoming a new parent and looking after a small baby can be stressful and exhausting. Sadly, the view of pregnancy and birth as a major rite of passage is rarely acknowledged in our society and the event may be experienced by the mother as a massive shock. In fact, shock can be helpful for personal growth because it breaks down stuck patterns and old habits, leaving us free to make new choices. Shock can free us and help us become more truly who we are. However, this kind of change is rarely easy and certainly not always welcome, especially if we do not understand what is happening and we have insufficient support. An initiation to a new state of being is a challenging process and it is normal for it to bring up difficult feelings. For new parents, this is a time of personal death and rebirth. There may be a necessary period of mourning, for instance for a different type of birthing, the loss of one's old self or one's previous life. All sorts of questions and unfamiliar feelings may arise. This is a natural part of the growth process. Women may feel totally overwhelmed by responsibility and have little idea or support in how to deal with these feelings. Huge expectations are placed on them of what a 'normal' woman and mother should be. Many women feel inadequate, guilty, and simply not good enough when faced with these expectations. They commonly do not have time to process their new state, and begin cooking, cleaning, and caring for others much too soon.

When all these factors are combined with exhaustion and a lack of social support, it is no surprise that the results can sometimes be devastating. Women often feel isolated and alone, they may develop persistent feelings of sadness and withdrawal, frequent tearfulness, fear and anxiety, trouble sleeping at night and feeling tired during the day, difficulty bonding with their baby and having frightening thoughts such as harming the baby, panic attacks and new phobias, a sense of unreality and feeling they are going mad, difficulty concentrating and making decisions, feelings of pointlessness and apathy, fears around their own health or that of the baby, not wanting to leave the baby with someone else, poor appetite, and lack of interest in sex. Signs and symptoms often develop gradually and are unrecognised by the woman herself, who typically feels guilty that she is not 'coping' as well as she feels she 'should'.

Risk factors include a family history of depression, previous history of mental illness, being raised in a dysfunctional family, sleep disturbance, a compromised or unwell baby, a poor relationship with one's partner, hypothyroid, isolation from family and friends, lack of emotional or financial support, and recent stressful life events, such as bereavement.

There is a need for support and counselling in a space of non-judgemental listening where women are free to talk about their feelings. Society expects new mothers to be ecstatic, and if a woman is unhappy it can be difficult for her to articulate this. It is important to look at her social circumstances in order to suggest a realistic plan of action for recovery. In practice, I prefer to avoid the term 'postnatal depression' because in my opinion it falsely medicalises a condition that is primarily sociological, related to society's unrealistic expectations of women and failure to honour rites of passage. In recent times I have been heartened to hear the condition being renamed 'unhappiness after childbirth' by certain medical professionals.[8] In the bigger picture, I hope that social conditions will shift in order to change the expectations placed on women, properly acknowledge important rites of passage, and provide appropriate care for new mothers. Postpartum doulas currently offer a much-needed service for a small number of women, and I look forward to a day when this kind of care is available to all, regardless of finances and individual circumstances.

It is crucial for a woman to have someone to talk openly to, whether a friend, family member, therapist, or other health practitioner. Herbalists can support women by encouraging them to talk, listening without judgement, and offering practical advice. Women often need reminding not to blame themselves and that being depressed does not mean they are a 'bad mother', neither does it mean they are going mad.

Simple steps to recovery include sufficient rest and sleep, making time for self, regular exercise such as daily walking, and a healthy diet ensuring adequate B vitamins especially B6, zinc, chromium, and essential fatty acids. Tryptophan-rich foods are helpful, including chicken, turkey, salmon, kidney beans, oats, lentils, chick peas, sunflower and pumpkin seeds, potatoes, walnuts, and avocado. Ensure healthy levels of magnesium and calcium. Some women swear by eating their placenta to offset postpartum depression (see page 216).

Herbal treatment

Hormone levels are a factor, notably low thyroid, but the endocrine system needs to be assessed and treated as a whole (see also 'Thyroiditis'). Hormone balance must be viewed in the context of a woman's life and the body-mind-spirit connections. It is crucial not to simply blame hormones and overlook the underlying causes of imbalance.

For herbal prescribing, the endocrine and nervous systems are usually the key areas to address. The hypothalamic-pituitary-adrenal (HPA) axis may need particular attention. Some of my most valued herbs for treatment here include Chaste Tree (*Vitex agnus castus*), Lady's Mantle (*Alchemilla vulgaris*), Passionflower (*Passiflora incarnata*), Skullcap (*Scutellaria lateriflora*), Vervain (*Verbena off.*), Oats (*Avena sativa*), St John's Wort (*Hypericum perforatum*), Lemon Balm (*Melissa off.*), Siberian Ginseng (*Eleutherococcus senticosus*), Rosemary (*Rosemarinus off.*), Rose (*Rosa* spp.), Roseroot (*Rhodiola rosea*), Valerian (*Valeriana off.*), Lavender (*Lavandula augustiflolia*), and Cramp bark (*Viburnum opulus*). See 'Emotional and Stress-Related Conditions of Pregnancy' Chapter 8 page 120 and 'Sleep Disorders' page 161 for further details.

Flower essences

Flower essences are a valuable part of treatment, for instance Rescue for shock and trauma, Lady's Smock for helping adjustment to change, Little Saints for feelings of overwhelm, Dog Rose for isolation, Nurturing Mother for exhaustion, Borage for grief and tearfulness, Motherwort to aid bonding.

Essential oils

Essential oils are effective for daily hand, foot, or full body massage, adding to bath or footbath, inhalations, use in spray, diffuser, or burner. Appropriate oils include Rose, Lavender, Bergamot, Geranium, Neroli, Rose, Ylang-Ylang (blend of 1–3).

Additional supports

It is important for a woman to make time for herself and choose activities that she enjoys. She may benefit from therapies such as massage, reflexology, hypnotherapy, craniosacral, psychotherapy, or cognitive behavioural therapy (CBT).

Infant massage provides numerous physical, psychological, and emotional benefits for babies and their mothers, and it has been shown that women who give their babies regular baby massage have less postpartum depression.[9]

Prolapse, pelvic organ prolapse (POP)

Postpartum prolapse occurs when the muscles and tissues supporting the pelvic region weaken and stretch under the pressure of pregnancy and childbirth, causing one or more of the pelvic organs to slip down from their normal position and protrude into the vaginal canal. There are various types of pelvic organ prolapse including Uterine prolapse, vaginal vault prolapse (prolapse of vaginal walls), cystocele (prolapse of bladder), urethrocele (prolapse of urethra), cystourethrocele (prolapse of both bladder and urethra), rectocele (prolapse of rectum), and enterocele (prolapse of small bowel). A prolapse is not life-threatening but can cause pain and discomfort, especially in later stages if the prolapse becomes exposed outside of the vagina.

It is estimated that more than 50% of women will develop prolapse symptoms at some point in their lives, with childbirth being a high risk factor.[10] For some women this occurs straight away as a postpartum prolapse, for others it may happen later in life, particularly after menopause.

Throughout pregnancy, the increased laxity of pelvic tissues plus the weight of the growing foetus contribute to extra pressure being exerted by the pelvic organs. The pushing and pressure of childbirth cause additional stretching of ligaments and fascia, especially if there is a long second stage, assisted delivery, or multiple deliveries.

Returning to normal activity too soon is another major cause of prolapse, or the premature return to high-impact exercise. Joint hypermobility is a contributory factor for some women.

Postpartum prolapse usually improves over time, particularly when relaxin levels drop after ceasing to breastfeed, reducing tissue laxity and helping the pelvis to stabilise.

Signs and symptoms of prolapse include urinary incontinence (usually manifesting as stress incontinence), frequent bladder infections, urinary frequency and urgency, dysuria, constipation, dyspareunia, feelings of pressure, dragging or heaviness in the pelvic area, lower back or pelvic pain, difficulty inserting a tampon or keeping one in place, a visible bulge of tissue protruding from the vagina, either permanently or on coughing or straining. Typically, symptoms get progressively worse on standing or throughout the day. Medical approaches for chronic prolapse include fitting a vaginal pessary or undergoing targeted surgery.

Physical therapy combined with herbs can work wonders for prolapse. Daily pelvic floor exercises are indicated (see Pelvic Floor Exercises page 42) and can usefully be combined with breathing exercises. If necessary, find a good physiotherapist to assist. Avoid caffeine, carbonated drinks, alcohol, and smoking. Maintain a healthy weight and avoid constipation and straining. Learn to lift heavy weights (including children) safely,[11] avoid too much high impact exercise, and treat any persistent cough that may otherwise cause or contribute to a weakening of the pelvic floor muscles.

Herbal treatment

Warm sitz baths can help cleanse and tone the pelvic tissues, promoting blood flow and encouraging the organs back upwards. Suggested herbs include Raspberry leaf (*Rubus idaeus*), Marigold (*Calendula off.*), Plantain (*Plantago lanceolata/major*), White Deadnettle (*Lamium album*), Rosemary (*Rosemarinus off.*), Horsetail (*Equisetum arvense*), Rose (*Rosa* spp.). Bathe two or three times per week.

For internal treatment, Raspberry leaf (*Rubus idaeus*), Milk Vetch (*Astragalus membranaceus*), Partridge berry (*Mitchella repens*) and Black Haw (*Viburnum prunifolium*) all promote pelvic tone, reducing prolapse and vaginal laxity.

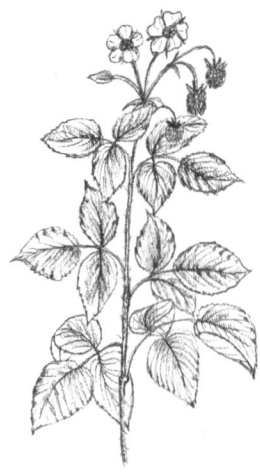

Scar tissue

Scarring and adhesions are key factors involved in a wide range of women's pelvic health issues. During childbirth, scar tissue can arise from injury or surgery. It may form after a tear, stitches, episiotomy, C-section, forceps or vacuum delivery, or simply from a vaginal birth, for instance if the baby was stuck in the pelvis for an extended time. Adhesions may also form, where thin sheets of scar tissue form between organs and tissues in the abdomen or pelvis, connecting the surfaces and causing pain from obstruction, stretching, or pulling at nerves. Women may have pre-existing pelvic scar tissue from gynaecological procedures or surgery, sexual abuse, or conditions such as endometriosis. See 'Caesarean Section' and 'Perineal Healing' for treatments to prevent scarring.

A scar is a physical representation of trauma. Memory is not only stored in the brain but also in our cells and tissues, and emotions experienced at the time of a physical trauma can be held as tissue memory in a scar.[12] In this way, scar tissue may hold the memory of an event, including emotions such as fear, anger, or sorrow. If these are not released, they can become locked into the scar tissue and remain as a damaging influence in the body, leading to manifestations such as physical pain and adhesions, as well as emotional manifestations where the trapped emotions may become re-activated by day-to-day events, for instance, causing emotional outbursts. I view this as a version of homeostasis, where the human organism is constantly attempting to restore a state of healthy balance. In this case, the body is doing its best to release unhealthy emotions from the cells. A full discussion of cellular memory[13] is outside the scope of this book, but it is highly beneficial to be mindful of this topic when treating women with perineal or C-section scars, or indeed any scarring. Plant medicine has a lot to offer in this area (see below).

Emotions commonly arise when scar tissue is touched for the first time. Physically, there is often numbness and sensitivity, frequently turning to tingling as sensation gradually returns. Over time, which may be short or long, old memories and emotions can spontaneously arise and be released. This can happen during a treatment, such as a gentle massage or herbal oil pack, or the release may be part of a less conscious process. What is important is that once the traumatic memories are cleared, the woman will feel a definite shift both physically and emotionally. Chronic pain may be relieved and her memory of the original trauma will be no longer associated with the same 'negative' emotions, with the result that she can now view the experience from a place of calm detachment. Often a woman receives some new insight, invariably she has the sense of freedom and a burden being lifted.

Herbal treatment

For perineal and C-section scarring, herbal oils, essences, heat, and gentle massage all make effective local treatments to soften scar tissue and release trapped emotional energy. Comfrey (*Symphytum off.*) and Rosehip (*Rosa canina* fructus) oils are both excellent to accelerate healing and aid tissue regeneration in the treatment of scars following surgery. Rosehip oil is rather unstable and the addition of vitamin E will reduce rancidification. Essential oils and essences can be added as required. Sandalwood essential oil is my favourite choice for scar tissue. Alternatives include Lavender, Neroli, and Frankincense. Birds Foot Trefoil and Comfrey essences both aid the release of tissue trauma and promote deep healing.

Herbs taken internally can facilitate the softening and breaking down of scar tissue with resultant release of tissue memory. Marigold (*Calendula off.*), tea or tincture, is superb for clearing pelvic and abdominal adhesions, and Marshmallow (*Althaea officinalis* radix) can be included to gently soften the energetic release of harsh cellular memory.

Scar breakdown oil

This oil is suitable for perineal or C-section scars and the same oil can be used both for massage and oil packs. Women can use the oil for twice daily massage and do the oil pack once or twice a week.

Rx Comfrey infused in Almond Oil 25, Rosehip Oil 5, vitamin E contents of one or two 250iu capsules, Sandalwood EO 10gtt, Comfrey Essence 3gtt.

For massage: Lie on back and apply oil with gentle touch, morning and night. Touch may need to be brief and as light as a feather in the beginning, generally becoming firmer over time. Be guided by intuition. To assist breakdown of scar tissue, when ready, make 20–30 small circular motions with fingertips.

For an oil pack: Soak a warm flannel or piece of cotton cloth in oil, lie on back and apply cloth to area of scarring. Cover with a layer of non-absorbent material, such as parchment paper or a thin sheet of plastic. Cover this with a towel and lastly a hot water bottle. Remain lying down for twenty minutes: relaxing, reading, meditating, listening to music, or whatever feels good. Remove the pack and massage any remaining oil into the scar. This is best done before bed.

Castor oil packs

Castor oil can penetrate deep into the body and has the ability to break down scar tissue, adhesions, and other abnormalities in the abdomen and pelvis. It reduces pain and inflammation, stimulates the lymphatic system, and promotes growth of healthy tissue. A Castor oil pack is an effective method to break down scar tissue but may be too strong for a woman in the twelve weeks postpartum, especially if she is breastfeeding. Regular use stimulates powerful detoxification generally requiring concurrent support of internal medicines. Castor oil packs can be something to consider for later if needed. The method is the same as the oil pack described above.

Sexual dysfunction

Childbirth brings many changes affecting sexual function in the postpartum period. Sexual function declines significantly in the fourth trimester due to factors such as perineal trauma, exhaustion, lack of vaginal lubrication, dyspareunia, stress, anxiety, and depression. Women may experience incontinence of urine, flatus or stool, pelvic organ prolapse, difficulty reaching orgasm, vaginal bleeding, or irritation after sex. They may have body-image issues and cultural influences can also play a part, with some cultures forbidding sexual intercourse for a period of time after childbirth.

No wonder that most women report very low libido for three months after giving birth.

This is normal and can also be the case for men, whose testosterone levels can drop by a third in the first six months after having a baby.[14] If a woman is tired and sore it may be helpful to find other ways to be close and loving for a while. Typically, a woman's libido increases significantly by 6 months postpartum, although it may not yet be back to pre-pregnancy levels. Fear of pregnancy can also be a factor, and unless another baby is wanted straight away, it is important to use contraception since there is a risk of conceiving even if breastfeeding. Sleep and good nutrition are vital for healing and restoration. B6 and zinc can be particularly beneficial for raising libido.

While a temporary reduction in libido is acceptable, women should not be left experiencing ongoing dyspareunia. If these symptoms remain untreated a woman may develop a fear of having intercourse and the issue can escalate, resulting in long-term physical and psychological damage.

Perineal trauma is a major factor in dyspareunia and needs immediate attention (see 'Perineal Healing'). Discomfort during intercourse may be helped by using a lubricant, especially in a breastfeeding woman where hormone levels can cause thinning and dryness of the vaginal tissues. Pelvic floor exercises can also make a significant difference to sexual function (see 'Pelvic Floor Exercises').

Herbal treatment for pain

Pasque Flower (*Anemone pulsatilla*) is my favourite herb for reproductive pain. However, it is said to be contraindicated in lactation, so caution is required in breastfeeding mothers.[15] Anemone relieves vaginal and pelvic sensitivity, while easing fear and apprehension. Ten drops of tincture daily, taken at night. Alternatives include Skullcap (*Scutellaria lateriflora*), Passionflower (*Passiflora incarnata*) and Vervain (*Verbena off.*), up to 5ml tds, singly or combined. Almond oil, 50ml with a drop of Lavender essential oil can be used as a lubricant.

Herbs for low libido

Postpartum tonics, as described above, will replenish blood and vital energy, support hormone balance and thereby aid sexual function. A healthy sex life depends on good ovarian, adrenal, and pituitary function, as well as psychological well-being.

Herbs I find of particular value to support and raise libido include Chaste Tree (*Vitex agnus castus*), Saw Palmetto (*Serenoa repens*), Damiana (*Turnera diffusa*), Siberian Ginseng (*Eleutherococcus senticosus*), Passionflower (*Passiflora incarnata*), Liquorice (*Glycyrhhiza glabra*).

Ylang-Ylang essential oil has aphrodisiac properties and can be incorporated into an oil for massage or used for inhalation or in an oil burner or diffuser. Rose EO may similarly be helpful.

Sleep (see 'Fatigue' above and herbal treatments listed under 'Sleep Disorders' page 161 Chapter 8 'Conditions of Pregnancy')
Stress Incontinence (see 'Incontinence')

Thyroiditis, postpartum

Postpartum thyroiditis is defined as thyroid dysfunction occurring in the first twelve months after having a baby, miscarriage, or termination. It is the most common endocrine disorder associated with pregnancy, an autoimmune condition believed to affect between 5 and 7% of postpartum women, and probably under-diagnosed.[16] Risk factors include type I diabetes, thyroid autoantibodies, history or family history of thyroid disease.

The exact cause is unknown, but the condition is precipitated by the postpartum immunological rebound that occurs after the immune system changes of pregnancy.

It can present with diverse clinical presentations and may lead to chronic hypothyroidism. Most commonly, there is an initial stage of hyperthyroidism, usually between one to six months after pregnancy, causing symptoms such as anxiety, tachycardia or irregular beats, irritability, sensitivity to heat, unexplained weight loss, tremor, insomnia, and excessive hair loss. This stage usually last two to four months and frequently goes undiagnosed. The thyroid may then return to normal, or the woman may develop a hypothyroid condition (between three to twelve months after the pregnancy) with typical symptoms such as weight gain, fatigue, depression, poor memory, dry skin, constipation, muscle pain, and aversion to cold. This second stage can last up to a year after the pregnancy and may then resolve spontaneously. A small group of women will be left with chronic hypothyroidism, and for any woman, a diagnosis of postpartum thyroiditis indicates a high risk of thyroid disease in later life, and may predispose to cardiovascular disease.

To treat or prevent postpartum thyroiditis, a woman needs a balanced diet of protein, healthy fats, and high-quality nutrient-dense carbohydrates with plenty of vegetables. Avoid processed foods and ensure high levels of vitamins and minerals, especially vitamin C, B vitamins, magnesium, zinc, and iron. Eat regular meals throughout the day, eating slowly and in a relaxed fashion. Take daily walks in the fresh air.

Selenium supplementation (100–200 ug daily) has been identified as potentially preventative of postpartum thyroiditis although more studies are needed.

Herbal treatment involves balancing the entire endocrine system. Adrenal balance is intimately connected to healthy thyroid function, and postpartum thyroiditis often reflects a situation of high stress and a degree of adrenal overactivity or exhaustion. It is vital to reduce stress and thereby limit the release of cortisol from the adrenals (see 'Emotional and Stress-Related Conditions'). The adrenals may need nourishing and restoring. Passionflower (*Passiflora incarnata*) and Pasque Flower (*Anemone pulsatilla*) can calm and soothe the adrenals, while Liquorice (*Glycyrrhiza glabra*) and Roseroot (*Rhodiola rosea*) can nourish. Siberian Ginseng (*Eleutherococcus senticosus*) is both restorative and relaxing for adrenals and thyroid, although caution is advised in prescribing Eleutherococcus to breastfeeding mothers in the first 6 weeks postpartum. Motherwort (*Leonurus cardiaca*), and Lemon Balm (*Melissa off.*) can calm an overactive thyroid, while Bladder Wrack (*Fucus vesiculosis*) and Irish Moss (*Chondrus crispus*) are nutritive. For women who are not breastfeeding, Bugleweed (*Lycopus virginicus/europaeus*) can be helpful to reduce excessive thyroid activity (contraindicated in lactation). Chasteberry (*Vitex agnus castus*) may also play a valuable role. All endocrine activity needs evaluation, as well as giving support to liver and digestive function.

Urinary Incontinence (see 'Incontinence')
Urinary Tract Infection (see 'Urinary Tract Infection' page 164 Chapter 8 'Conditions of Pregnancy')
Uterine Contractions (see 'Afterpains')
Uterine Infection (see 'Endometritis')
Vulvar Varicosities (see 'Varicose Veins' page 168 Chapter 8 'Conditions of Pregnancy')

Notes

1. Labyrinths may be seen as womb-like representations of the Divine Feminine, facilitating transformation and rebirth. They can be used as a form of meditation to relax the mind into a focused and peaceful state. To finger-walk a labyrinth, simply place your finger at the entrance to the labyrinth, set your intention, (in this case to step fully into a new phase as a mother), and trace the path of the labyrinth with your finger. Pause in the centre, and when you are ready, retrace your steps outward.

    You can find a guided labyrinth walk on my website: https://derrynagittah.ie as well as labyrinth cloths that can be used for finger-walking, hand-made by Mongolian women for the Jampa Ling Tibetan Buddhist centre, Ireland: https://derrynagittah.ie/collections/other-products/products/hand-stitched-labyrinth-cloths [last accessed 27/7/21].

    The '*Labyrinth Wisdom Cards*' by Tony Christie (Cork: Gaois Publications, 2012) are a suggested Oracle deck.
2. Sophie Messenger, *Why Postnatal Recovery Matters* (London: Pinter and Martin, 2020).
3. Ghana, Samieh, Sevil Hakimi, Mojgan Mirghafourvand, Fatemeh Abbasalizadeh, and Nasser Behnampour. "Randomized controlled trial of abdominal binders for postoperative pain, distress, and blood loss after cesarean delivery." *International Journal of Gynecology & Obstetrics* 137, no. 3 (2017): 271–276.
4. Elizondo, Guillermo, Donato Saldivar, Homero Nanez, Luis E. Todd, and Jesus Z. Villarreal. "Pituitary gland growth during normal pregnancy: an in vivo study using magnetic resonance imaging." *The American Journal of Medicine* 85, no. 2 (1988): 217–220.
5. 'Closing the Bones' ceremony brought to the West by Dr Rocio Alarcon, ethnopharmacologist and healer from Ecuador https://www.iamoe.org/about-rocio [last accessed 8/6/21].
6. Webb S, Sherburn M, Ismail K M K. Managing perineal trauma after childbirth. *BMJ* 2014; 349: g6829 doi:10.1136/bmj.g6829

7. U. Halbreich, S. Karkun / Journal of Affective Disorders 91 (2006) 97–111, Cross-cultural and social diversity of prevalence of postpartum depression and depressive symptoms.
8. Murray Enkin et al. *A guide to effective care in pregnancy and childbirth* (Oxford: Oxford University Press, 2000), 436.
9. See International Association of Infant Massage https://www.iaim.net [last accessed 6/6/21].
10. Bump RC, Norton PA. Epidemiology and natural history of pelvic floor dysfunction. Obstet Gynecol Clin North Am. 1998 Dec; 25(4):723–46. doi: 10.1016/s0889-8545(05)70039-5. PMID: 9921553.
11. The UK National Health Service (NHS) suggests holding a load close to your waist and avoid bending your back.
12. For more information about tissue memory and cellular consciousness, see the work of neuroscientist Candace Pert, PhD, including her groundbreaking book *Molecules of Emotion: The Science Behind Mind-Body Medicine*, Scribner, New York, 1997.
13. Cellular memory has been highlighted in recent decades after stories emerged from transplant recipients, describing how they had acquired the memories and personality characteristics of their donor. This has been particularly notable in patients following heart transplantation, where recipients have reported acquiring memories from the donor's life, changes in food or music preferences, cravings, altered attitudes, habits, and behaviours. In one widely publicised case, an eight year old heart transplant recipient helped to solve the brutal murder of her donor after having vivid nightmares of being murdered.

    The topic of memory transfer is only recently being explored by science. There are various hypotheses but little is understood. Young children may often recall events that occurred before their conception or from other lifetimes they claim to have lived. Some children remember communicating with their parents prior to being conceived and spiritual hypnotherapy with individuals of all ages has uncovered memories of the afterlife and of life between lives. Memory is a complex phenomenon, transcending biology and physical perception.
14. In *The Male Brain* by Louann Brizendine, she reports that a father's testosterone levels drop by up to one third after his baby is born. The lower a father's testosterone levels fall, the more he dotes on his baby.
15. Simon Mills and Kerry Bone, *Essential Guide to Herbal Safety* (Missouri: Churchill Livingstone, 2005), 523.
16. Alex F. Muller, Hemmo A. Drexhage, Arie Berghout, Postpartum Thyroiditis and Autoimmune Thyroiditis in Women of Childbearing Age: Recent Insights and Consequences for Antenatal and Postnatal Care, *Endocrine Reviews*, Volume 22, Issue 5, 1 October 2001, 605–630.

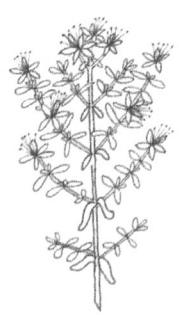

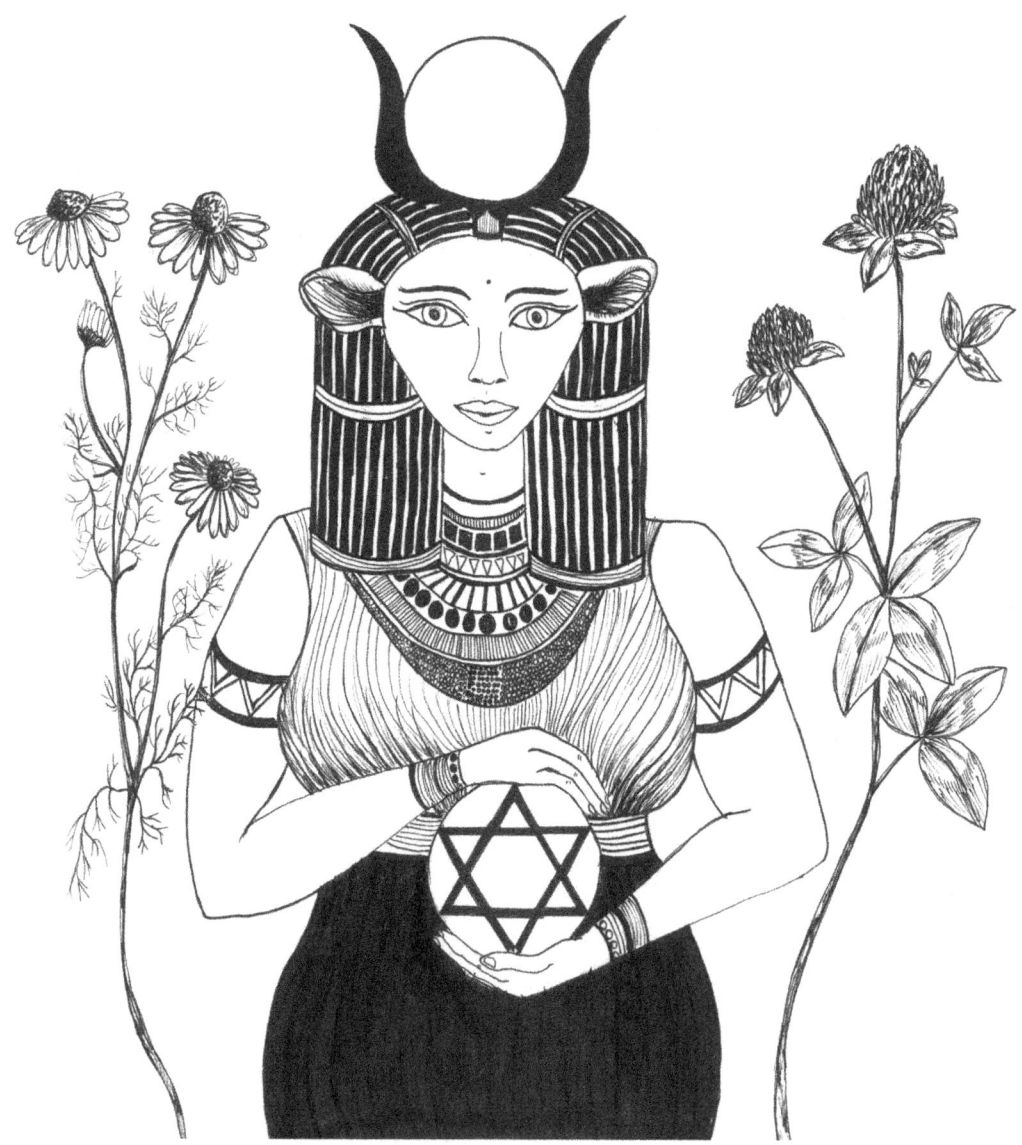

Hathor. Primordial Mother Goddess of love, pleasure and maternal care. A protector of women, she celebrates music and beauty, promoting gratitude.
Red Clover (*Trifolium pratense*). Brings nourishment, centredness, wisdom and good fortune.
Chamomile (*Chamomilla recutita*). Purveyor of inner peace and joy.

CHAPTER 14

Lactation

Benefits of breastfeeding

Breastfeeding is widely acknowledged to be the best and most complete form of nutrition for healthy full-term infants. Breast milk contains the ideal balance of vitamins, proteins, fats, and other macronutrients and is more easily digested than formula. The World Health Organisation recommends that mothers breastfeed exclusively for the first six months of a baby's life, with continued breastfeeding in addition to solid foods for at least the first two years.

As well as its nutritional benefits, breastfeeding offers a host of other advantages. Physical contact between mother and baby during the early postpartum period promotes bonding, helps prolong the lactation stage, and may help adapt the mother's gastrointestinal tract to the increased energy demands of lactation. For the mother, breastfeeding accelerates uterine involution and repositioning, as well as reducing the risk of uterine haemorrhage. It decreases the risk of ovarian and breast cancer, cardiovascular disease, and type 2 diabetes. It also helps her regain her pre-pregnancy weight and provides long-term anti-stress effects, reducing blood pressure and cortisol levels during feeds. It also gives immense pleasure and emotional satisfaction to most women.

Breastfeeding regulates and enhances the physiological systems of mother and baby.

For the newborn infant, as well as providing optimal nutrition, breast milk contains antibodies from the mother that protect against infection from viruses and bacteria. Other anti-infective factors it provides include immunoglobulins (IgA, immunoglobulin A, in particular), white blood cells, whey protein (lysozyme and lactoferrin), and oligosaccharides. Thirteen weeks of breastfeeding increases the baby's protection against gastro-enteritis for up to twenty-four months. Fifteen weeks exclusive breastfeeding lowers the baby's risk of respiratory illnesses and asthma, allergies, ear or urinary tract infections. Breastfeeding supports healthy growth and development, including improved neurodevelopment and behaviour ratings, improved dentition, and a reduced risk of obesity and type 2 diabetes in adulthood.

Preterm babies who receive human milk experience additional benefits, including a reduced risk of necrotising enterocolitis (NEC), enteral feed intolerance, chronic lung disease, retinopathy of prematurity, neurodevelopmental delays, and re-hospitalisation.

Lactation and lactogenesis

Lactation describes the production of breast milk and its secretion from the mammary gland after delivery. **Lactogenesis** is the process of developing the ability to secrete milk and involves the maturation of the breast alveoli.

The steps of lactation have been classified as follows:

Stage I (Lactogenesis—secretory differentiation) | Beginning in mid-pregnancy to day two or day three postpartum, the breasts develop the capacity to secrete breast milk, including the secretion of colostrum.
Stage II (Lactogenesis—secretory activation) | Beginning around day two or three postpartum until around day eight, breast milk volume increases rapidly and then abruptly levels off.
Stage III (galactopoiesis—maintenance) | From approximately day nine postpartum and onwards, the volume of breast milk produced is maintained through a supply and demand mechanism.
Stage IV (involution) | Regression and atrophy post lactation, on average, forty days after the last breastfeed, when breast milk secretion ceases.

Hormone changes involved in lactation

As outlined in Chapter 13 (see page 237 'Hormonal changes after birth'), when progesterone and oestrogen levels drop following delivery, prolactin levels rise and its secretory activity is enhanced directly or indirectly by growth hormone, thyroxine, glucocorticoids, and insulin. When the baby suckles, oxytocin and prolactin are released from the pituitary, passing through the maternal circulation to the breast, where prolactin stimulates milk production and oxytocin stimulates milk ejection ('letdown') at the nipple.

Oxytocin release is further triggered by skin-to-skin contact with the baby and increases in response to physical touch. Letdown can also be induced simply by the presence of the baby or the infant's cry, and it is inhibited by factors such as pain, breast engorgement, or other adverse conditions. The optimal environment for oxytocin flow is quiet, dark and intimate, in an atmosphere where the mother feels safe. High levels of cortisol are known to delay lactogenesis while low levels and decreased stress improve breastfeeding. Oxytocin also stimulates uterine contractions as part of the process of involution of the uterus postpartum.

Together, oxytocin and prolactin aid milk release and further milk production, thereby setting up an important feedback loop and helping to establish breastfeeding.

Copious milk production starts around fifty to seventy-three hours after delivery (the milk 'comes in'). In primiparous women, this is slightly delayed, and early milk volume is lower. Lower milk volume is also observed in women who have caesarean births compared with those who deliver vaginally. Late onset of milk production has also been seen in women with retained placental fragments, diabetes, and stressful vaginal deliveries. With retained placental fragments, milk production could be inhibited by the continued secretion of progesterone and would continue to be inhibited until removal of the remaining placental fragments.

While breastfeeding, the mother's body continues to secrete relaxin, which contributes to looser ligaments and may delay recovery from prolapse.

Once lactation is established and maintained, production is regulated by the interaction of both physical and biochemical factors. If milk is not removed, elevated intramammary pressure and accumulation of a feedback inhibitor of lactation reduce milk production and initiate mammary involution. If breast milk is removed, the inhibitor is also removed, and secretion resumes. In this way, the quantity of milk produced is perfectly regulated to match the baby's needs.

Hormones involved in the maintenance stage include growth hormone, glucocorticoids, thyroid hormones, insulin, parathyroid hormone, oxytocin, and prolactin.

Finally, the involution of mammary glands (lobules) occurs with the cessation of lactation and requires a combination of lactogenic hormone deprivation and local autocrine signals. Full regression does not occur, and pregnancy causes a permanent increase in the size and number of lobules.

Following lactation, there is always the potential for the mammary glands to produce milk in response to regular nipple stimulation. It is also possible for someone who has never been pregnant to lactate. Some adoptive and non-gestational mothers stimulate milk production by using a breast pump every two to three hours, before the baby comes. In addition, some transgender men, transgender women and non-binary individuals choose to breastfeed or chestfeed their babies. For some people, it may be relatively easy to produce milk, while others will need medical support, such as hormone treatment to induce lactation. Research is needed to understand the effects of treatments on quality and quantity of milk produced.

Breast milk stages

In the first few weeks after a baby is born, breast milk progresses through three main stages: colostrum, transitional breast milk, and mature breast milk.

Colostrum is the first milk a breastfed baby receives, containing more protein, minerals, and fat-soluble vitamins (A and K) than mature milk. It is a high-density milk, rich in white blood cells and antibodies to protect the newborn from infection and disease. It is especially high in secretory IgA, which helps to protect the mucous membranes in the throat, lungs, and intestines of the infant. Colostrum also contains immune and growth factors and other bioactives that help to activate the baby's immune system, promote gut function, and pave the way for a healthy gut microbiome in the first few days of life. It contains lactoferrin, a protein that has immune properties and helps with the absorption of iron. Colostrum has a mild laxative effect, encouraging the passing of the newborn's first stool (meconium), which clears excess bilirubin and helps prevent jaundice.

After two to six days, high-protein **transitional milk** is produced. This is produced in a larger quantity than the colostrum, gradually transitioning to **mature milk** over the course of about two weeks. Compared to colostrum, mature milk is lower in protein but higher in fat and milk sugars. Mature milk contains around 90% water to meet the baby's fluid requirements. The fat content in milk increases throughout each feed. At the beginning of a feed, 'foremilk' is produced, which is thin and watery and will quench the baby's thirst, providing proteins, lactose, water, and other nutrients. Later in the feed comes the 'hindmilk', which tends to be thicker and creamier in appearance, providing up to two or three times more fat. The hindmilk provides much of the energy of a feed. Other components in mature milk include human growth factors, cortisol, insulin, thyroxine, and prolactin.

Mature milk adapts to the development of the baby and has a different composition at different times of day. For instance, breast milk contains low levels of tryptophan (precursor to melatonin) in the morning and much higher levels at night. This may help the infant to establish their circadian rhythm of being awake during the day and asleep at night. A mother's prolactin levels also rise at night.

Establishing breastfeeding

Breastfeeding is a learned skill. For some women, establishing breastfeeding is a wonderfully easy and pleasurable experience, whereas for others, it can require enormous amounts of time and patience for the mother and those who assist her. Breastfeeding may take three or four weeks to get established, requiring determination, perseverance, and encouragement, preferably with the help and support of a midwife or another woman experienced at breastfeeding. In particular, mothers may require assistance with learning how to position and attach the baby to ensure they are able to feed the baby comfortably and that the infant is able to successfully transfer milk. Optimal breastfeeding attachment, or latching, aims to ensure an adequate transfer of milk and therefore sufficient drainage of the breast for continued milk supply and prevention of nipple pain.

The main reasons women give for discontinuing breastfeeding are nipple trauma, breast engorgement, mastitis, and insufficient milk. Most of these problems can be prevented if a woman has emotional and practical support, and by unrestricted breastfeeding by a baby who has been well positioned from the start. Breastfeeding is facilitated by early contact between mother and baby, and the baby needs to eat and sleep according to his or her own individual rhythms. Duration of suckling should not be limited. Breastfeeding is enhanced if the mother is relaxed, unhurried, and confident of her ability to breastfeed. Women can be reassured that breast size does not affect a mother's ability to produce sufficient milk.

Establishing breastfeeding can be particularly important for a baby who is sick or premature in order to provide extra immunity and enhance growth and development. If a baby is too small or ill to breastfeed, expressing breast milk from the start will help maintain the mother's milk supply.

Those who care for women during pregnancy and childbirth have a vital role to play in enabling a woman to breastfeed successfully. In hospital settings it is still common to hear of new mothers who have been told that their milk supply is insufficient and the baby needs a 'top up' with formula. This undermines a mother's confidence, and once a bottle has been given it can be more difficult to establish breastfeeding, because the baby finds it less work to suck from a bottle teat. It is crucial that mothers receive encouragement at this time. Valuable support can also be found from organisations such as La Leche League,[1] which provides information and support to women who want to breastfeed their babies. The importance of supporting women at the start of lactation has been highlighted by the recent COVID-19 pandemic, which has had a significant impact on many aspects of neonatal care, including breastfeeding support services for pregnant women and mothers.[2] Reports show an unprecedented decline in breastfeeding rates.[3] With health care systems under considerable pressure, changes in clinical practice, and a reduction in supporting staff, new mothers are not receiving the support they need in the early critical days of lactation, leading to breastfeeding problems at home and early weaning. Medical professionals are worried that restoring hospital practices that promote breastfeeding may be difficult.[4]

It goes without saying that if a woman is unable or chooses not to breastfeed, for whatever reason, it is important that she receives support and knows that bottle feeding can still be very satisfying for her baby.

Nutrition for breastfeeding mothers

A mother who is fully breastfeeding requires a minimum of 500 additional calories per day. Breastfeeding women need a nourishing and well-balanced diet with plenty of protein, adequate iron, unrefined carbohydrates, essential fatty acids, and an abundance of fresh fruit and vegetables.

During lactation, there is an increased requirement for energy, protein, all the vitamins (except B_6), calcium, phosphorus, magnesium, zinc, copper, and selenium. A daily supplement of at least 10 micrograms of vitamin D should be considered as a precaution, especially from October–March. It is worth considering taking a multivitamin and mineral supplement designed specifically for breastfeeding mothers.

B6 should not be supplemented at more than 50mg daily, since it may suppress levels of prolactin.

On average, babies of vegan mothers tend to be smaller than other babies and vegan women must pay particular attention to their nutrient needs (see Chapter 3 'Nutrition').

Maize, oats, barley, peas, beans, and pulses can all help enrich and increase milk supply, while leafy green vegetables, green beans, carrots, sweet potatoes, asparagus, and apricots will promote and sustain lactation. The omega-3 fatty acids in oily fish are important for infant brain development.

A breastfeeding mother can allow her hunger and thirst to regulate her food and fluid intake. She will need plenty of fluids and may drink copious amounts of water and herb teas. Slimming diets should be avoided.

Freezing and thawing breastmilk can give it a soapy taste, which some babies may not like, and the foods a breastfeeding mother eats will contribute to the flavour of her milk. Therefore, a diet high in fruit and vegetables exposes the infant to the flavours of these foods and may help the child to more easily accept the taste of fruit and vegetables when they begin eating solids.

Contaminants in breastmilk

The taste and quality of breastmilk are affected by a host of factors such as medications, hormones, smoking, and alcohol. Women should avoid alcohol, cigarettes, and caffeine which can overstimulate an infant. Breastfeeding mothers should also avoid the combined oestrogen-progesterone contraceptive pill, since it can adversely influence both the quality and quantity of milk.

Breast milk tends to attract heavy metals and other contaminants due to its high-fat and protein content, and a wide variety of harmful substances can be passed from the mother into her milk. Compounds that have been identified include bisphenol A (BPA, a plastic component), PBDEs (used in flame retardants), perchlorate (used in rocket fuel), perfluorinated chemicals (PFCs, used in floor cleaners and non-stick pans), phthalates (used in plastics), polyvinyl chloride (PVC, commonly known as vinyl), and the heavy metals cadmium, lead, and mercury as leading offenders. This has caused widespread concern. However, research suggests that airborne pollutants in city air represent a much larger toxic load for nursing infants and emphasises the need to reduce the indoor air sources of these compounds.

Formula milk cannot be viewed as a 'pure' alternative either. Many formulas contain corn syrup, hydrogenated oils and genetically modified ingredients, all of which have potential harmful effects. Furthermore, in recent studies, formula milks have been found to contain high levels of toxic metals such as lead, arsenic, cadmium and mercury.[5]

It seems to me, despite breast milk's vulnerability to chemical contamination, the profound benefits of breastfeeding far outweigh the risks. Breastfeeding women are advised to eat a diet as 'clean' and organic as possible (see Chapter 3 'Nutrition'), avoid exposure to toxic chemicals and look for safer alternatives to products, such as cleaning supplies, food storage, and personal care products that contain toxic substances.

Prescribing herbs to breastfeeding mothers

Herbs have a long history of supporting breastfeeding mothers. Not only do they assist the mother, many herbs can pass through her breast milk and benefit her baby. Well-established herbal medicines provide a valuable way to nourish and support both mother and child.

Galactagogues have traditionally been used to help ensure a rich and plentiful milk supply and each galactagogue herb offers its own unique additional gifts, such as Fennel (*Foeniculum vulgare*) helping to treat and prevent colic in the newborn, and Vervain (*Verbena off.*) supporting the nervous system (see 'Insufficient Milk Supply' below for further discussion of galactagogues). Other herbs offer their virtues in different ways, such a Raspberry leaf (*Rubus idaeus*) and Nettle (*Urtica dioica*) bringing nutritive support to both mother and baby.

Engorgement

Physiological breast engorgement

When the milk comes in between days two and six post-partum, normal breast filling occurs and the breasts become heavy and swollen without pain. When milk production increases rapidly during these first few days post-partum, physiological breast engorgement can occur with more milk being made than the baby can remove. This results in lymphatic and vascular congestion and oedema of the glandular breast tissue. Oedema is caused by a build-up of milk, blood, and other fluids in the breasts. The breasts can become swollen, hot, hard, and tender, with redness, shiny skin, and diffuse oedema, often causing the nipples to become taut and flattened. Symptoms are usually bilateral and while there may be a slight rise in temperature (<38.4°C), systemic symptoms are absent, unlike in mastitis. However, engorgement may lead to mastitis if left untreated. Pathological engorgement may also occur throughout the time of breastfeeding, typically resulting from restrictions on feeding frequency and duration, and from problems positioning the baby at the breast.

Management of engorgement

The key to managing breast engorgement is promoting the frequent and effective removal of milk from the breast. Women are encouraged to empty their breasts (either by feeding or by the use of a breast pump) as often as possible, typically every two to three hours to maintain milk supply. Empty one breast fully before offering the other. Prior to feeding, the areolar region can be gently massaged with fingertips to temporarily move excess fluid away from the nipple and improve the baby's latch.

Herbal treatment for engorged breasts

Cabbage leaves (green or white) or Rhubarb leaves are all effective for external use to relieve the pain and swelling of engorgement. For tough leaves, remove the hard spine, soften leaves between your hands, on a radiator or by using an iron on low heat setting, and place them inside bra. If cooling is required, leaves can be refrigerated and applied chilled to draw heat from the breast. Change when limp.

Alternatively, apply a hot compress of Comfrey (*Symphytum off.*), Marigold (*Calendula off.*), or Cleavers (*Galium aperine*), singly or combined. Heat is better for softening but if there is a lot of excess heat a cooling effect can be obtained by applying chilled compresses or by freezing the herb tea into ice cubes and applying as an ice pack to relieve discomfort.

Drink Marigold or Cleavers tea along with using the compress. Lady's Mantle (*Alchemilla vulgaris*) lotion can be used prophylactically to tone the breasts.

Essential oils of Lavender, Rose, or Geranium also make a good compress or can be added to a bath to help relieve discomfort.

Insufficient milk supply

Insufficient milk supply is one of the most commonly given reasons for ceasing breastfeeding early. In particular, inexperienced mothers often worry that they are not producing enough milk, especially if they have a fretful baby who is difficult to soothe. Concerns are often unfounded, but lack of confidence and anxiety only serve to make matters worse. In fact, a mother's milk supply is generally fine as long as a baby is gaining weight and producing wet nappies, and soft and yellow stools.

Some babies may feed very often because they have a strong desire to be in close contact with their mother. If this occurs, the mother will generally start to produce the right amount of milk if her baby is well positioned and actively drinking milk from her breast. Mothers often worry about changes in feeding patterns but these are usually normal. Babies have growth spurts at different times. When a baby goes through a growth spurt, he or she will feed more frequently for a while in order to increase the supply for their new energy needs. If a baby reduces breastfeeding times, it can mean that they have become more efficient at draining the breast.

Signs of low milk supply

If there is insufficient milk, babies may have delayed bowel movements, decreased urinary output, jaundice, weight loss from birth, and lethargy. The baby may appear sleepy or frustrated at the breast, or may suckle for short periods only.

Low milk supply can be caused by certain medical conditions that prevent a baby from breastfeeding effectively, such as cleft palate, metabolic or neurological issues. These are rare and once excluded, maternal factors are usually the cause.

Primary lactation insufficiency occurs in up to 5% of mothers, resulting from inadequate glandular tissue due to issues such as breast abnormalities, breast or nipple surgery (either medically indicated or cosmetic). Women who have had breast augmentation may experience issues with lactation and breastfeeding, but this depends on the location of the incision, for instance, armpit incisions are more favourable for normal breastfeeding than incisions around the areola.

Secondary lactation insufficiency, which is far more common, is usually a result of inappropriate feeding routines or use of supplementary milk leading to diminished milk synthesis and eventually an insufficient supply.

How to increase milk supply

The key to increasing milk supply is frequent and effective milk removal, which stimulates increased milk production. Mothers may need help with positioning and attachment. They need to feel physically and psychologically comfortable and to have unrestricted skin-to-skin contact during breastfeeding. Milk supply will increase if there is increased frequency of breastfeeding, usually with no more than three hours between breastfeeds and feeding eight-twelve times a day.

Women who are combination feeding (part breast and part formula), can increase their milk supply by giving the baby less formula. Use of a dummy (pacifier or soother) may reduce the amount of milk a mother produces. For women who are expressing their milk, for instance using a pump, it can be helpful to use relaxation techniques while expressing, such as music or deep breathing. A daily glass of Guinness is often recommended to increase milk supply.

Herbal treatments

Herbal galactagogues give additional support by promoting milk production. I typically include galactagogues as part of a new mother's postpartum tonic (see page 200). These are usually sufficient, but if desired, she can drink additional galactagogue teas such as Fennel (*Foeniculum vulgare*), Vervain (*Verbena off.*), Fenugreek (*Trigonella foenum graecum*), Nettle (*Urtica dioica*), Aniseed (*Pimpinella anisum*), Dill (*Anethum graveolens*) and Caraway (*Carum carvi*). Fennel tea is my usual herb of choice here since it also tones the digestive system and helps prevent and treat infant colic. Lavender essential oil also helps increase milk production, and can be used for massage, inhalation, diffusion, or in a burner, increasing oxytocin levels and enhancing milk supply. Oatstraw (*Avena sativa*) tea can be included as a nourishing tonic to lift the spirits and ensure abundant milk supply. Marshmallow root (*Althaea officinalis* radix.) improves the quality of milk.

Oversupply of milk

Some women experience an oversupply of milk and leaking breasts, most commonly occurring in the first four-six weeks. Women produce more milk than the baby needs, leading to potential stress for mother and baby. This problem is frequently linked to switching breasts too early and it helps to pay particular attention to positioning and attachment, and let the baby decide the duration of feeding. It can help to allow the baby to completely finish one breast before swapping to the second. If engorgement occurs, follow the advice for 'Engorgement'. Oversupply of milk requires the proper establishment of the supply and demand mechanism and is unaffected by the prescription of herbal galactagogues. Herbal galactagogues are not contraindicated at usual dosages since they promote healthy milk production but do not overstimulate.

Nipples, sore or cracked

In the early days of breastfeeding, many mothers experience a phase of painful, sore nipples. Nipple pain that extends beyond the first few days warrants further attention, as if left untreated, it can lead to other breast problems such as engorgement or mastitis. Sore and cracked nipples are among the main reasons why women give up breastfeeding. Causes of nipple pain include poor positioning and attachment, failure to release suction before removing the baby from the breast, skin sensitivity, climate variables, and high intra-oral baby vacuums. Pain may occur with or without infection. If a woman has moderate or severe nipple inversion it can make breastfeeding difficult, but good positioning and deep latch techniques help tremendously. For women with inverted nipples, it is crucial to get skilled help with positioning and latch-on such as that provided by practitioners from La Leche League International. Women can be reassured that if they persevere, breastfeeding will eventually become pain free. This knowledge can offer a light in the darkness for a woman who is going through the experience of nipple pain.

Management of sore or cracked nipples

Pay careful attention to latch and positioning. Avoid excessive washing of nipples; especially avoid using soap which strips natural oils. If nipples leak milk, keep them dry between feeds by using breast pads to prevent them getting soggy. Expose nipples to fresh air as much as possible. Start each feed on a different side.

Some women find nipple shields helpful for protection, best used only after other options have been tried. If a woman is using them, ensure they are positioned correctly and are the right size. Avoid tight clothing, such as underwired bras, to minimize pressure on the breast. If breastfeeding is too painful, it may help to express temporarily for twenty-four hours, with gradual reintroduction of breastfeeding as pain subsides. Ensure high levels of vitamin C in the diet.

A widely used remedy is to express a little breast milk and rub one or two drops onto the sore or cracked nipple. Repeat before and after every feed. Alternatively, the contents of a vitamin E capsule or Evening Primrose (*Oenothera biennis*) oil can be applied after feeds.

Herbal treatments

Marigold (*Calendula off.*) infusion is effective applied as a lotion before and after feeds, followed by the application of a soothing healing cream or ointment such as Marigold,

Chamomile (*Chamomilla recutita*), Comfrey (*Symphytum off.*), Marshmallow (*Althaea off.*), or Slippery Elm (*Ulmus rubra*) after feeds. This can be gently wiped off with Marigold infusion prior to the next feed.

If there is scabbing on the nipple, apply the Marigold infusion as a warm compress to soak and soften the scab prior to breastfeeding. If pain relief is needed, apply Marigold infusion as a cold compress or cool pack either before or after a feed. Chamomile infusion can be substituted for Marigold, or dilute Oak bark (*Quercus robur/petraea*) decoction as a toning astringent.

Blocked ducts

A blocked or plugged duct is a condition where a blockage in a milk duct results in insufficient drainage of the duct, causing a build-up of milk behind the blockage. Signs and symptoms may be gradual. A blocked breast duct may appear as a tender lump the size of a pea or larger, and occasionally presents with a small white blister on the nipple. The breast may be sensitive and the tender lump may or may not be palpable with defined margins. The baby may be fussy when feeding from the affected breast, since the flow of milk can be reduced. Left untreated, the lump can become inflamed, progressing to infection, engorgement, and mastitis (see 'Mastitis' below).

It is not always clear why blocked ducts occur, but insufficient breast drainage is most likely the cause. Poor drainage may be caused by poor attachment and positioning, tight clothing around the breast, long periods between breastfeeds, or scarring from surgery.

Management of blocked ducts

Feed frequently, paying particular attention to positioning and attachment. Feeding with the affected side first and trying different feeding positions may help clear the blockage, as well as temporarily expressing after each feed. Rest as much as possible and avoid tight clothing.

Herbal treatments

Apply a warm compress of Chamomile or Marigold infusion just before feeding, massaging the affected area towards the nipple and continuing the massage during breastfeeding. Alternatively, massaging the affected area can be done under a warm shower or in a warm bath with essential oils of Lavender or Chamomile in the water.

Cool compresses of Chamomile, Marshmallow, or Fennel tea can be applied after breastfeeding if required to ease pain and inflammation.

Mastitis

Mastitis is an inflammation of the breast that may or may not be accompanied by infection. In lactating women, mastitis mostly occurs during the first six weeks post-partum, however, it can also occur at any other point during lactation, and is essentially caused by an accumulation of milk, and frequently linked with insufficient rest. Worldwide, up to 20% of breastfeeding mothers develop lactation mastitis (puerperal mastitis).[6] Non-infectious mastitis is due to an inflammatory response caused by an accumulation of milk in the breast. Infectious mastitis occurs when accumulated milk enables bacteria to grow, usually *Staphylococcus aureus*. Meticillin-resistant *Staphylococcus aureus* (MRSA) infection is increasing, and can be more common in women who have had a C-section.

Risk factors for mastitis include poor attachment, milk accumulation due to insufficient number or duration of feeds, pressure on the breast such as tight clothing, nipple damage, breast trauma, and blocked milk ducts. Feeding may have been reduced due to partial formula feeding, changes in regime such as the baby starting to sleep through the night, rapid weaning, or painful breasts.

Sudden cessation of breastfeeding in a woman with infectious mastitis increases the risk of breast abscess which can lead to surgical incision and drainage. Between 0.4 to 11% of lactating mothers develop a breast abscess and most of these are as a complication of lactation mastitis.[7]

Signs of mastitis

Mastitis typically presents as a tender, warm or hot, red, swollen, wedge-shaped area of a single breast, usually accompanied by fever (>38.5°C) and occurring at least a week postpartum (as opposed to engorgement, which typically presents on the second or third day of breastfeeding. See 'Engorgement'). Women can develop flu-like symptoms such as rigors, muscle pain, lethargy, depression, nausea, and headache. The affected area feels firm and hot and there may be swelling of axillary lymph nodes. If a breast abscess has developed, there will be a fluctuant tender lump, with overlying erythema.

Diagnosis of mastitis is usually clinical and it is not possible to differentiate clinically between infectious and non-infectious mastitis. Detection of pathogens in breast milk is not always possible, and the results of milk culture may not be a useful guide for therapy, especially since the pathogens involved may be contaminants or skin flora. The presence of MRSA is increasing and milk may need to be cultured if infection is severe or recurrent, or has been acquired in hospital.

Management of mastitis

Women need emotional support as well as practical help. They can be encouraged to continue breastfeeding and reassured that mastitis does not interfere with the ability to breastfeed. In order to improve milk removal, it can be helpful to ask a skilled person to observe a feed to assess and advise on feeding pattern, positioning, attachment, and sucking behaviour. If feeding is too painful or the affected breast still feels full after a feed, express milk until symptoms subside. Increase frequency of breastfeeds and feed on the affected side first while symptoms persist. Gently massage the breast before feeding.

Herbal treatment

Mastitis can deteriorate rapidly and needs immediate treatment, responding well to frequent breastfeeding, herbs, and rest. Apply soothing, warm poultices of Marshmallow root (*Althaea off.* radix), Slippery Elm (*Ulmus rubra*), and Comfrey (*Symphytum off.*) powders, singly or combined, between feeds, or make a poultice from fresh Chamomile (*Chamomilla recutita*) flowers and Comfrey leaves. Raw grated cabbage leaves also make a reliable poultice.

Alternatively, warm compresses of Chamomile and Comfrey can be applied. The woman can apply the poultice or compress while soaking in a warm bath containing Lavender or Chamomile essential oils.

To relieve pain, take Valerian (*Valeriana off.*) 20 drops hourly, plus Rescue essence, and apply cold compresses of Chamomile or Marshmallow after feeding.

Rest is crucial, preferably in bed, drinking plenty of herb teas such as Chamomile, Cleavers (*Gallium aperine*), Marigold (*Calendula off.*), and Fennel (*Foeniculum vulgare*).

In all cases, raw Garlic (*Allium sativum*) is recommended to be taken internally as a powerful anti-infective, one clove three or four times daily, crushed into food, water, or honey.

If infection is suspected, for instance if the woman has an infected nipple injury, or if she has a fever or is in any way acutely unwell, give Echinacea (*Echinacea* spp.) at 5–10ml every three hours. Give Echinacea prophylactically rather than risk deterioration of mastitis.

With herbal treatment, mastitis can be expected to start to resolve within twelve hours.

For breast abscess (practitioner only treatment) apply warm poultices of Cleavers, Marshmallow, and Linseed combined.

Candida infection, candidiasis, thrush

A breastfeeding mother can develop thrush affecting the nipple, areola, and/or breast. This can cause severe pain and is another reason why women stop breastfeeding early. Signs and symptoms include itching or burning nipple pain, shiny or flaking skin on the nipple or areola, painful breasts without tender spots or sore lumps, stabbing pains behind the areola.

The mother may experience severe pain in both breasts or nipples, usually after a period of pain-free breastfeeding. Pain is bilateral and may be experienced both during and between feeds. It is usually of sudden onset following a period of pain-free breastfeeding. Pruritis is common and breast pain alone is not usually associated with thrush.

Differential diagnosis includes skin diseases, such as eczema, psoriasis, impetigo, herpes, and bacterial infection, as well as breast pain from other causes such as engorgement, blocked ducts, mastitis, circulatory problems (Raynaud's syndrome), or incorrect positioning/latch. Thrush is often linked to previous nipple damage and is more likely if the woman has candida affecting another part of her body (commonly the vagina), if another family member has candida such as athlete's foot, or if mother or baby have recently been treated with antibiotics or corticosteroids. Thrush is also associated with the use of bottles in the first two weeks postpartum, diabetes, anaemia, and use of a dummy.

Thrush spreads easily, so mother and baby need concurrent treatment even if symptom free (see 'Candida' page 287 Chapter 15 'Care of the Newborn'). The baby's mouth may be infected and sore, making him or her fussy during and after feeds, and nappy rash can be another indication of candida infection in the baby.

Management

Pay careful attention to hygiene, scrupulously washing hands, especially after nappy changing or using the toilet. Use separate towels, washing them frequently at 60°C. Wear a clean cotton bra every day and keep nipples as dry as possible. Add 200ml vinegar to baths and final rinses in washing machines, since thrush cannot thrive in acidic conditions.

Herbal treatments

Follow advice for 'Candidiasis' page 115 in 'Conditions of Pregnancy'.
Marigold infusion can be applied as a lotion to nipples and areolar areas.

Weaning

Weaning typically refers to the introduction of solid foods into a baby's diet. This commonly starts when the baby is around six months old, causing milk production to reduce slowly over time as the baby gradually takes less breastmilk. In certain circumstances, such as the death of an infant, a mother may need to wean her body from making milk straight away. Sage tea, red or garden (*Salvia miltiorrhiza/off.*), is most effective at arresting milk production. Drink three or four cups daily, 2 teaspoons per cup. To ease the process and prevent engorgement, milk can be expressed or pumped, removing just enough milk to reduce pressure in the breasts but not enough to empty them so that they produce more milk. Sage infusion or diluted tincture is also used topically as a lotion or compress to reduce milk supply. The amount of time to arrest milk production varies from mother to mother.

Alternative weaning herbs include Rosemary (*Rosemarinus off.*), Peppermint (*Mentha piperata*), and Herb Robert (*Geranium robertianum*).

Notes

1. La Leche League International https://www.llli.org [last accessed 22/6/21].
2. A selection of recent research on the effects of COVID-19 on mothers, babies and families can be found at https://www.unicef.org.uk/babyfriendly/news-and-research/baby-friendly-research/coronavirus-research/ [last accessed 1/2/22].
3. Latorre G, Martinelli D, Guida P, Masi E, De Benedictis R, Maggio L. Impact of COVID-19 pandemic lockdown on exclusive breastfeeding in non-infected mothers. Int Breastfeed J. 2021 Apr 17;16(1):36. doi: 10.1186/s13006-021-00382-4. PMID: 33865408; PMCID: PMC8052849.

    See also https://www.medela.com/dam/medela-com/Project-Hero/PDF-and-Images/preserving-breastfeeding-in-the-age-of-covid-19.pdf?uuid=jcr:5f04c85b-8bd1-4ab6-a313-fbc5ef732815 [last accessed 1/2/22].
4. Riccardo Davanzo, neonatologist at institute for maternal and child health, Trieste, Italy has said that due to marked changes in breastfeeding care, there is a risk of "long-run inertia" and it will be difficult to restore hospital practices promoting breastfeeding. This would be detrimental not only to the health of the infant but also to the overall public health situation.

    Ricardo Davanzo et al. "Breastfeeding and coronavirus disease-2019: Ad interim indications of the Italian Society of Neonatology endorsed by the Union of European Neonatal & Perinatal Societies." Maternal & child nutrition 16, no. 3 (2020): e13010.
5. Report from the US House Committee on Oversight and Reform: https://oversight.house.gov/sites/democrats.oversight.house.gov/files/2021-02-04%20ECP%20Baby%20Food%20Staff%20Report.pdf [last accessed 1/2/22].
6. Wilson E, Woodd SL, Benova L; Incidence of and Risk Factors for Lactational Mastitis: A Systematic Review. J Hum Lact. 2020 Nov 36(4):673–686. doi: 10.1177/0890334420907898. Epub 2020 Apr 14.
7. Dener C, Inan A. Breast abscesses in lactating women. World J Surg. 2003 Feb;27(2): 130–3. doi: 10.1007/s00268-002-6563-6. PMID: 12616423.

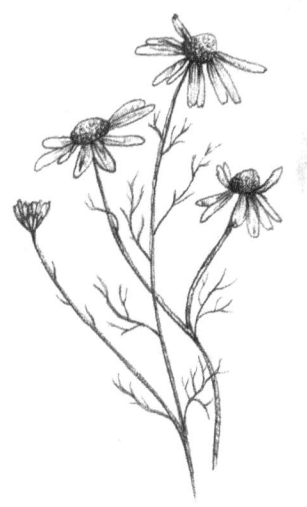

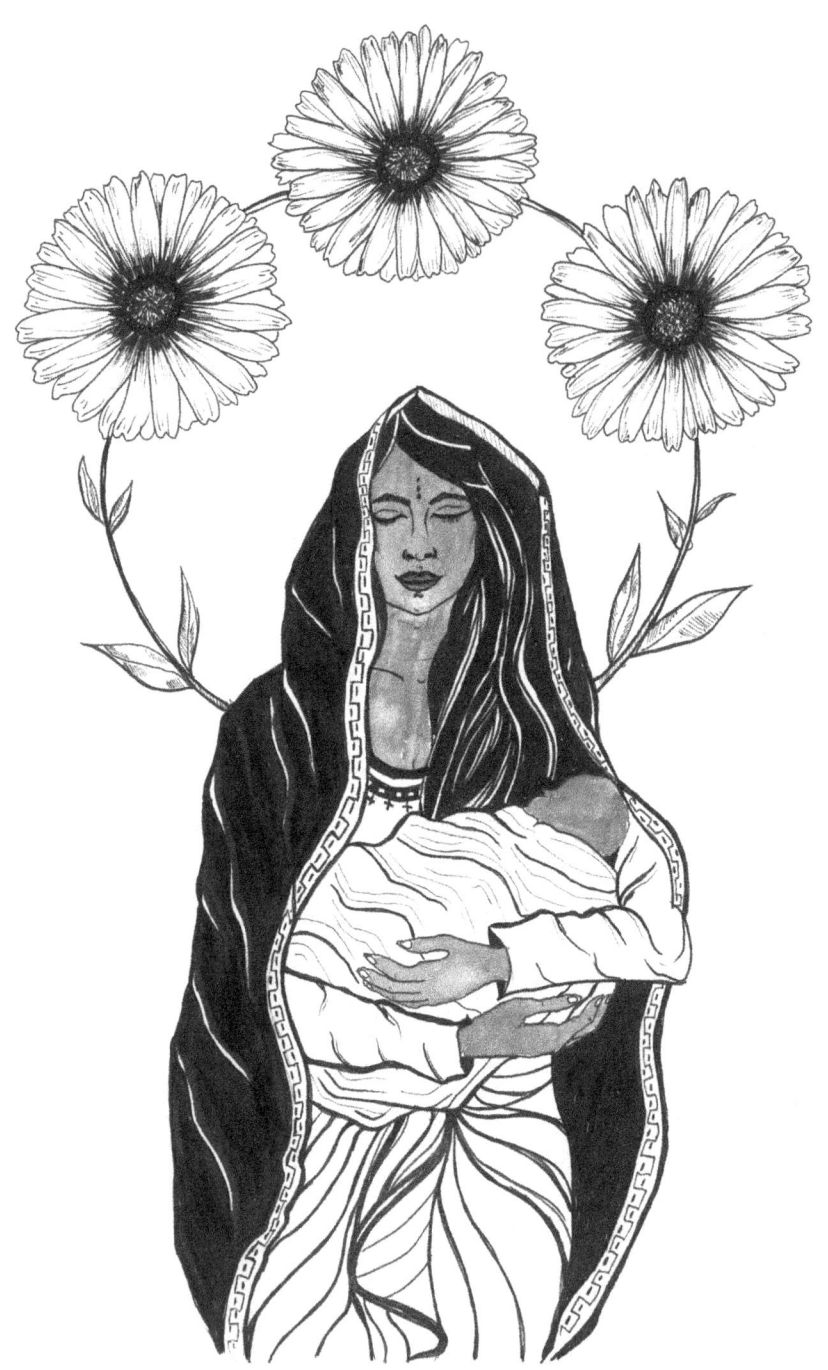

Black Madonna. Earth Mother Goddess, source of Heaven and Earth with creative power. Protector of children.
Marigold (*Calendula off.*) The gold of the Sun. She who purifies, uplifts, and heals.

CHAPTER 15

Care of the newborn

Adapting to life outside the womb

A newborn baby goes through remarkable adjustments in the first days and weeks of life outside the womb. This sensitive, sentient being finds itself in a completely new environment. Their body systems are still developing, and they are learning to breathe, digest food, and focus their eyes, coping with cold, light, hunger, and physical separation from their mother. This adaptation is a truly amazing feat involving a host of new sensations, experiences, and bodily functions.

Certain health issues may commonly arise in the first three months of life, frequently linked to the baby's immature state and the process of adaptation. A baby is also highly sensitive to however its mother is feeling. Herbs offer effective treatment and support for many of these early conditions. Plant medicine can be offered in a variety of ways for babies, including herbal baths, washes, lotions, creams, and ointments. A breastfeeding mother can take herbs and pass them on to her baby through her milk and infants can be given herbs directly as weak infusions. Other methods of application include hand and foot baths, compresses, poultices, and tepid sponging. A limited number of essential oils can be diluted in a base oil for massage, or used in a burner, bath, spray or diffuser. Use in a burner/diffuser is the gentlest method. Vibrational essences can particularly assist during this time of intense adjustment, being easily added to baths, massage oils, creams, room sprays, or placed directly on the skin.

Most common conditions of the newborn are not serious and babies tend to recover very quickly. A new mother may have unfounded anxiety for her baby, especially when the baby's behaviour patterns are as yet unknown. However, a mother's intuition is strong and should always be taken seriously. Newborns are at higher risk of infections in the first month, particularly the first seven days.

Signs of serious illness can include:
Fits, convulsions, not breathing, unconsciousness
Wheezing, grunting, or whistling sounds while breathing
Difficulty breathing, rapid breathing
Severe drowsiness
Blue or very pale
Unexplained bleeding from any part of body
Stiff neck and irritability
Worsening of jaundice
Other signs to watch out for: signs of obvious pain, continual or unusual screaming or crying, poor feeding where it is an abrupt change in normal pattern.

A–Z of common conditions of the newborn

In the sections below, the herbs listed can be given directly to infants, unless stated otherwise. **Where teas are suggested for babies, use ¼ teaspoon herb per cup, infuse 10 minutes, covered, dosage 10–30ml tds/qds, given in teaspoonful doses or added to a bottle of milk or water.** Babies are highly sensitive individuals.

Allergies, Intolerances

Babies are sensitive creatures and their adjustment to the outside world is not always smooth. An increasing number of babies experience allergies or intolerances either to food or to something in their environment. In clinical practice, herbalists regularly see babies having these reactions and whose symptoms respond either to dietary elimination, changes in the external environment, or both. This subject could fill an entire book and is important to summarise here since allergy is frequently associated with many of the common conditions of the newborn.[1]

Cow's milk protein allergy

Cow's milk protein allergy or intolerance (CMPA/I) is the most common food allergy in babies, currently estimated to affect around 7% of babies. In bottle-fed infants, symptoms usually develop before one month of age, often within one week of the introduction of a cow's milk-based formula. The most common body systems affected are the skin, the gut, and the respiratory system, with the majority of babies having two or more affected systems. Symptoms include atopic eczema (typically a scaly, red skin rash), recurrent wheeze, intermittent or frequent diarrhoea, constipation, vomiting, runny nose, nasal congestion, dry skin, urticaria or other rashes, recurrent nappy rash, red and itchy eyes, ear infections, green stools with mucus or blood. Babies may be fretful, have difficulty feeding, colic, sleeplessness, dark circles under their eyes, or long periods of inconsolable crying. Symptoms may be immediate, occurring minutes after milk intake, or they may occur within the next few hours or even days.

Many of these sensitive babies will go on to develop adverse reactions to other foods, and 50–80% are thought to develop some form of inhalant allergy before puberty. Gastrointestinal symptoms tend to decline as the child gets older but these children have a significantly increased risk of persistent CMPA, asthma, rhinoconjunctivitis, and other atopic disease.

Cow's milk allergy in breastfed babies

Breastfed babies may also be sensitive to cow's milk protein in their mother's diet, resulting in the same range of symptoms as can occur in bottle-fed babies, although severe atopic eczema is a predominant symptom in exclusively breast-fed infants.[2] The severity of a food reaction generally depends upon the degree of the baby's sensitivity and the amount of dairy eaten by the mother. The baby may react within minutes, but symptoms are more likely to appear between four and twenty-four hours after exposure. Symptoms can be ongoing and harder to spot if the mother is having a regular intake of dairy products.

Babies with a family history of allergy are at highest risk, and in these cases, it is recommended that mothers limit their dairy consumption during pregnancy and continue after the baby's birth.

Other suspect foods for breastfeeding mothers

While cow's milk protein is the most common food allergen for babies, other likely suspects include wheat, eggs, shellfish, soya, corn, peanuts, tomatoes, and citrus, especially oranges. Also suspect any food that a family member is allergic to, any food the mother recently ate a large amount of, or anything that the mother either craves or consciously dislikes but may be eating while breastfeeding (and/or ate while pregnant) for the benefit of her baby.

Note that CMPA is an allergy to one or more proteins contained in cow's milk. This is different to lactose intolerance which is a digestive reaction to the sugar present in the milk. Therefore, in CMPA it does not help to switch to lactose-free dairy products.

Cooking dairy products may reduce but will not eliminate the allergens. A baby with a dairy allergy may also react to beef.

Bottle fed babies

For bottle fed babies it is generally straightforward simply to try a different formula. Multiple options exist, including formula milks based on goat's milk, sheep's milk, soy, or specially formulated hypoallergenic milks. A significant percentage of babies with cow's milk protein allergy will also react to soy. Many dairy-allergic babies also react to goat's milk or sheep's milk. Try one new milk at a time.

Elimination diets for mothers of breastfed babies

In many cases, it is obvious what food a baby is reacting to, but other times it may be more complex, with several foods or something unexpected being involved. If so, it is helpful to keep a food and symptom diary with a record of foods eaten by the mother, timing of feeds and the baby's behaviour/symptoms.

Eliminate suspect foods for two to three weeks to see if symptoms improve (it takes up to three weeks to eliminate dairy from the body). If improvement is seen, re-introduce slowly, one by one, with five days between each new food and leaving cow's milk products until last. Start with small amounts, gradually increasing over the five days. If the baby has an adverse reaction, stop the food immediately and allow time for the baby's symptoms to calm down completely before reintroducing another food. Any foods that cause a reaction are best excluded for several weeks before a retrial, or left off completely if the reaction was severe. Avoid processed foods, artificial preservatives, colourings, flavourings, refined sugar, alcohol and coffee, as well as pharmaceutical drugs, and contact with cigarette smoke.

A baby's symptoms usually begin to improve within five to seven days of eliminating a problem food but occasionally it takes two to three weeks or longer. Sometimes symptoms may worsen for up to seven days before they improve.

If the baby has only a mild sensitivity, the mother may be able to limit the amount she eats, rather than exclude it totally. However, where an infant has a strong reaction to a food, avoiding the allergen totally can help prevent the development of a lifelong or life-threatening allergy. Take note of any reactions that do occur, especially strong reactions, since these foods should not be introduced early on in weaning and may need to be avoided longer-term. Many babies grow out of food sensitivities as their body systems mature and children have often outgrown them by three years old. However, some allergies and sensitivities persist and may indicate the need for treatment of other imbalances or weaknesses in the body, particularly digestive.

When weaning does occur, avoid all the most common suspect foods and anything already identified or that either parent is allergic to. All common allergens are best avoided until the child is at least one year old.

Herbal treatment for food allergy and intolerance

Infants can be given small amounts of gentle herb teas to soothe and support the digestion, and moderate the allergic response. Teas include Chamomile (*Chamomilla recutita*), Marshmallow (*Althaea off.*), or Fennel (*Foeniculum vulgare*). Breastfeeding mothers are encouraged to drink gentle herb teas to assist the baby's digestion, such as Chamomile, Marshmallow, Fennel, Slippery Elm (*Ulmus rubra*), and Lemon Balm (*Melissa off.*). Essential oils of Chamomile or Lavender, 1% dilution in almond oil, can be used for baby massage, in the bath or in a burner or diffuser.

Care of breastfeeding mothers

While avoiding allergens, ensure the mother is eating a balanced, nutrient-dense diet, including plenty of iron and calcium. Having a baby with allergies can be highly stressful and the mother may benefit from sedatives, such as Passionflower (*Passiflora incarnata*) or Valerian (*Valeriana off.*).

In most cases, exclusive breastfeeding is still preferable to bottle feeding, offering many benefits including protection against allergy in the longer-term and recommended for six months minimum. However, in severe cases of allergy, where the baby is having strong reactions to multiple foods in the mother's diet, this may cause such difficulty for mother and baby that it may be preferable to switch to a hypoallergenic formula.

Environmental allergies and sensitivities

Most allergies in babies are caused by foods but some allergies and sensitivities originate from the environment. Though less common in newborn babies, allergies to dust, animal hair, feathers, moulds, pollens, and other inhaled allergens can trigger allergy symptoms affecting the respiratory system. More commonly, infants react to environmental allergens through contact with the skin, causing issues such as contact dermatitis, hives, or urticaria. Possible allergens include shampoos, soaps, detergents, fabric conditioner, perfumes, baby wipes, wool, and bedding. Mothers are advised to use cotton fabrics and unperfumed cleaning products that are as mild as possible. Chamomile or Lavender tea may be drunk by mother and baby to mitigate the allergic response.

Bronchial conditions see Respiratory illness page 295.

Candida Infection, Thrush

See also Chapter 14 'Lactation', 'Candida infection' page 279.

Candida or thrush may occur in the mouth or appear as a red, angry nappy rash in a newborn infant. Usually there is an infective 'loop' between mother and child and both need treatment, even if symptom-free.

Oral candida causes creamy white lesions, usually on the baby's tongue or inner cheeks. Sometimes this spreads to the roof of the mouth, gums, and tonsils, or the back of the throat. When wiped off the lesions leave red sore areas, which may bleed. The baby's mouth may be sore and uncomfortable, making the baby fussy during and between feeds. They may slip on and off the breast and may make a clicking sound.

Oral candida can also spread to the nappy area causing a pimply red rash. This usually has bright red, shiny patches with clearly defined borders, and may also affect the skin folds. A mass of red pustules may appear beyond the outer edge of the rash.

Bottle-fed babies are more likely to develop thrush and taking antibiotics will predispose. A woman with thrush should avoid freezing expressed milk since freezing does not kill yeast cells and the stored milk may reinfect the baby.

Herbal treatments

For oral thrush:
Wash out the baby's mouth with swabs of Marigold (*Calendula off.*) or Garlic (*Allium sativum*) infusion.
Breastfeeding mothers can take plenty of raw Garlic in their diet.
For candida nappy rash:
Wash with Marigold infusion and apply Marigold cream. See also 'Nappy rash'.
Immune system restoratives may be indicated in persistent cases, such as Marigold, Echinacea (*Echinacea* spp.), or Thyme (*Thymus vulgaris*) tea, taken by mother or baby.

Colic

Colic is a broad term describing excessive and frequent crying in a baby who appears to be otherwise well, defined as incessant crying for around three hours a day that cannot be comforted. Estimated to affect one in five babies, it typically starts around two weeks old and usually ends by four months of age. It can occur at any time, often happening at the same time each evening. It seems that babies are experiencing acute spasmodic pain with contractions of the immature intestines or trapped gas, frequently causing them to draw up their knees, arch their back or clench their fists. Some babies cry for many hours during the day or night, leaving both baby and mother exhausted. Colic can be extremely distressing for mothers, listening to their baby crying and unable to comfort them, often feeling helpless, inadequate, and increasingly desperate to stop the crying. Mothers in this situation need help and support in dealing with stress.

Causes are not fully understood but colic is largely associated with the immaturity of the baby's digestive system. Food sensitivities can play a part, whether allergies/intolerances or simply foods that pass through the breast milk and may be hard for a baby to deal with, such as excess fruit or brassicas. Keep a food diary to identify possible triggers (see 'Allergies'). Other factors can include an over-abundant milk supply, reflux, or problems latching onto the breast causing air to be swallowed. A baby may be suffering the after-effects of a traumatic birth, or may be affected by being in an environment of stress or tension. Colic is more common in premature babies.

Management

Different things help different babies but most infants are more settled if they have skin-to-skin contact with their mother and can feed whenever they need to. Simply holding and carrying the baby may help, or holding him or her in different positions.

Sit the baby upright during feeds and wind after feeding. Avoid over-stimulating the baby with loud noise, bright colours, or a crowded room. Playing relaxing music, or movement and motion may help, for instance a walk in the buggy or pram, or a car journey.

Herbal treatments

Teas: Give 20–30ml of a carminative, digestive tea before feeds. Suitable carminatives are Fennel seed (*Foeniculum vulgare*), Dill (*Anethum graveolens*), Caraway (*Carum carvi*) or Aniseed (*Pimpinella anisum*), Caraway being the strongest. Repeat after feeds if necessary. Hydrosols are also effective. Add Catnip (*Nepeta cataria*) and Chamomile (*Chamomilla recutita*) to ease the nervous system and aid restful sleep. Give 20–30ml Slippery Elm (*Ulmus rubra*) in warm water to soothe and calm digestion.

Baths: A warm relaxing bath together can calm both mother and baby, and some babies who are refusing to feed will naturally latch on in warm water. Add full strength herb teas, selecting from Fennel, Chamomile, Catnip, Lemon Balm (*Melissa off.*), Dill, Caraway, Aniseed, and Lavender (*Lavandula* spp.), singly or combined.

Massage: Some babies with colic will enjoy a gentle baby massage. Avoid massage directly after a feed. Chamomile and Lavender EO, 2% dilution in base oil, make a soothing oil for colic.

Craniosacral treatment or chiropractic adjustment is valuable for disturbances resulting from cranial or other physical trauma.

Constipation

Formula fed babies are more likely to be constipated than those exclusively on breast milk. It is unusual for breastfed babies to be constipated, and for some, it can be normal to go for several days without passing a stool. As long as the baby is not in discomfort or distress, this is not a problem. If there appears to be discomfort, consider the possibility of sensitivity to something in the mother's diet (see 'Allergy').

Formula milk is less easily digested than breast milk and can lead to constipation with hard stools that may be blood-tinged. The baby may have a tight belly and be straining while passing stools.

For babies with constipation, ensure they are drinking enough fluids. Give diluted prune juice or water from cooking prunes for a gentle laxative effect.

Teas: Combine Fennel (*Foeniculum vulgare*), Chamomile (*Chamomilla recutita*), and Liquorice (*Glycyrrhiza glabra*) root, giving 25ml at night.

Baths: A warm bath can help a baby's muscles relax and facilitate a bowel movement. Add Chamomile or Lavender, tea or essential oil (1% dilution in a dispersant) to the bath.

Massage: Gentle abdominal massage may stimulate a bowel movement. Combine Chamomile or Lavender EO at 1% in a base oil, massaging in a clockwise direction. Can be repeated several times throughout the day, particularly beneficial before a warm bath. Also helpful rubbed on soles of feet.

Cradle cap, seborrhoeic dermatitis

Seborrhoeic dermatitis (or 'seborrhoeic eczema') is common in infants, usually occurring before three months and resolving spontaneously by six to twelve months. This is thought to be caused by hyperactivity of sebaceous glands responding to residual circulating maternal hormones shortly after birth. It most frequently affects the scalp as 'cradle cap', sometimes the nappy area, less often the eyebrows, forehead, temples, folds around the nose, and area behind the ears. Very rarely, it becomes generalised which may indicate the development of atopic eczema, especially if there is a family history of atopy.

Cradle cap causes crusty or oily scaly patches on a baby's scalp. It is not usually itchy, but can cause thick, white, or yellow scales that are difficult to remove. Gentle brushing with a soft brush can help to loosen the scales. To assist removal, gently massage sunflower, wheatgerm, or coconut oil into the scalp. Leave to soak for at least two hours before using a mild baby shampoo and tepid water to wash the scalp. Oak bark (*Quercus robur/petraea*) decoction or distilled Witch Hazel (*Hamamelis virginiana*) rubbed into the scalp or applied as a compress can astringe and slow down oil production. Heartsease (*Viola tricolor*) infusion may be drunk by a breastfeeding mother or given directly to the baby

In the nappy area, the skin may become red, inflamed, and flaky, generally affecting the groin although it may spread. See 'Nappy Rash' for treatments.

Croup see Respiratory illness page 295.

Diarrhoea, infantile diarrhoea

Loose stools can be normal and diarrhoea is unusual in breast-fed babies. However, if a baby is unwell, with frequent, watery stools, and/or vomiting, he or she may have gastroenteritis. This is more likely to occur in a bottle-fed baby. Give plenty of fluids since babies can quickly become dehydrated. Diarrhoea may also be linked with stress and tension. Persistent diarrhoea may be associated with allergy (see 'Allergy').

Diarrhoea can cause severe nappy rash (see 'Nappy Rash'). Seek help if acute, frequent diarrhoea persists in a baby for more than twenty-four hours.

Herbal treatments

Teas: Agrimony (*Agrimonia eupatoria*), Meadowsweet (*Filipendula ulmaria*), Raspberry leaf (*Rubus idaeus*), or Cinnamon (*Cinnamonum zeylandicum/verum*). Add Chamomile (*Chamomilla recutita*), Lemon Balm (*Melissa off.*), Limeflowers (*Tilia europaea*), or Catnip (*Nepeta cataria*) if tension is a factor.

Give Slippery Elm (*Ulmus rubra*) in warm water to soothe the bowel.

Ear infections, otitis media

An upper respiratory infection can lead to otitis media causing pain and swelling of the eardrum. Signs of pain include rubbing or pulling at ears, crying more than usual, and trouble sleeping. Fever may be present. Left untreated, the eardrum may burst, causing pus to drain out and relieving pain. Treat with Echinacea (*Echinacea* spp.) and Garlic (*Allium sativum*) as for 'Infections'. If the eardrum is intact, make ear drops with Mullein (*Verbascum thapsus*) infused oil 50ml and Lavender EO 1gtt, put into outer ear and plug with cotton wool before bed. Frequent ear infections may be associated with CMPA/I (see 'Allergies').

Eczema, atopic dermatitis

The terms 'atopic eczema' and 'atopic dermatitis' are used interchangeably. They describe a chronic and relapsing inflammatory skin condition causing itchy, dry, inflamed, cracked skin, and the most common dermatitis in babies. Atopic dermatitis often affects hands, wrists, knee and elbow creases, cheeks, scalp, and behind the ears. The trunk is frequently affected in babies. In severe cases the whole body can be inflamed. Intense itching may break the skin causing areas of wetness or bleeding, and leading to infection, skin thickening or permanent scarring.

Onset is usually between ages three and six months but can be at any time. There is skin barrier dysfunction, frequently associated with environmental and food allergies (see 'Allergies'), and family history of atopy. Exacerbating factors include dry skin, irritants, stress, allergies, infection, sweating, and climate conditions such as extremely dry or hot and humid. Severe itch can cause disturbed sleep and irritability.

Management

Avoid soap, detergents, any products with harsh chemicals, wool, or man-made fabrics or clothing; also avoid low humidity or rapid changes in temperature. Check for allergies, avoid dust or sand, cigarette smoke, long, hot baths or showers. Keep baby's fingernails short to reduce skin damage from scratching. Baby can wear cotton mittens at night.

Herbal treatments

Frequent application of moisturising emollient ointments to soothe, heal, and calm itching.

Chickweed (*Stellaria media*) and Marshmallow (*Althaea off.*) ointment is highly effective. Also Comfrey (*Symphytum off.*) can be used, or Marigold (*Calendula off.*) if infection is present. For large areas, use a soothing, anti-pruritic, anti-inflammatory oil, such as Chickweed, Comfrey, Marigold, or St John's Wort (*Hypericum perforatum*) infused oils with 10% Avocado oil and 1% Lavender EO. For weeping skin, apply cool compresses of Oak bark (*Quercus robur/petraea*) decoction.

To calm nerves and relieve itch, add Oats (*Avena sativa*) in muslin bag under hot tap for baths, or 3gtt Lavender EO. Add 1 cup cider vinegar as extra for itch. Pat dry gently and moisturise well. Heartsease (*Viola tricolor*) or Red Clover (*Trifolium pratense*) infusion can be added to baths, 1 cup, and taken internally 10–30ml tds.

Eye conditions

Babies can have a normal discharge resulting in a collection of dried mucus, usually cream coloured, in the corner of the eye. Often due to an irritant entering the eye from dirty hands. Wipe away with water.

Blocked tear duct or 'sticky eye'

A blocked tear duct is present in 10% of newborns. The main symptom is a constant watery eye, without swelling of the eyelid or redness of the eye. Tears fill the eye and run down the face. The wet eye may get secondary infections that cause the eyelids to become matted with pus.

Conjunctivitis

Conjunctivitis is a bacterial or viral infection of the eye. In bacterial infection the main symptom is eyelids stuck together with pus (yellow or green discharge) after sleep. Can affect one or both eyes. After being wiped away, the pus recurs during the day. Eyelids are often puffy. The whites of the eye may or may not be red or pink. In viral conjunctivitis, the main sign is pinkness of the sclera and watery eyes. Usually bilateral. Most viruses do not cause pus in the eyes.

Herbal treatment

For all these conditions, infusions of Elderflower (*Sambucus nigra* flos), Marigold (*Calendula off.*), Chamomile (*Chamomilla recutita*), Fennel (*Foeniculum vulgare*), or Eyebright (*Euphrasia off.*) are used to wash the baby's eyes, straining thoroughly through muslin or a coffee filter. Wet a sterile cotton ball with cooled infusion and gently wipe the baby's eye from the inside corner to the outside corner. Use a new cotton ball for each wipe. Dry the eye using a different cotton ball, wiping from the inside corner out. Repeat at least three or four times daily. If discharge is profuse, add a good pinch of Golden Seal (*Hydrastis canadensis*) powder to the infusion. Breastfeeding mothers can eat raw Garlic (*Allium sativum*) to assist clearing infection.

Infections and fevers

Most fevers in infants (above 38°C) are caused by viral infections, such as colds or other upper respiratory infections. About 10% are caused by potentially more serious bacterial illness, such as blood infections or meningitis. If fever persists more than twenty-four hours or if you are concerned about other signs of infection (see 'Signs of Serious Illness' above), immediate medical intervention may be required.

Infant fever management

If the baby's temperature is raised, remove excess clothing and bed coverings. Wearing a vest and nappy, and being covered by a sheet may be sufficient. Keep a febrile infant in a well-ventilated room that is neither very hot nor very cold. Ensure plenty of fluids such as breast milk, herb teas (below), water, or diluted juices.

Herbal treatments for infections and fevers

For fever, the baby's body can be cooled with tepid sponging, using lukewarm Elderflower (*Sambucus nigra*) and Yarrow (*Achillea millefollium*) tea, or diluted vinegar (1part vinegar to 2 parts water). These liquids may also be used as a compress on the forehead and abdomen, or wrapped around the baby's feet.

For fevers, colds, and runny nose, give teas of Elderflower, Catnip (*Nepeta cataria*), and Yarrow to the baby and to breastfeeding mothers. Add Hyssop (*Hyssopus off.*) or Red Clover (*Trifolium pratense*) for cough, Limeflowers (*Tilia europaea*) or Chamomile (*Chamomilla recutita*) for irritability. Any of these teas can be added to a warm bath. Include Thyme (*Thymus vulgaris*) infusion in the bath if there is lung involvement, see also 'Respiratory illness'.

For infection, with or without fever, a breastfeeding mother can consume plenty of raw Garlic (*Allium sativum*), and Garlic can be crushed into vegetable oil and applied to the soles of the baby's feet (take care not to burn the baby's delicate skin, wipe off immediately if redness is seen).

Use Eucalyptus or Lemon EO in a burner or diffuser, or in a room spray to moisten the air. Include Lavender or Chamomile EO to bring calm.

If a baby has a blocked nose that prevents feeding, Elderflower tea nose drops can loosen thick nasal mucus. Nasal passages may be suctioned with a rubber-bulb syringe.

After thirty-five years of practice, Echinacea (*Echinacea* spp.) is still my number one herb for treating and preventing infection, with garlic a close second. These are frequently prescribed together. In babies I have witnessed these two plants perform amazing accomplishments, including restoring the health of a critically ill four week old baby, hospitalised with a drug-resistant infection, who responded within four days to daily Echinacea tincture and Garlic juice (aa 5ml) given by nasogastric tube. For less severe infections at home, give Echinacea, 10–20gtt bd/tds, well diluted with water or formula. Breastfeeding mothers can take Echinacea 5–10ml tds/qds to treat their babies.

Jaundice, neonatal jaundice

Jaundice is estimated to affect 60% of babies, including 80% of those born prematurely. It usually starts at between two to three days old and lasts from ten to fourteen days, characterised by yellowing of skin, whites of eyes, palms, and soles of feet. It is more common in breastfed babies, and can last a month or more. Neonatal jaundice is usually harmless, caused by the breakdown of the baby's red blood cells by the liver which are no longer required once the baby is breathing oxygen. The breakdown of red blood cells results in a build-up of bilirubin which the newborn's immature liver may be slow to process. In most cases, this gradually corrects itself without treatment. Around 5% of babies have a blood bilirubin level high enough to need treatment, mainly phototherapy where the baby is placed under a light to help break down bilirubin. Parents can assist this process at home by exposing the baby to indirect sunlight or natural light, for instance by putting the baby on the bed just in a nappy. Breastfeeding mothers can support the baby's liver by drinking Dandelion (*Taraxacum off.*) root decoction, 2 cups daily.

In a small number of cases, jaundice can be the sign of an underlying health condition such as infection or liver problems. This may often be the case if jaundice develops within the first twenty-four hours after delivery.

Nappy rash

Many babies develop nappy rash. It may be mild with red patches, or the entire nappy area can be inflamed and sore, with red raw areas, spots, pimples, and blisters. It may lead to secondary bacterial or herpes infection, and the baby may be uncomfortable and distressed.

Causes include skin sensitivity, candida (see 'Candida'), food sensitivity (see 'Allergies'), leaving nappies on too long before changing, inadequate drying of the baby's skin after washing, reaction to antibiotics, early atopic eczema, seborrhoeic dermatitis, diarrhoea, and teething.

Management

Prevention is the best treatment. Change wet or dirty nappies promptly, using cotton wool and dilute Marigold (*Calendula off.*) infusion to clean the whole nappy area gently but thoroughly, wiping from front to back. Pat dry after washing, avoid vigorous rubbing, whenever possible leave off the nappy so skin is exposed to air. Do not use soap, bubble bath, talcum powder, alcohol-based baby wipes, or scented products.

Herbal treatments

Apply a protective barrier ointment after drying the skin. Marigold is particularly helpful being soothing, healing, and anti-infective. Comfrey (*Symphytum off.*), Marshmallow (*Althaea off.*), Plantain (*Plantago lanceolata/major*), Chickweed (*Stellaria media*), and Chamomile (*Chamomilla recutita*) are all suitable. Alternatively, apply infused oil of Marigold, Plantain, Comfrey, or St John's Wort (*Hypericum perforatum*), using Sunflower oil and incorporating 10% Avocado oil to help soothe inflammation. Chamomile or Lavender EO 1% can be added.

Reflux

Reflux and regurgitation of milk can affect up to 40% of babies and usually resolve by twelve to eighteen months. Reflux is primarily caused by immaturity of the baby's digestive tract, and is also associated with food allergy such as CMPA (see 'Allergies'). Typical onset around eight weeks, improving over time as the oesophagus develops. Signs of reflux include regurgitation of milk during or after feeds, refusing feeds, gagging or choking, crying during feeds, persistent hiccups or coughing, and frequent ear infections.

Hold babies upright rather than lying down, especially during feeds. Check for allergy involvement, and check positioning and attachment if breastfeeding. Fennel (*Foeniculum vulgare*) tea or Slippery Elm (*Ulmus rubra*), 20–30ml given to babies before feeds will ease.

Respiratory Illness

Respiratory illness is common in infancy; including colds, flu, croup, and bronchiolitis, which can all cause lethargy and poor feeding. See 'Infections and Fevers' for treatment of colds and flu. Upper respiratory infection is most commonly viral and may spread to the chest, or infection may directly affect the lower airways, such as a bacterial pneumonia. Asthma often starts as a nocturnal cough although too early to diagnose in first twelve weeks of life. In rare cases, respiratory illness may develop into a serious acute condition.

Chest infections, bronchitis

A chest infection usually begins as the common cold. Cough is typically accompanied by nasal discharge, watery at first, becoming thicker and coloured after several days. There may be slight fever and general malaise. Cough can be dry or productive, with wheeze, rapid or shallow breathing, and a rapid heartbeat.

Give the baby warm Hyssop (*Hyssopus off.*) infusions tds/qds to help clear obstructed airways. Breastfeeding mothers can take Echinacea (*Echinacea* spp.) 5–10ml tds/qds and plenty of raw Garlic (*Allium sativum*) (at least three cloves daily). Give bottle-fed babies Echinacea 10–20gtt bd/tds, diluted. Give Thyme (*Thymus vulgaris*) baths and apply chest rub two or three times daily to chest and soles of feet, using infused oil of fresh Thyme, with 1% dilution essential oils of Chamomile and Lavender. Burn or diffuse Eucalyptus EO in the baby's room.

Croup, laryngotracheobronchitis

Usually viral, causes swelling of the trachea and larynx, with hoarseness, harsh cough, and characteristic high-pitched sound on inhalation. Humidity and steam help greatly, especially at night. Boil a kettle continuously in the bedroom or take the baby into the bathroom and turn on hot water to create a steamy atmosphere. Give infusions of Catnip (*Nepeta cataria*), Hyssop, or Red Clover (*Trifolium pratense*) with addition of 10 drops Echinacea tds. Give prophylactic Thyme baths before bed, followed by chest rub as for chest infections.

Bronchiolitis

Inflammation of the bronchioles, caused by a range of viruses including the respiratory syncytial virus (RSV), which typically occurs in the winter months. For many healthy infants, RSV causes symptoms of the common cold, but some babies develop bronchiolitis, characterised by rapid shallow breathing, chest retraction, wheezing, difficulty feeding, and intermittent but persistent cough. The baby may have fever and flaring of nostrils. Most cases are mild and clear within two to three days, some need hospital treatment. Early signs resemble common cold with runny nose and cough, further signs developing over next few days. Treatment as for bronchitis.

Sleep problems, restlessness, and wakefulness

It is normal for sleep patterns to take a while to establish after birth and every baby is different. Massage and a relaxing herbal bath before bed will help, and avoiding stimulation if the baby wakes during the night, such as bright lights or playing with the baby.

Massage oil: Lavender, Chamomile, Geranium, or Rose EO 1% dilution in base oil

Baths: Infusions of Chamomile (*Chamomilla recutita*), Lavender (*Lavandula augustifolia*), Rose (*Rosa spp.*), Limeflowers (*Tilia europaea*), Lemon Balm (*Melissa off.*). Oatmeal (*Avena sativa*) in bag. Catnip (*Nepeta cataria*) and Thyme (*Thymus vulgaris*) for irritability with coughs or colds. EO Lavender for restlessness.

Vibrational essences: Chamomile essence 3gtt in a relaxing room spray, or added to massage oil, bath, or placed directly on skin. Other essences will help in individual circumstances (see Chapter 16).

Umbilical care

The baby's cord will have been cut and clamped. The clamp is released after a few hours and it usually takes from one to two weeks for the cord stump to fall off, although it can happen earlier or up to a week later. The cord stump can be cleaned with Marigold (*Calendula off.*) infusion or dilute tincture. This can be continued after the stump falls off until the navel is completely healed and dry.

Vomiting

Occasional vomiting is normal in a baby, with causes including indigestion, coughing, and crying. However, if a baby is suddenly and repeatedly vomiting, it may be due to infection. She or he may also have diarrhoea. Give Meadowsweet (*Filipendula ulmaria*) tea and teaspoonful doses of Slippery Elm (*Ulmus rubra*) to settle her stomach. Chamomile (*Chamomilla recutita*) or Lemon Balm (*Melissa off.*) tea are also beneficial. Give plenty of fluids to ensure the baby is not dehydrated. Breast milk provides ideal rehydration.

Vomiting is also associated with food allergy (see 'Allergies') or may be projectile vomiting from pyloric stenosis which usually manifests at between two and twelve weeks old. Pyloric stenosis typically requires surgery.

Welcoming the newborn

Herbs to welcome and bless a new baby

Herbs have traditionally been associated with the blessing of babies. A plant may simply be hung on the baby's cradle, made into an amulet or pouch, or incorporated as part of a more elaborate ritual or ceremony. A blessing plant with symbolic meaning makes a beautiful and thoughtful gift for a new baby.

Many parents like to hold a ceremony to bless their newborn infant and welcome them to their family and the Earth. This may be part of a religious ceremony, such as a Christening, or it may be performed as part of a baby naming ceremony. The latter is where parents gather with family and friends to welcome and name the baby, stating their love and commitment, acknowledging the role of family and friends and offering blessings for the child's future. This is held wherever the parents choose and might include readings, poems, music, parental promises and the appointment of 'guide-parents'. In addition to these more formal events, some parents like to perform their own simple and intimate baby blessing, often carried out soon after the baby's birth. In all these cases, herbs can play an appropriate role. Some traditional baby blessing plants and practices are listed below.

Baby blessing herbs

Birch	Place a Birch twig bundle tied with red ribbon in the corner of the baby's room, bringing blessings of vitality and radiant health
Cloves	Make a blessing bag of Cloves as a protection charm to be hung in a corner of the baby's room to keep them safe from harm
Hawthorn	Include Hawthorn in a bag or bouquet to be hung up above or near the baby's cradle to bring protection and good-luck

Peony	Peony root is traditionally used as a protection necklace for a baby. Thread the peony root beads onto yellow or gold thread. The necklace can be hung in a corner or over the door in the baby's room
Vervain	Used in baby blessings to bring luck and good health, and with the aim of making the child both happy and clever
Yarrow	Tie a small bunch of Yarrow with a ribbon and hang near the baby's cradle for love and protection

Notes

1. Allergies and intolerances are technically different entities, but for simplicity I am calling them all 'allergies', since in infants this does not alter the general herbal approach.
2. Høst A. (1994). Cow's milk protein allergy and intolerance in infancy. Some clinical, epidemiological and immunological aspects. *Pediatric allergy and immunology: official publication of the European Society of Pediatric Allergy and Immunology*, 5(5 Suppl), 1–36.

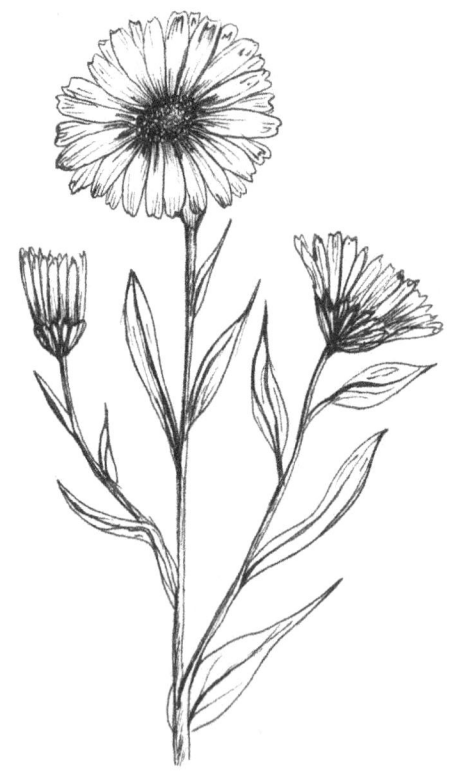

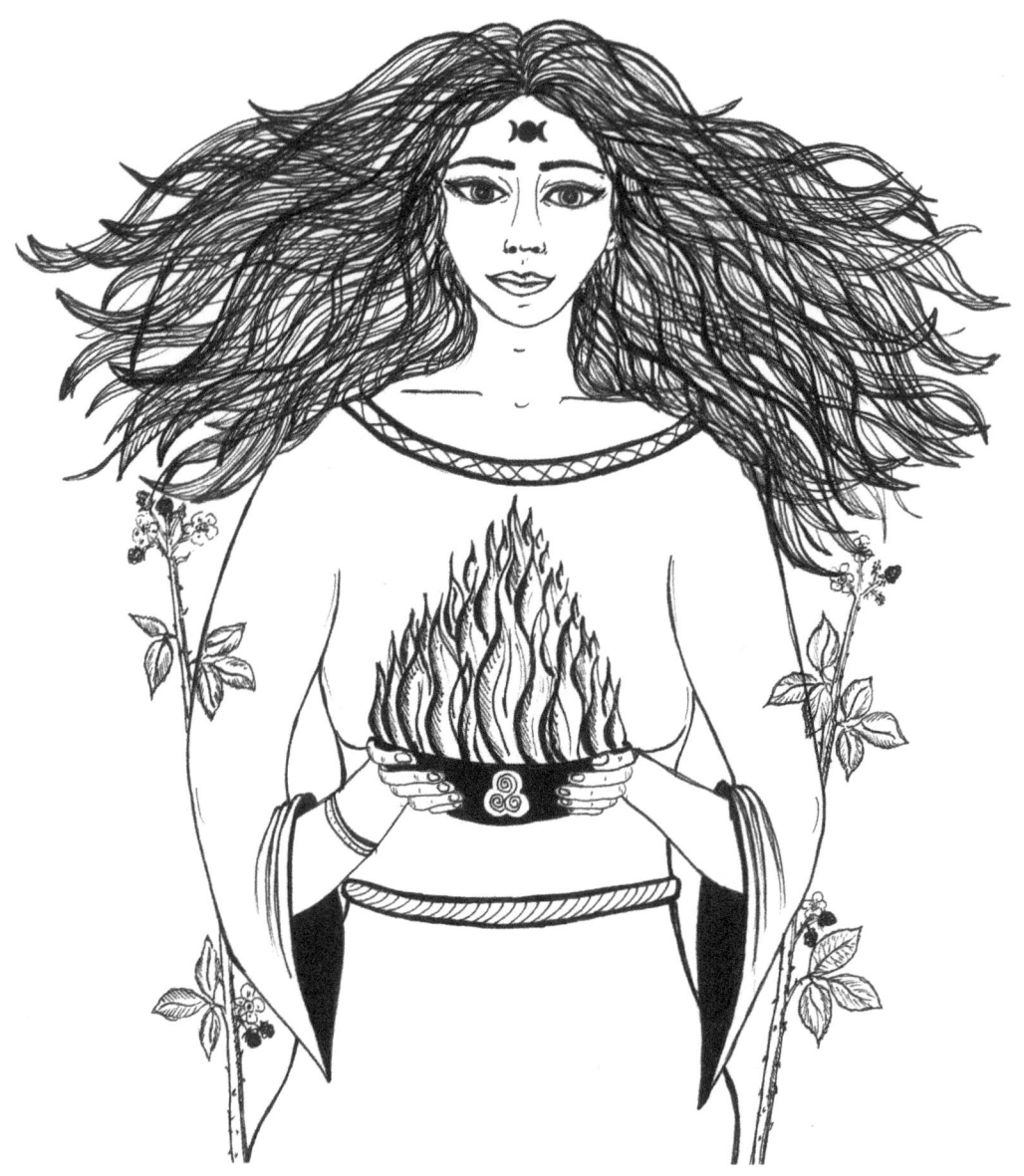

Brigid. Goddess of healing, creativity and smithcraft. Keeper of the Sacred Flame and holy wells. Bringer of inspiration.
Blackberry, Bramble (*Rubus fructicosus*). The tenacious, resilient one who strengthens boundaries and takes decisive action.

CHAPTER 16

Vibrational essences

What are vibrational essences?

Vibrational essences play a unique role in healthcare and can be a valuable addition to a herbalist's tool kit. Flower essences were first popularised by Dr Edward Bach in 1930's when he produced the Bach Flower Remedies, aimed at treating emotional and psychological disturbances. His Rescue Remedy is well known globally as a remedy for shock and trauma.

Since that time, interest in flower essences has grown and inspired essence makers all around the world. Today, in addition to the original thirty-eight remedies of Dr Bach, thousands of essences are available globally, all relevant to our rapidly changing world and addressing emotional, mental, spiritual, and physical needs. Many of these vibrational essences incorporate not only flowers, but additional energies, such as those from leaves, minerals, animals, and aspects of the environment.

Medicine for the soul

Vibrational essences are medicine for the soul. Bach described disease as a conflict between the personality and the soul, stating that "health depends on being in harmony with our souls". He went on to explain that "we each have a Divine Mission, and our souls use our minds and bodies as instruments to do this work, so that when all three are working in unison the result is perfect health and perfect happiness".[1]

Vibrational medicine is a form of energy medicine, viewing physical matter as networks of complex and inter-related energy fields. Water is the universal carrier of vibrational imprints, and essences are water extracts carrying the vibrational imprint of whatever they are made from. During the process of flower essence making, the water starts to resonate with the vibration of the flower and this resonance remains held in the water. A flower essence can be described as a vibrational expression of the plant or the perfect light of the flower, held within the sacred space of the water. The essence is a high vibrational electrical solution imprinted with the unique energy patterns of the flower and encapsulating its healing virtues, the gifts the flower is bringing to the world.

Essences are not the only way to access these unique virtues, for instance, you might experience them simply by sitting with the plant, or even from a tincture that has been made with care and intent. However, vibrational essences offer a remarkably simple and efficient way to preserve and administer the subtle gifts of a plant, readily opening a gateway to the plant's consciousness and deeper non-physical qualities.

How do essences work?

Vibrational essences work according to the principle of resonance. The energetic structure of an essence resonates with and amplifies particular qualities within a person's soul. The closer an essence matches the person's energetic condition, the more effective it will be. On the other hand, if there is no particular resonance, the essence will not have an impact, thereby eliminating any risk of overdosage or adverse effect.

Essences bring out our highest potential. They help us become responsible for our soul life and deepen our capacity for human love. From a spiritual perspective we are 'coming home' when we take an essence.

Vibrational essences in pregnancy and lactation

Vibrational essences are safe for use in pregnancy, lactation, and for people of all ages, including the newborn. They have no harmful side effects and can be prescribed by herbalists and non-herbalists alike. Essences do not push or suppress, and you will not cause harm by choosing the 'wrong' essence, it will simply not be effective. Pregnant and lactating women and babies have heightened sensitivity and may only require a single dose to receive significant benefit.

Gentle medicine for mind, body, emotions, and spirit

Vibrational medicine directly addresses core issues that may be holding the soul back from following its true path. Working gently yet profoundly, essences treat underlying energy patterns, impacting on physical, emotional, mental, and spiritual levels. They provide a powerful way to address fears, anxieties, and stuck patterns, to heal and prevent illness, and to transform consciousness.

Using essences in herbal practice

I have loved essences ever since being introduced to the Bach Rescue Remedy as a teenager. During my herbal training, herbalist Chris Hedley taught me how to dowse for essences with a pendulum, a method I found outstandingly effective and helpful. When I set up in herbal practice, it was natural for me to incorporate essences in my work, and I have found them to be a valuable aspect of herbal medicine, as well as helping to give me a deep appreciation of the consciousness and soul properties of plants. Initially I prescribed the Bach remedies, gradually adding others, such as those from the Flower Essence Society (FES[2]) and I have been making my own since 1987. Nowadays, I use all my own essences and these are the ones referenced in this text because they are the ones I am using routinely in clinical practice. However, a wide variety of wonderful essences exists worldwide, and you can easily make your own (see 'Resources' for books describing methods of making essences). With so many essences available, you are advised to do your own research, follow your inner guidance and work with whatever appeals to you most. While not necessarily applicable for every patient, they can add another dimension to your herbal practice.

Choosing essences for a patient

Numerous techniques exist in order to choose the most suitable essences for an individual, including self-selection. The simplest method, starting out, can be to read the descriptions or indications and select what fits the patient (see below for a list of indications for the essences in this book). Trust your intuition.

For me, dowsing with a pendulum has been my most trusted method of selection for nearly forty years. I simply ask to know the best essences for the patient's soul at this time. This method, once mastered, is particularly advantageous when selecting essences for babies or anyone who is not able to articulate their needs or deeper feelings. It allows me to find the specific essences required for the most beneficial effect.

Dowsing offers a way to uncover hidden soul issues, providing a diagnostic aid as well as revealing the most appropriate treatment. When a patient sees the essences that emerge from dowsing, it can enhance their own self-awareness and assist them in following their soul's path. For instance, a woman whose baby is overdue may discover a previously unrecognised psychological block that is preventing her from going into labour. A full discussion of the use of essences is outside the scope of this book, but if they are calling you, I would encourage further exploration. Vibrational essences offer profound support for pregnant women and their babies.

Internal use of essences

Essences are usually sold as 'stock' bottles, preserved in an alcohol base such as brandy or occasionally vinegar. An essence may be taken neat, two or three drops under the tongue, or diluted in a glass of water or other beverage (including herb tea or tincture) and sipped as required. Alternatively, one or more essences can be made up into a treatment bottle. This is prepared by adding two to three drops of your chosen 'stock' remedy or remedies to a 30ml dropper bottle filled with natural spring water and a little brandy or cider vinegar to help its keeping qualities. Take four drops under the tongue, or in any convenient way, four times daily or as required. A 30ml bottle will last around three weeks. In crisis, take the prepared remedy as frequently as needed. A breastfeeding mother can take the essences to pass on to her baby, or two drops (neat or diluted 'stock') can be added to the baby's bottle. When taking drops from a treatment bottle, care must be taken not to touch the pipette directly on the tongue since this may contaminate the liquid.

Typically, between one and five essences are taken at once but there are no rules. Equally, duration of treatment is variable. As mentioned above, effects can be instant. This may mean that only one dose is required, or it may be that continued use is of benefit to consolidate and integrate change. Sometimes essences are given sequentially, each one having a 'key' effect that unlocks accessibility to the next level, for instance, when breaking down stuck patterns. Suffice to say, there is no time limit to treatment.

Topical application

Essences may be given in a wide variety of different ways, including topical application by rubbing them directly on the skin or adding them (2 drops of each chosen essence) to creams, ointments, lotions, oils, and baths. All these methods are suitable for pregnancy, lactation, and for babies.

Sprays

Room or aura sprays make a highly effective and simple method of application, easy to administer in most situations, including a hospital delivery room. Any individual essences can be made into sprays, diluted in water, hydrosol or even herb tea. The sprays I make are usually a synergistic blend of essences, hydrosols and essential oils. A typical room spray recipe is 50ml of chosen hydrosol, 2gtt of each required stock essence, 3gtt of an appropriate essential oil and 5gtt of soya lecithins[3] as an emulsifying agent. This can be used as a spray around the body to suffuse the auric field and to transform the atmosphere in rooms, cars, and other indoor and outdoor spaces.

Below is a selection of sprays particularly beneficial for pregnancy and birth:

Sacred Birthing *Motherwort, Nurturing Mother, Primrose, Skullcap, Arnica essences in a base of Damask Rose hydrosol and Rose essential oil*

A general purpose birthing spray bringing vibrations of deep peace, love, confidence, and empowerment to mother and child.

Affirmations: "I open to this wondrous experience with confidence and love", "I am in my power", "I open myself to birth my beautiful baby".

Sacred Space *Airmid, Angelica, Self-Heal, St John's Wort, Yarrow essences in a base of Agua Florida*[4]

A combination that cleanses and protects sacred space, inviting in helpful energies.

Affirmation: "This space is/I am cleansed and protected, sparkling with light", "I am in a safe, protected and sacred space".

Mother Goddess *Lady's Smock, Meadowsweet, and Derrynagittah Lily in a base of Damask Rose hydrosol and Rose essential oil*

A spray that connects with the Goddess as Mother, carrying vibrations of pure love, abundance, nurturing, beauty, gentleness, and creativity.

Affirmations: "The love of the Mother Goddess is with me", "The Divine Mother in me shines through", "I am a beautiful, loving Mother".

Happy Healthy Baby *Dog Rose, Nurturing Mother, Calendula in a base of Lavender hydrosol and Lavender essential oil*

Affirmations (spoken to the baby by the person using the spray): "You are loved and beautiful", "You are so very welcome and loved", "You are thriving and peaceful, soothed and content".

Indications/key qualities of essences referenced in this book

Essence	Indications/Key Qualities
Airmid	Hopelessness, overwhelm. Promotes trust and healing
Angelica	Feeling unsafe, insecure. Brings protection, angelic energies
Arnica	Recovery from shock and trauma
Banishing Guilt	Guilt
Bird's Foot Trefoil	Emotional wounding. Aids release of tissue trauma
Borage	Grief, low mood, tearfulness. Gives courage
Brigid's Blessing	Self-doubt, indecision. Brings trust, inspiration, decisive action
Bugarach	Feeling scattered, soul loss. Aids group harmony
Calendula	Low mood, depression, polluted atmospheres. Brings joy
Chamomile	Relieves fear and anxiety. Promotes calm courage
Comfrey	Tissue trauma. Promotes strength and healthy growth
Derrynagittah Lily	Whenever mothering is needed. Love, nurturing, gentleness
Dog Rose	Isolation. Brings a sense of feeling supported, never alone
Elecampane	Shame, feeling betrayed. Restores the heart
Forget-me-not	Helps us understand our spiritual connection with others
Forgiveness	Blame. Facilitates forgiveness of self and others
Lady's Smock	Feeling restricted. Brings protection, regulates timing
Lapis	Anger, rage, feelings of revenge. Helps with letting go
Little Saints	Difficulty coping, overwhelm. Steadiness in times of turmoil
Lousewort	Difficulty expressing feelings, shame. Raises self-worth
Marshmarigold	Difficulty letting go. Strengthens boundaries
Motherwort	Lack of confidence. Eases grief, promotes bonding

Mugwort	Disturbing dreams, resistance to change. Eases transitions
Nurturing mother	Exhaustion, lack of trust. Nurtures, soothes, promotes labour
Oak	Exhaustion, despair. Brings strength, courage, joy
Pink Heart Crystal	Loss, betrayal and heartbreak. Restores the heart
Plantain	Generational grief. Transforms old family patterns
Primrose	Any stuck condition, stalled labour. Initiation to a new level
Rescue	Assists recovery from shock and trauma. Restores auric field
Rosemary	Obsessive thoughts, disassociation. Centering and alertness
Sacred Waters	Stuck emotional patterns. Brings acceptance and flow
Skullcap	Blocked creative energy. Facilitates self-expression
St John's Wort	Vulnerability, anxiety. Feeling confident and protected
Tulsi	Anger, soul loss. Disperses anger in stressful situations
Valerian	Emotional distress, tension. Relieves pain, aids restful sleep
Vervain	Stress, perfectionism. Relaxation and loving acceptance of self
White Buffalo	Hopelessness, disharmony. Especially indicated for children

Essences, in all their forms, work well in combination with affirmations or positive statements to enhance their effect. This helps the mind and personality to align with the soul. It can be helpful to suggest that a person repeat the affirmation whenever they use the essence. Below is a list of indications with suitable essences and suggested affirmations.

Indications, suggested essences, and affirmations

Indication	Essence	Affirmation
Adjusting to change	Lady's Smock, Primrose	I am ready for change.
Anger	Lapis, Blackthorn	I let go of blame and bitterness.
Anxiety	Lady's Smock, Vervain	All is well. I live my life effortlessly.
Confidence, lack of	Motherwort	I am ready for anything.
Dark thoughts	Diviner's Sage	I have inner peace.
Dislike of one's body	Vervain	I look on the bright side. I love my (pregnant) body.
Expectations	Lapis	I go with the flow and trust the Universe.
Depression, low mood	Calendula	My heart is light and full of joy.
Disturbing dreams	Mugwort, Vervain	My sleep is calm and restful.

Exhaustion	Nurturing Mother	I am strong and energetic. I let go of struggle.
Fear/Terror	Chamomile	I am serene and courageous.
Fears for the baby	Lady's Smock	My baby is strong and healthy.
Fear of childbirth	Skullcap	My baby and I take this journey together to an awesome delivery.
Feeling alone, isolation	Dog Rose, Meadowsweet	I am never alone.
Feeling unsupported	Lady's Smock	I am supported and loved.
Grief/tearfulness	Borage, Pink Heart Crystal	My heart is soothed. I reclaim my joy.
Guilt	Banishing Guilt	I always did the best I could.
Healthy growth, to assist	Comfrey	My baby and I are thriving and strong.
Hopelessness, despair	White Buffalo	I hold onto hope in uncertain times.
Overwhelm, Inner turmoil	Little Saints	I remain strong under extreme stress.
Mother child bonding	Motherwort	My baby and I are always connected in love.
Shock and trauma	Arnica, Rescue, St John's Wort, Year of 21	I am calm, soothed, and steady.
Trust, lack of	Nurturing Mother	I trust my intuition. I trust in life itself.
Vulnerability	St John's Wort, Angelica	I am confident and protected. I know I am safe.

A complete list of my essences and their actions can be found at https://derrynagittah.ie/pages/what-are-vibrational-essences

Notes

1. Julian Barnard (editor), *Collected Writings of Edward Bach*. Bath: Ashgrove Press, 1994, 90–91.
2. www.flowersociety.org [last accessed 2/2/22].
3. Available from specialist suppliers, see Resources.
4. Agua Florida "Water of the Flowers" is a grain alcohol blend with citrus, herbs and spices, originating from South America.

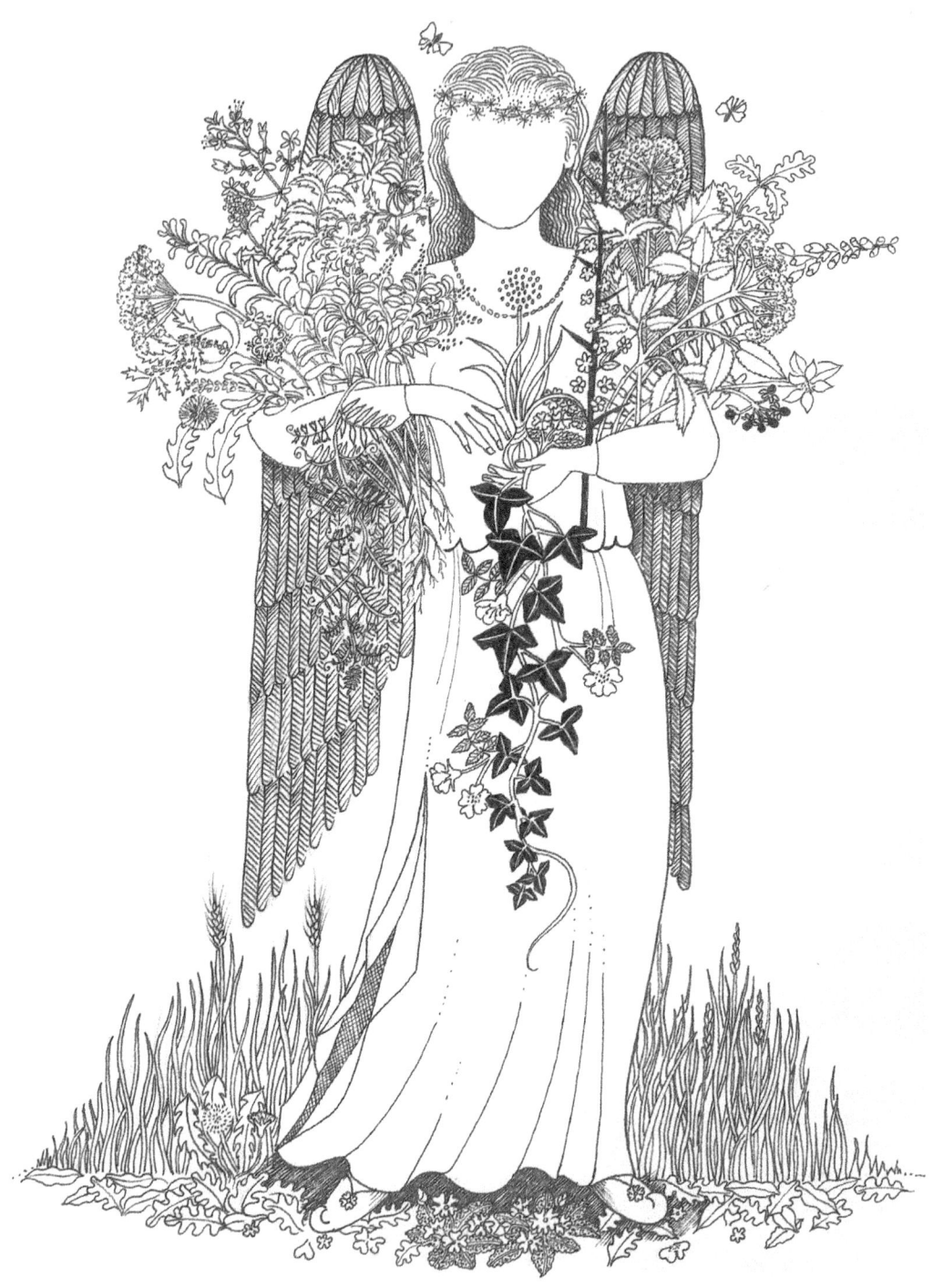

GLOSSARY OF HERBAL ACTIONS

Adaptogen	Increases the body's resistance and ability to cope with physical, chemical, and biological stresses
Alterative (depurative, blood-cleansing)	Restores proper function, health and vitality by helping the body to assimilate nutrients and eliminate waste
Analgesic	Pain relieving
Antacid	Prevents or corrects acidity, especially in the stomach
Anthelmintic	Destroys or expels parasitic worms
Anti-allergic	Prevents or relieves allergy
Anti-arthritic	Prevents or reduces joint inflammation
Anti-atheromatous	Prevents or reduces atheroma
Antibacterial	Helps the body destroy or resist bacteria
Anti-bilious	Reduces poor digestion from liver dysfunction
Anti-catarrhal	Counteracts build-up of excess mucus in the body
Anticoagulant	Prevents formation of blood clots
Antidepressant	Relieves or prevents depressed states of mind
Anti-emetic	Relieves or prevents nausea and vomiting
Antifungal	Helps body destroy or resist yeasts and other fungal organisms
Anti-haemorrhagic	Prevents or arrests haemorrhage
Antihidrotic	Reduces or prevents sweating

Antihistamine	Reduces damaging effects of histamine in allergic reactions
Anti-hypothyroid	Relieves or prevents underactive thyroid
Anti-inflammatory	Combats excessive inflammation
Antilithic	Prevents or reduces formation or development of calculi
Anti-microbial	Helps the body destroy or resist pathogenic organisms
Anti-neoplastic	Prevents, inhibits or halts the development of a neoplasm (tumour)
Antiobesic	Prevents or reduces obesity
Antioxidant	Protects the body against free-radical damage
Anti-platelet	Decreases platelet aggregation and inhibits clot formation in the arterial circulation
Anti-rheumatic	Alleviates or prevents rheumatic disease
Anti-sclerotic	Reduces hardening of tissues, especially arteries
Antiseptic	Helps the body destroy or resist pathogenic organisms
Anti-spasmodic	Prevents or reduces spasm
Antithrombotic	Prevents or reduces thrombosis
Anti-tussive	Prevents or reduces cough
Antiviral	Helps the body resist viral infection
Anxiolytic	Relieves anxiety
Aperient	Gentle digestive stimulant
Aphrodisiac	Increases sexual excitement and libido
Aromatic	Having a distinctive aroma
Astringent	Contracts, firms and strengthens tissue, reducing secretions and discharges
Bitter	Stimulating tonic for digestive system
Bronchodilator	Causes dilation of the bronchi
Cardiotonic	Increases efficiency and improves contraction of heart muscle
Carminative	Stimulates peristalsis in the digestive system and relaxes the stomach. Promotes expulsion of gas from the digestive tract
Cell proliferant	Increases cell proliferation and tissue growth
Cholagogue	Stimulates secretion of bile in the liver and release from the gall bladder. Laxative effect
Choleretic	Increases secretion of bile from the liver
Cicatrisant	Promotes wound healing and healthy cell regeneration
Decongestant	Relieves congestion

Demulcent	High in mucilage. Soothes, relaxes and protects irritated or inflamed tissue
Deobstruent	Removes obstructions in the tissues and eliminative organs
Diaphoretic	Promotes perspiration and aids elimination through the skin
Digestive	Aids digestive function
Diuretic	Increases secretion and elimination of urine
Dopaminergic	Increases dopamine-related activity in the brain
Emetic	Causes vomiting
Emmenagogue	True emmenagogues stimulate and normalise menstrual flow Term is sometimes used more broadly to describe tonics to the female reproductive system
Emollient	Applied externally, softens, soothes and protects the skin
Expectorant	Helps the body to remove excess mucus from the respiratory system
Febrifuge	Helps the body to bring down a fever
Galactagogue	Increases the flow of milk during lactation
Haemostatic	Arrests bleeding
Hepatic	Tones and strengthens the liver, improving function
Hepatoprotective	Protects the liver
Hypnotic	Powerful relaxant and sedative, helps induce sleep
Hypoglycaemic	Reduces elevated blood sugar levels
Hypotensive	Reduces elevated blood pressure
Immune modulator	Helps the body to resist and adapt (see Adaptagen)
Immunostimulant	Promotes immune activity
Laxative	Promotes evacuation of the bowels
Lymphatic	Supports health and activity of the lymphatic system
Nervine	Benefits, tones and strengthens the nervous system. May relax or stimulate
Neuralgesic	Reduces or prevents nerve pain
Oestrogenic	Promotes oestrogen release or has an action similar to that of oestrogen
Ophthalmic	Has an affinity for the eyes, relieves eye diseases
Oxytocic	Promotes oxytocin release or has an action similar to that of oxytocin, stimulates uterine contractions
Pancreatic	Aids the health and function of the pancreas
Parturient	Aids the process of giving birth

Partus preparator	Prepares the body for healthy childbirth
Progesterogenic	Promotes progesterone release or has an action similar to that of progesterone
Psychotropic	Affects mood, thoughts or perception
Purgative	Promotes cleansing, especially by the bowels
Refrigerant	A cooling agent
Rubefacient	Stimulates dilation of capillaries and local irritation when applied externally
Sedative	Calms the nervous system, reduces effects of stress and nervousness
Sialagogue	Stimulates secretion of saliva from salivary glands
Spasmolytic	Prevents or reduces spasm
Splenic	Aids the health and function of the spleen
Stimulant	Quickens and invigorates the physiological function of the body
Stomachic	Rtimulating tonic that aids stomach function
Styptic/haemostatic	Reduces or stops external bleeding
Sympathomimetic	Produces effects characteristic of stimulation of the sympathetic nervous system
Tonic	Strengthens and invigorates either specific organs or the whole body
Trophorestorative	Nutritive restorative, usually for an organ or system
Vasoconstrictor	Contracts blood vessels
Vasodilator	Dilates blood vessels
Vasoprotective	Protects blood vessels
Vulnerary	Wound healing when applied externally

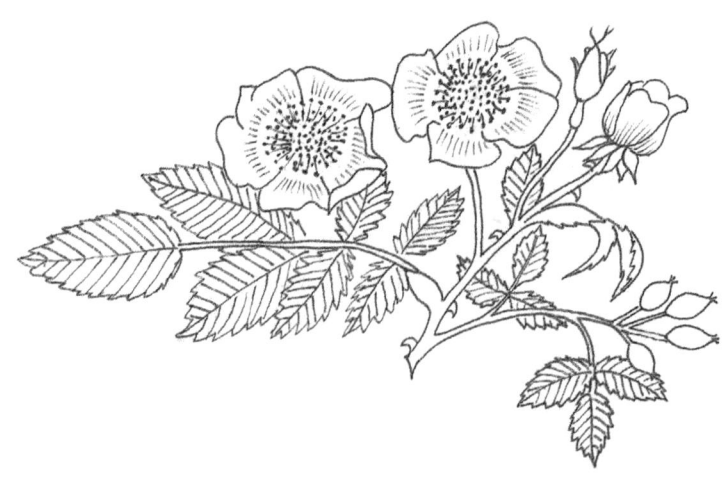

RESOURCES

Herbal suppliers

For tinctures, fluid extracts, dried herbs, creams, ointments, essential oils, and other herbal products. [websites last accessed 27/7/21]

Rutland Biodynamics www.rutlandbio.com

Avicenna www.avicennaherbs.co.uk also stocks emulsifying agents such as soya lecithins for making sprays as well as a wide range of hydrosols

Planta Medica www.plantamedica.co.uk (for UK) www.plantamedicaeurope.eu (for EU countries)

BIBLIOGRAPHY

Essential oils

Pam Conrad, *Women's Health Aromatherapy.* London: Singing Dragon, 2019.
Nikki Darrell, *Essential Oils: Their Therapeutic use in Herbal medicine, Aromatic Medicine and Aromatherapy; A Concise Manual.* Cork: Veriditas Hibernica, 2014.

General interest

Phyllida Anam-Aire, *A Celtic Book of Dying.* Forres, Scotland: Findhorn Press, 2005.
Susan Boulet, *Goddess Knowledge Cards.* CA: Pomegranate, 2003.
Louann Brizendine, *The Male Brain.* New York: Reuters, 2010.
Brenda Davies, *Journey of the Soul.* London: Hodder and Stoughton, 2002.
Wayne W. Dyer and Dee Garnes, *Memories of Heaven.* London: Hay House, 2015.
Sandra Ingerman, *Soul Retrieval: Mending the fragmented self.* San Francisco: Harper Collins, 1991.
Elizabeth Kubler Ross, *On Death and Dying.* New York: Scribner Book Co, 2014.
Amy Sophia Marashinsky, *The Goddess Oracle.* Stamford, CT: U.S. Games Systems, inc., 2006.
Robert Schwartz, *Your Soul's Gift, The Healing power of the Life you Planned before you were born.* London: Watkins, 2012.
Franklyn Sills. *Foundations of Craniosacral Biodynamics.* Berkeley: North Atlantic Books, 2012.

Herbs for pregnancy

Anne McIntyre, *Herbal for Mother and Child*. London: Thorsons, 1992.
Carol Rogers, *The Women's Guide to Herbal Medicine*. London: Hamish Hamilton, 1995.
Denise Tiran and Sue Mack, *Complimentary Therapies for Pregnancy and Childbirth*. London: Balliére Tindall, 1995.
Susun S. Weed, *Wise Woman Herbal for the Childbearing Year*. New York: Ash tree Publishing, 1986.

Herbal medicine and plants

Julian Barker, *The Medicinal Flora of Britain and Northwestern Europe*. West Wickham, Kent: Winter Press, 2001.
Thomas Bartram, *Encyclopedia of Herbal Medicine*. Christchurch, Dorset: Grace Publishers, 1995.
James Green, *The Herbal Medicine-Makers Handbook*. Berkeley, CA: Crossing Press, 2000.
Christopher Hedley & Non Shaw, *The Herbal Book of Making and Taking*. London: Aeon, 2020.
David Hoffman, *Holistic Herbal*. Forres: Findhorn Press, 1983.
Christopher Menzies-Trull, *Herbal Medicine Keys to Physiomedicalism Including Pharmacopoeia*. Newcastle, UK: FPHM, 2003.
Maurice Mességué, *Of Men and Plants*. London: Weidenfeld and Nicolson Ltd, 1972.
Christina Oakley Harrington, *The Treadwell's Book of Plant magic*. London: Treadwells Books, 2020.

Herbal safety

Sue Evans et al, 'Report on the safety of the oral consumption of the pyrollizidine alkaloid containing herbs *Symphytum officinale, Tussilago farfara* and *Borago officinalis*' https://nimh.org.uk/wp-content/uploads/2020/04/PA_Report2019.pdf [last accessed 6/7/21]
Zoe Gardner and Michael McGuffin, *American Herbal Products Association's Botanical Safety Handbook*. Boca Raton, FL: CRC Press, 2013.
Simon Mills and Kerry Bone, *The Essential Guide to Herbal Safety*. Missouri: Churchill Livingstone, 2005.

Pregnancy and childbirth, lactation

Cathy Ashwin & Michelle Anderson, *Myles Pocket Reference for Midwives*. London: Elsevier, 2017.
Nim Barnes, *How to Conceive Healthy Babies the Natural Way*, London: New Generation Publishing, 2016.
Murray Enkin et al, *A guide to effective care in pregnancy and childbirth*, Oxford: Oxford University Press, 2000.
Patrick Holford & Susannah Lawson, *Optimum Nutrition Before, During and After Pregnancy*. London: Hachette Digital, 2004.

La Leche League International, *The Womanly Art of Breastfeeding*. New York: Random House, 2010.
Ina May Gaskin, *Ina May's Guide to Childbirth*. London: Vermilion, 2003.
Sophie Messager, *Why Postnatal Recovery Matters*, London: Pinter & Martin, 2020.
Suzannah Olivier, *Eating for a perfect pregnancy*. London: Pocket Books, 2001.
Aviva Jill Romm, *The Natural Pregnancy Book*. Berkeley, CA: Ten Speed Press, 1997.
Nicky Wesson, *Alternative Maternity*, London: Macdonald & Co., 1989.

Vibrational essences

Julian Barnard (editor), *Collected Writings of Edward Bach*. Bath: Ashgrove Press, 1994.
Julian & Martine Barnard, *The Healing Herbs of Edward Bach*. Bath: Ashgrove Press, 1988.
Patricia Kaminski, *Flowers that Heal*. Dublin: Newleaf, 1998.
Sue Lily, *The Essence Practitioner*. London: Singing Dragon, 2015.
Nora Weeks and Victor Bullen, *The Bach Flower Remedies Illustrations and Preparations*. Saffron Walden, Essex: C.W. Daniel, 1964. Gives traditional making methods

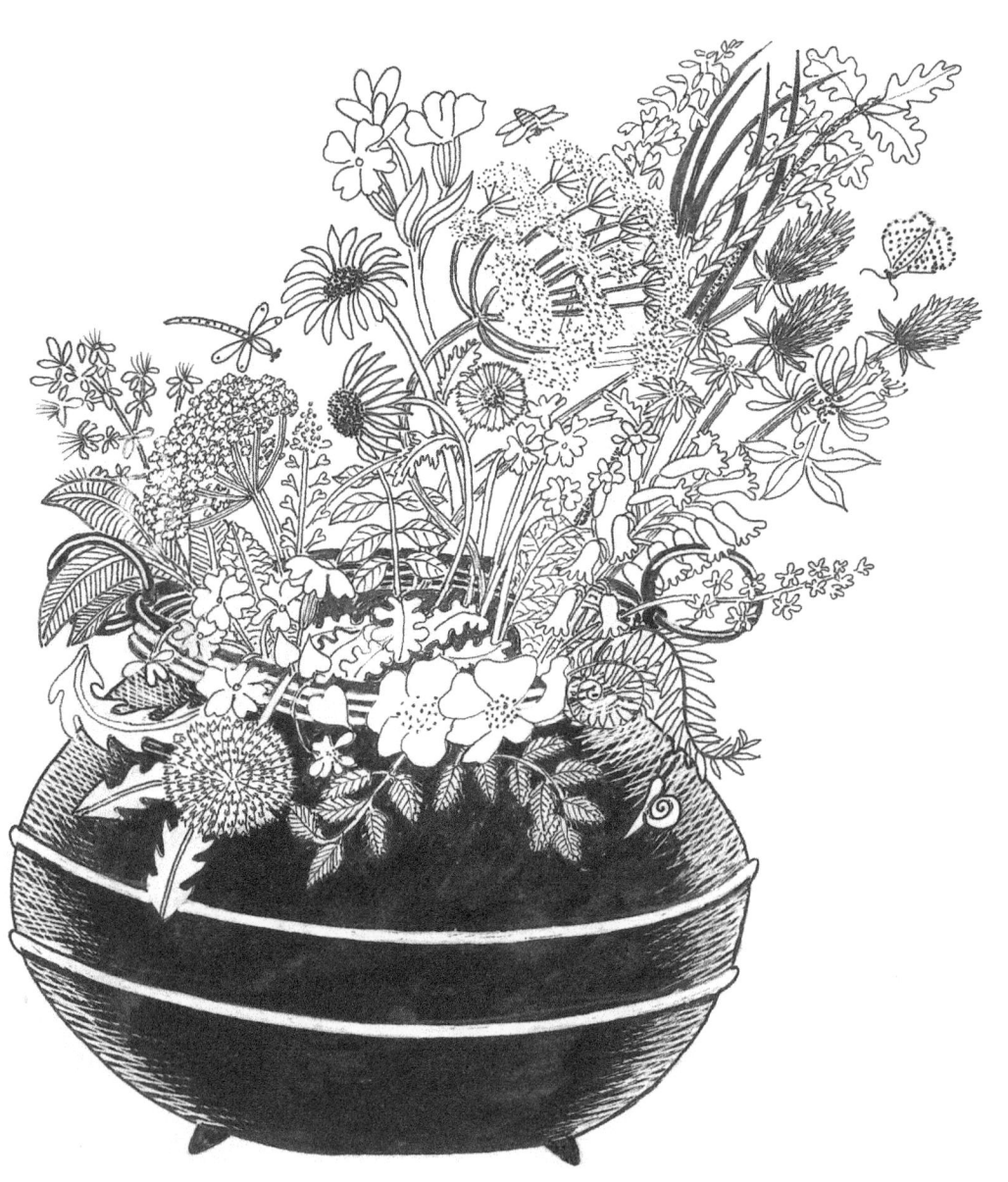

ACKNOWLEDGEMENTS

With grateful thanks to the plant world for their generosity, support, teachings, and amazing medicine. Thanks to the Divine Feminine, ever-present in this work.

Gratitude to my colleagues, the herbalists, past and present, who have assisted in the care of childbearing women and passed their wisdom on for future generations. Thanks to all my teachers, and particular thanks to Janet Hicks for her inspiration and encouragement at the beginning of my journey. Thanks to all the women who have entrusted themselves to my care over the years. Thanks for giving me the opportunity to learn and to do the work I love.

Gratitude to the wonderful team at Aeon for their support and hard work, and to Nikki for initiating the process. Thanks to my loving family and friends for their unwavering support.

Thanks to India for her beautiful illustrations and for graciously sharing my journey with the plants and Goddesses. Thanks to Juliet for extensive herbal proof-reading and advice, to Julie Ann for advice on essential oils and to Anita for the proof-reading of Healing After Loss. Particular thanks to Marion, for practical help and support in more ways than I can possibly list. Thank you, Marion, you are an absolute treasure.

Last but not least, acknowledging the three Sacred Laws, introduced to me by métis Medicine Woman, Arwyn DreamWalker: 'All things are born of Woman, Nothing shall be done to harm the Child, Love is all there is'.

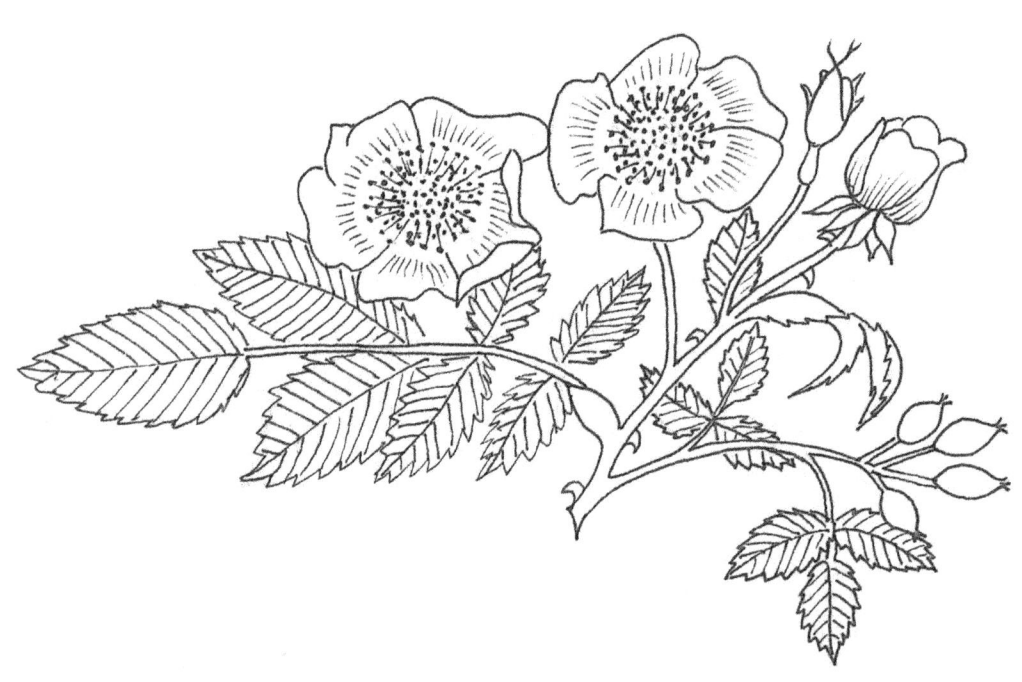

AUTHOR BIOGRAPHY

Carole Guyett MNIMH trained at the School of Herbal Medicine in Tunbridge Wells, UK and has been a practising medical herbalist for more than 35 years. She has worked extensively in the areas of fertility, pregnancy, and birthing, and has experience of teaching obstetrics and gynaecology to herbal students and practitioners. Carole is also trained as a medicine woman and practices sacred plant medicine. Carole lives in Ireland where she runs apprenticeships, workshops, and sacred ceremony. She is author of *Sacred Plant Initiations*.

INDEX OF GODDESS ILLUSTRATIONS

Airmid, Assorted herbs, 72
Artemis, Mugwort, 224
Bast, Valerian, 188
Black Madonna, Marigold, 282
Brigid, Bramble, 300
Demeter, Oats, 28
Flora, Dog Rose and Daisy, 50
Gaia, Raspberry, iii, 18
Hathor, Red Clover and Chamomile, 266

Hecate, Garlic, 206
Hygeia, Vervain, 40
Isis, Motherwort, 102
Kwan Yin, Lotus and Willow, 236
Minerva, Geranium, 58
Morgan le Fay, Apple, xvi
Morrigan, Deadly Nightshade, 174
Sheela na Gig, Elder, 211
White Shell Woman, Corn, xii

INDEX

AA. *See* arachidonic acid
abdominal pain and cramps, 104. *See also* pregnancy conditions
    Braxton Hicks contractions, 104
    false labour pains, 104–105
    in 1st trimester, 104
    herbs to slow down contractions, 105
    labour, 105
    light spotting, 104
    motherwort, 104–105
    preterm labour, 105–106
    in 2nd and 3rd trimesters, 104
abortion, spontaneous. *See* miscarriage
ABV. *See* alcohol by volume
Achillea millefolium. *See* yarrow
acid
    reflux. *See* heartburn
    urine, 165
acute. *See also* miscarriage
    cystitis, 164
    pyelonephritis, 164
    threatened miscarriage, 137–139
adaptogen, 309
adjuncts to herbal treatment, 203. *See also* labour and birth
Aesculus hippocastanum. *See* horsechestnut
AFP. *See* alpha-fetoprotein

after birth. *See also* labour and birth; postpartum care
    hormonal changes, 237–238
    preparation, 196
after-care, 232. *See also* herbs for labour and delivery
afterpains, 244–245. *See also* postpartum care
AFV. *See* amniotic fluid volume
Agrimonia eupatoria. *See* agrimony
agrimony (*Agrimonia eupatoria*), 74
Agropyron repens. *See* couchgrass
Agua Florida, 307
Alchemilla vulgaris. *See* lady's mantle
alcohol by volume (ABV), 70
alcohol in tinctures, 4, 60–62
alfalfa (*Medicago sativa*), 89
allergy, 106, 298
    cow's milk, 284–285
    food, 30
    herbal treatment, 286
Allium sativum. *See* garlic
alpha-fetoprotein (AFP), 24
alterative, 309
alternative induction herbs, 203
Althaea officinalis. *See* marshmallow
amniocentesis, 24
amniotic fluid volume (AFV), 130

INDEX

amniotomy, 220
anaemia, 106, 245. *See also* postpartum care; pregnancy conditions
    haemodilution and blood volume expansion, 106–107
    herbalist's role, 108
    herbs and dietary advice, 108–110
    iron-rich herbs, 109
    iron tonic, 109–110
    screening for, 107–108
    symptoms of nutritional anaemia, 108
    types, 107
analgesic, 309
anal sphincter damage, 253
Anemone pulsatilla. *See* pasque flower
Anethum graveolens. *See* dill
Angelica archangelica. *See* garden angelica
Angelica sinensis. *See* Chinese angelica
Angelica sinensis. *See* Dong Quai
Angelica sinensis, 200
aniseed (*Pimpinella anisum*), 91
antacid, 309
antenatal
    care, 19
    screening, 23–25
antepartum haemorrhage (APH), 103, 113
anthelmintic, 309
anti-allergic, 309
anti-atheromatous, 309
antibacterial, 309
anti-bilious, 309
anti-catarrhal, 309
anticoagulant, 309
anti-D, 23
antidepressant, 309
anti-emetic, 309
antifungal, 309
anti-haemorrhagics, 152, 309
antihidrotic, 309
antihistamine, 310
anti-hypothyroid, 310
anti-infective
    factors, 267–268
    oils, 199
anti-inflammatory, 310
antilithic, 310
anti-microbial, 310
anti-neoplastic, 310
antiobesic, 310
antioxidants, 38, 310. *See also* nutrition

antiphospholipid syndrome (APS), 136, 143–144
anti-platelet, 310
anti-rheumatic, 310
anti-sclerotic, 310
antiseptic, 310
    uterine tonics, 250
anti-spasmodic, 310
antithrombotic, 310
anti-tussive, 310
antiviral, 310
anxiety, 120–122. *See also* emotional and stress-related conditions
    in labour, 226
    postpartum, 248
anxiolytic, 310
aperient, 310
APH. *See* antepartum haemorrhage
aphrodisiac, 310
apothecary's rose (*Rosa gallica*), 92
APS. *See* antiphospholipid syndrome
Arabin® pessary, 117
arachidonic acid (AA), 38
Arctium Lappa. *See* burdock
arnica (*Arnica montana*), 76
Arnica montana. *See* arnica
aromatic, 310
Artemisia vulgaris. *See* mugwort
ashwagandha (*Withania somnifera*), 100, 195
assisted birth, 220. *See also* labour and birth
assisted pregnancies, 25
assisted reproduction, 137, 144
Astragalus membranaceus. *See* milk vetch
astringent, 250, 310
athletic, 203
atopic dermatitis, 160, 284, 285, 291. *See also* skin disorders
    herbal treatments, 291–292
    management, 291
atopic eczema, 160, 284–285, 291. *See also* skin disorders
atopic eruption of pregnancy, 160
Avena sativa. *See* oats

baby blessing herbs, 297–298. *See also* newborn care
baby's cord stump, 232. *See also* herbs for labour and delivery
back/pelvic pain, 111, 245. *See also* postpartum care; pregnancy conditions

general advice for, 111
    herbal baths, 112
    herbal treatment, 111
    internal treatment, 112–113
    massage oils, 112
    ointments, 112
    rubbing oils and liniments, 112
bacterial vaginosis (BV), 167. *See also*
    pregnancy conditions
Ballota nigra. *See* Black Horehound
Baptisia tinctoria. *See* wild indigo
Barosma betulina. *See* buchu
basic food hygiene, 33. *See also* nutrition
baths, 66–67. *See also* herbal pharmacy
    herbal, 112
Bellis perennis. *See* daisy
beth root (*Trillium erectum*), 97–98
bilberry (*Vaccinium myrtillus*), 98
birth, assisted, 220. *See also* labour and birth
birth attendants, 22–23
birthing balls, 41, 218. *See also* exercise and
    lifestyle; labour and birth
birthing options, 189–190. *See also* labour and
    birth
birthing pack, 197. *See also* labour and birth
    basics, 197
    calendula lotion, 200
    chaste tree dosage in lactation, 200–201
    essential oils, 199
    ginseng 'energy sticks', 198
    herbs for, 225
    labour drops, 197–198
    massage oils, 198–199
    practitioner birthing kit, 233
    postnatal tonic, 200
    raspberry leaf tea, 198
    room spray, 199–200
    tinctures for relaxation, 198
birth trauma, 245–247. *See also*
    postpartum care
bisphenol A (BPA), 272
bitter, 310
blackberry (*Rubus fructicosus*), 93
Black Cohosh (*Cimicifuga racemosa*), 81–82, 196,
    234
black elder (*Sambucus nigra*), 94
Black Haw (*Viburnum prunifolium*), 99–100, 137,
    139, 195
Black Horehound (*Ballota nigra*), 77, 148
bladder, overactive, 252

bladder wrack (*Fucus vesiculosis*), 84
bleeding, 113, 247. *See also* postpartum care;
    pregnancy conditions
    in first 20 weeks, 113
    later in pregnancy, 114
blocked ducts, 277. *See also* lactation
    sticky eye, 292
blood volume expansion, 106–107
Blue Cohosh (*Caulophyllum thalictroides*),
    79–80, 234
bottle fed babies, 285. *See also* newborn allergies
BPA. *See* bisphenol A
bramble (*Rubus fructicosus*), 93
Braxton Hicks contractions, 56–57, 104.
    See also trimester
breast changes, 114–115. *See also* pregnancy
    conditions
breast engorgement, 273. *See also* lactation
    herbal treatment, 274
    management of, 273
    physiological, 273
breastfeeding, 267. *See also* lactation
    benefits of, 267–268
    elimination diets, 286
    establishing, 270–271
    herbs to, 273
    mother care, 287
    nutrition for, 271–272
    suspect foods, 285
breast milk. *See also* lactation
    contaminants in, 272–273
    stages, 269–270
breech presentation, 192–193. *See also* labour
    and birth
bronchiolitis, 296. *See also* respiratory
    illness
bronchitis, 295. *See also* respiratory illness
bronchodilator, 310
buchu (*Barosma betulina*), 78
burdock (*Arctium Lappa*), 76
burial ceremony, 180–181. *See also* healing
    after loss
butternut bark (*Juglans cinerea*), 88
BV. *See* bacterial vaginosis

cabbage leaves, 274
caesarean section (C-section), 221–222, 247.
    See also labour and birth;
    postpartum care
    post-operative pain and healing, 248

wound care, 247–248
vaginal birth after (VBAC), 192
caffeine, 33. *See also* nutrition
calcium, 37. *See also* nutrition
calendula lotion, 200. *See also* birthing pack
Calendula officinalis. *See* marigold
Candida albicans, 115–116. *See also* pregnancy conditions
candida infection, 115–116, 279–280, 287–288. *See also* pregnancy conditions
candidiasis, 115–116, 279–280, 287–288. *See also* pregnancy conditions
Capsella bursa pastoris. *See* shepherd's purse
Capsicum minimum. *See* cayenne pepper
capsules, 65. *See also* herbal pharmacy
caraway (*Carum carvi*), 79
cardiotocography. *See* electronic foetal monitoring
cardiotonic, 310
Carduus marianus, Silybum marianum. *See* milk thistle
carminative, 310
carpal tunnel syndrome (CTS), 116. *See also* pregnancy conditions
Carum carvi. *See* caraway
Cassia acutifolia/angustifolia spp. *See* senna
castor oil packs, 260. *See also* scar tissue
castor oil plant (*Ricinus communis*), 92
catmint (*Nepeta cataria*), 90
catnep (*Nepeta cataria*), 90
catnip (*Nepeta cataria*), 90
Caulophyllum thalictroides. *See* Blue Cohosh
cayenne pepper (*Capsicum minimum*), 79
CBT. *See* cognitive behavioural therapy
cell proliferant, 310
cellular memory, 264
Centella/Hydrocotyle asiatica. *See* gotu cola
cerclage. *See* transvaginal cervical 'stitch'
cervical ectopy, 117
cervical insufficiency, 117
cervical polyps, 117
cervicitis, 117–118
cervix conditions, 117. *See also* pregnancy conditions
cervical ectopy, 117
cervical insufficiency, 117
cervical polyps, 117
cervicitis, 117–118
cervix ripening, 202, 209. *See also* labour and birth
Cetraria islandica. *See* Iceland moss

chamomile, 121
Chamomilla recutita. *See* German chamomile
Chaste Tree (*Vitex agnus castus*), 100, 137, 200–201. *See also* birthing pack
cheeses, 34. *See also* nutrition
chest infections, 295. *See also* respiratory illness
chickweed (*Stellaria media*), 95
childbirth, 207. *See also* labour and birth
conscious, 190
fear of, 190–191
herbs to prepare for, 194–196
mystery of, 207–208
preparation for, 193–194
Chinese angelica (*Angelica sinensis*), 76
chloasma, 160. *See also* skin disorders
cholagogue, 310
choleretic, 310
chorionic villus sampling (CVS), 24
chromium, 37. *See also* nutrition
chronic conditions, 20
cicatrisant, 310
Cimicifuga racemosa. *See* Black Cohosh
cinnamon (*Cinnamonum zeylandicum/verum*), 82
Cinnamonum zeylandicum/verum. *See* cinnamon
CITES, 2, 16
cleavers (*Galium aperine*), 85
clinical shock. *See* shock, clinical
Closing the Bones, 247
CMPA/I. *See* cow's milk protein allergy or intolerance
cognitive behavioural therapy (CBT), 257
colic, 288
herbal treatments, 289
management, 288–289
COMA. *See* Committee on Medical Aspects of Food and Nutrition Policy
comfrey leaf, 112
Commiphora molmol. *See* myrrh
Commiphora myrrha. *See* myrrh
Committee on Medical Aspects of Food and Nutrition Policy (COMA), 39
common comfrey (*Symphytum officinale*), 95–96
common lime (*Tilia europaea*), 97
compresses, 68. *See also* herbal pharmacy
conception, 51–52. *See also* pregnancy stages
conjunctivitis, 292
connecting with one's baby, 46–47. *See also* exercise and lifestyle
conscious childbirth, 190. *See also* labour and birth

constipation, 118, 248, 289–290. *See also* postpartum care; pregnancy conditions
   herbal treatment, 118–119
contemporary Western herbal medicine, 1
contractions, 226–228. *See also* herbs for labour and delivery
cooling herbs, 156
cornsilk (*Zea mays*), 100–101, 131, 165
corticotrophin-releasing hormone, 56. *See also* third trimester
costovertebral angle (CVA), 164
couchgrass (*Agropyron repens*), 74–75
cow's milk, 29–30. *See also* newborn allergies
   allergy in breastfed babies, 285
   protein allergy, 284–285
cow's milk protein allergy or intolerance (CMPA/I), 284
cradle cap, 290
cramp bark (*Viburnum opulus*), 99, 121, 140
cramps. *See* abdominal pain and cramps
cramps, leg. *See* leg cramps
craniosacral therapy, 203
Crataegus monogyna/oxacanthoides. *See* hawthorn
cravings, 32. *See also* nutrition
croup, 296. *See also* respiratory illness
crowning, 215. *See also* labour and birth
C-section. *See* caesarean section
CTS. *See* carpal tunnel syndrome
Chamaelirium luteum. *See* False Unicorn
Curcuma longa. *See* turmeric
curled dock (*Rumex crispus*), 93
cuts, 232. *See also* herbs for labour and delivery
CVA. *See* costovertebral angle
CVS. *See* chorionic villus sampling
cystitis, 165. *See also* urinary tract conditions

D & C. *See* dilation and curettage
daisy (*Bellis perennis*), 78
damask rose (*Rosa damascene*), 92
damiana (*Turnera diffusa*), 98
dandelion (*Taraxacum officinale*), 96–97
DBP. *See* diastolic blood pressure
decoctions, standard, 60. *See also* herbal pharmacy
decongestant, 310
decosahexanoic acid (DHA), 38
deep vein thrombosis (DVT), 168
demulcent, 311
deobstruent, 311

depression, 122–123, 228. *See also* emotional and stress-related conditions
dermatitis, 160, 284–285, 291. *See also* skin disorders
dermatoses of pregnancy, 172
DHA. *See* decosahexanoic acid
diaphoretic, 311
diarrhoea, 290–291
diastasis recti, 242
diastolic blood pressure (DBP), 171
digestive, 311
dilatation. *See* dilation
dilation, 170
dilation and curettage (D & C), 117
dill (*Anethum graveolens*), 76
Dioscorea villosa. *See* wild yam
dispersant, 69
diuretic, 311
dizziness and fainting, 119. *See also* pregnancy conditions
dog rose (*Rosa canina*), 92
Dong Quai (*Angelica sinensis*), 76
dopaminergic, 311
dosages for pregnancy, lactation, and newborn, 73
dried herb additions, 166
DVT. *See* deep vein thrombosis

ear infections, 291
early miscarriage, 175. *See also* healing after loss
Echinacea angustifolia, pallida, and *purpurea*. *See* purple cone flower
eclampsia. *See* pre-eclampsia/eclampsia
ectopic pregnancy, 119–120, 175. *See also* healing after loss; pregnancy conditions
ECV. *See* external cephalic version
eczema, 160, 284–285, 291. *See also* skin disorders
   herbal treatments, 291–292
   management, 291
effacement, 209, 222
EFM. *See* electronic foetal monitoring
eggs, 34. *See also* nutrition
eicosapentanoic acid (EPA), 38
elder, (*Sambucus nigra*), 94, 178. *See also* healing after loss
elecampane (*Inula helenium*), 88
electronic foetal monitoring (EFM), 219
Eleutherococcus senticosus. *See* Siberian ginseng
elevator, 42. *See also* exercise and lifestyle

embryonic stage, 53. *See also* first trimester
emetic, 311
emmenagogue, 311
emollient, 311
emotional and stress-related conditions, 120, 248. *See also* postpartum care; pregnancy conditions; sleep disorders
    for fear, anxiety, stress, tension, 120–122, 248
    herbal treatment, 120
    for mood and emotional well-being, 122–123, 249
    sedative and pain relieving, 249
emulsifying agents, 65, 70, 304
endangered plants, 2
endometritis (uterine infection), 249. *See also* postpartum care
    herbal treatment, 249–250
entonox, 217
environmental allergies and sensitivities, 287. *See also* newborn allergies
EOs. *See* essential oils
EPA. *See* eicosapentanoic acid
Ephedra, 170
Ephedra sinica. *See* ma huang
epidural analgesia, 217–218. *See also* labour and birth
episiotomy, 220–221, 232, 245, 248, 259. *See also* labour and birth; postpartum care
epistaxis, 149. *See also* pregnancy conditions
epithelioid trophoblastic tumour (ETT), 125
Equisetum arvense. *See* horsetail
essential fatty acids, 38. *See also* nutrition
essential oils (EOs), 11, 68, 199. *See also* herbal pharmacy; herbal prescribing and safety
    baths with, 69–70
    contraindicated in pregnancy, lactation, and newborn, 15
    inhalation of, 69
    methods of application of, 69
    safe for external use for newborn infants, 14
    safe for external use with lactating women, 13–14
    safe in pregnancy, 12–13
    skin application of, 69
    sprays with, 70, 304
    to be used with caution, 14
ETT. *See* epithelioid trophoblastic tumour
Euphrasia officinalis. *See* eyebright

exercise and lifestyle, 41
    birthing balls, 41
    connecting with one's baby, 46–47
    elevator, 42
    exercise, 41–42
    herbal baths, 48
    massage and essential oils, 47–48
    pelvic floor exercises, 42
    progressive muscle relaxation, 45
    relaxation, 43–47
    rest, 43
    rhythmic breathing, 44
    sex, 43
    swimming or floating, 41
    yoga, 41
exhaustion, 123–124. *See also* pregnancy conditions
    herbs for, 228
    postpartum, 250
expectorant, 311
external cephalic version (ECV), 192
eyebright (*Euphrasia officinalis*), 84, 159
eye conditions, 292

fainting. *See* dizziness and fainting
false labour pains, 104–105
False Unicorn (*Chamaelirium luteum* (cultivated)), 80–81, 106, 137–138, 195
    root, 139
fatigue, 123–124, 250–251. *See also* postpartum care; pregnancy conditions
fear, 120–122. *See also* emotional and stress-related conditions
    of childbirth, 190–191
    herbs for, 226
febrifuge, 311
fennel (*Foeniculum vulgare*), 84
fenugreek (*Trigonella foenum graecum*), 97
FES. *See* Flower Essence Society
feverfew (*Tanacetum parthenium*), 96
fevers, 293
fibre, 38. *See also* nutrition
Filipendula ulmaria. *See* Meadowsweet
first trimester, 53. *See also* pregnancy stages; trimester
    embryonic stage, 53
    foetus, 54
    placenta, 54
    progesterone, 53
    relaxin, 53–54

spiritual and energetic adjustment, 54–55
two-way communication, 55
fish, 34. *See also* nutrition
flower essences, 6, 21. *See also* vibrational essences
Flower Essence Society (FES), 303
flower waters, 65–66. *See also* herbal pharmacy
"flowing fountain, the", 208
Foeniculum vulgare. See fennel
foetus, 54. *See also* labour and birth; trimester
    catecholamines, 209
    growth, 55
    monitoring, 219
folic acid, 35. *See also* nutrition
fomentations, 68
food allergy, 30. *See also* nutrition
footbaths, 67. *See also* herbal pharmacy
formula milk, 272. *See also* lactation
Fucus vesiculosis. See bladder wrack

galactagogues, 273, 275, 311
Galega officinalis. See Goat's Rue
Galium aperine. See cleavers
gamma-linoleic acid (GLA), 38
garden angelica (*Angelica archangelica*), 76
garlic (*Allium sativum*), 75
GBS. *See* group B streptococcus
Gelsemium sempervirens. See yellow jasmine
genital herpes. *See* herpes—genital
Gentiana lutea. See yellow gentian
Geranium robertianum. See herb Robert
German chamomile (*Chamomilla recutita, Matricaria chamomilla/recutita*), 81
gestational. *See also* pregnancy conditions; pregnancy stages
    age, 52–53
    diabetes, 124
    herbal diabetes treatment, 124–125
    rhinitis. *See* rhinitis
gestational trophoblastic disease (GTD), 125. *See also* pregnancy conditions
gestational trophoblastic neoplasia (GTN), 125
GI. *See* glycaemic index
ginger (*Zingiber officinalis*), 101, 148
ginseng (*Panax Ginseng*), 90. *See also* birthing pack
    energy sticks, 198
GLA. *See* gamma-linoleic acid
Glechoma hederacea. See ground ivy
glycaemic index (GI), 124

glycerites, 62. *See also* herbal pharmacy
Glycyrrhiza glabra. See liquorice
Goat's Rue (*Galega officinalis*), 85, 124
goldenrod (*Solidago virgaurea*), 95
golden seal (*Hydrastis canadensis*), 86–87
'golden triangle', 5–6
goodbye, saying, 183. *See also* healing after loss
gotu cola (*Centella/Hydrocotyle asiatica*), 80
grief, 228–229. *See also* herbs for labour and delivery
grieving, stages of, 185. *See also* healing after loss
ground ivy (*Glechoma hederacea*), 86
group B strep. *See* group B streptococcus
group B streptococcus (group B strep; GBS), 126. *See also* pregnancy conditions
    general measures for, 126
    herbal treatment, 126–127
GTD. *See* gestational trophoblastic disease
GTN. *See* gestational trophoblastic neoplasia
guelder rose (*Viburnum opulus*), 99
guided visualisation
    connecting with one's baby, 46–47
    inner sacred mother goddess, 26–27
    preparation for childbirth, 193–194
gums, 127. *See also* pregnancy conditions

haemodilution, 106–107
haemoglobin (Hb), 106
haemorrhage, retroplacental. *See* placental abruption
haemorrhoids, 168–170. *See also* pregnancy conditions
haemostatic, 311
hair loss, 159, 251–252. *See also* postpartum care
Hamamelis virginiana. See witch hazel
handbaths, 67. *See also* herbal pharmacy
happy healthy baby, 305. *See also* sprays
hawthorn (*Crataegus monogyna/oxacanthoides*), 82
Hb. *See* haemoglobin
hCG. *See* human chorionic gonadotrophin
headaches, 127. *See also* pregnancy conditions
    herbal treatment, 128, 229
healing after loss, 175
    for bereaved parents, 178–183
    burial ceremony when no body, 180–181
    early miscarriage, 175
    elder, 178
    heart oil, 177
    helpful plants, 179–180

332   INDEX

herbal bath ceremony for letting go, 182–183
herbal support for grief and loss, 176–178
herbs for grief, 176–177
massage oil, 177–178
medicine bundle, 180
practitioner self care, 184–185
rescue essence, 185
'rescue' spray, 178
Rose (*Rosa* spp.), 176
rose bath to heal wounded heart, 181
rosemary, 178
saying goodbye to loved one, 183
smudge, 185
soul loss, 185
spiritual perspectives on pregnancy loss, 184
stages of grieving, 185
stillbirth, 176
termination, 175
vibrational essences, 178, 185
yew, 179
heartburn, 128. *See also* pregnancy conditions
heart oil, 177. *See also* healing after loss
heartsease (*Viola tricolor*), 100
HELLP syndrome, 108, 153
hepatic, 311
hepatoprotective, 311
herbal bath, 48. *See also* exercise and lifestyle
ceremony, 182–183
herbal care of pregnant woman, 19
antenatal care, 19
antenatal care schedule, 21–22
antenatal screening and prophylaxis, 23–25
birth attendants, 22–23
chronic conditions treatment, 20
herbal consultation, 20–21
inner sacred mother goddess, 26–27
in-vitro fertilisation and assisted pregnancies, 25
journey to motherhood, 25–27
reasons to see herbalist, 19
in uncomplicated pregnancy, 21–22
herbalist's remit, xv
herbal legislation, 7. *See also* herbal prescribing and safety
herbal pharmacy, 59
baths, 66–67
capsules, 65
compresses, 68
creams, 65

decoctions, 60
essential oils, 68–70
flower waters, 65–66
footbaths and handbaths, 67
glycerites, 62
honeys, 63
hot water extracts, 59–60
infused oils, 63–64
liniments, 64
lotions, 68
ointments, 64
pessaries and suppositories, 66
poultices, 68
sitz baths or hip baths, 67
steam inhalations, 66
syrups, 63
tinctures, 60–62
vaginal steaming, 67–68
vinegars, 62
herbal prescribing and safety, 1
alcohol in tinctures, 4
caution in pregnancy and lactation, 10–11
considerations in prescribing herbs, 3–4
contraindicated in pregnancy and lactation, 8–10
endangered plants, 2
essential oils, 11–15
flower essences and vibrational essences, 6
general approach to herbal prescribing, 3
heightened sensitivity of pregnancy, 4
herbal legislation, 7
herbal safety, 7–8
laxative herbs, 10
physiomedicalism and non-native herbs, 1–2
prescribing guidelines, 6
principles in obstetric care, 2–3
principles of herbal practice, 2
synergy in herbal prescription, 5
therapeutic relationship, 5–6
tinctures and powders, 4
tincture strength and quality, 5
trust in process, 6
use of nutritional supplements, 7
use of whole plant, 5
herbal treatment, 103
atopic dermatitis, 291–293
back/pelvic pain, 111
bacterial vaginosis, 167
blocked ducts, 277
Candida albicans, 115–116

candida infection, 115–116, 279–280, 287–288
candidiasis, 115–116, 279–280, 287–288
colic, 289
constipation, 118–119, 248, 289–290
diarrhea, 290–291
eclampsia, 154
emotional and stress-related conditions, 120–122, 248
endometritis, 249
for engorged breasts, 274
eye conditions, 292
for food allergy and intolerance, 286
fourth trimester, 242
gestational diabetes, 124–125
group B streptococcus, 126–127
gums, 127
headaches, 128
heartburn, 128
hypertension and hypertensive disorders, 133
hypoglycaemia, 134–135
incontinence, 252
for infections and fevers, 293
insufficient milk supply, 275
induction, 202–203
mastitis, 279
nappy rash, 294–295
nausea & vomiting, 147–149
nipples, sore or cracked, 276–277
oedema, 150–151
oligohydramnios, 131
for pain, 261
perineal healing, 254
polyhydramnios, 132
postpartum depression, 256
prolapsed, 258
pruritis, 156–157
restless legs syndrome, 158
sleep disorders, 162
stretch marks, 163–164
thrush, 280, 287–288
urinary tract conditions, 165–166
vaginitis, 167
varicose veins and haemorrhoids, 169
vulvovaginal, 115–116
herb Robert (*Geranium robertianum*), 85–86
herbs
    alternative induction, 203
    for anxiety, 226
    atopic dermatitis treatment, 291–292
    baby blessing, 297–298. *See also* newborn care
    for back and pelvic pain, 112–113
    bath, 112
    bath ceremony for letting go, 182–183
    for birthing pack, 225
    to breastfeeding mothers, 273
    for childbirth, 194–196
    for colic, 289
    constipation treatment, 118–119
    consultation, 20–21
    contraindicated in pregnancy and lactation, 8–11
    cooling, 156
    creams, 65
    and dietary advice, 108–110
    for digestive weakness, 148
    dried herb additions, 166
    for exhaustion, 228
    for eye treatment, 292
    for food allergy and intolerance, 286
    galactagogues, 275
    for grief, 176–177
    hayfever, 106
    for hypertension, 132–133, 229
    hypoglycaemia, 134–135
    infused oils, 63–64
    iron-rich, 109
    kidney support, 166
    for labour, 203
    laxative herbs, 10
    to lift depression, 122–123
    for low libido, 261–262
    nipple sore or crack, 276–277
    non-native, 1–2
    ointments, 64
    oligohydramnios treatment, 131
    pelvic organ prolapse treatment, 258
    perineal treatment, 254
    polyhydramnios treatment, 132
    for postpartum care, 242
    practice principles, 2
    practitioner birthing kit, 233
    pre-eclampsia/eclampsia treatment, 152
    for pregnancy and childbirth medicine, xiii–xiv
    pruritis treatment, 156–157
    in recurrent miscarriage, 144
    safety, 7–8
    sexual dysfunction, 261–262
    sleep disorders, 162
    stress treatment, 120
    tea, 3

treatment for group B streptococcus, 126–127
uterine restorative formula, 143
warming teas, 148, 242
weaning, 280
herbs for labour and delivery, 225
anxiety and fear, 226
birthing kit, 233
birthing pack, 225
to bring to delivery, 225
care of baby's cord stump, 232
contractions, 226–228
depression, low mood, 228
exhaustion, 228
for first stage, 225–230
grief, 228–229
headache, 229
hypertension, 229
immediate after-care, 232–233
leg cramps, 229
mother child bonding, 231
nausea, 229
pain, 229–230
panic, 230
perineal care, 230
postpartum haemorrhage, 231
retained placenta, 231–232
rigid os, 230
for second stage, 230–231
shock, clinical, 232
tears, cuts, episiotomy, 232
for third stage, 231–232
uncomplicated 1st stage, 225
vulvar varicosities and haemorrhoids, 231–233
herpes
genital, 129
gestationis. *See* pemphigoid gestationis
simplex infection, 129
hip baths, 67. *See also* herbal pharmacy
holy basil (*Ocimum tenuiflorum/sanctum*), 90
honeys, 63. *See also* herbal pharmacy
hops (*Humulus lupulus*), 86
hormone
changes in early pregnancy, 52–54
changes in labour, 208–209
changes in lactation, 268–269
changes in second trimester, 55–56
changes in third trimester, 56
foetal catecholamines, 209
changes in fourth trimester, 237–238

involved in maintenance stage, 269
oxytocin, 208–209
pain-relieving endorphins, 209
prolactin, 209
relaxin, 209
horsechestnut (*Aesculus hippocastanum*), 74
horsetail (*Equisetum arvense*), 83–84
hot water extracts. *See* standard infusions
HPA. *See* hypothalamic-pituitary-adrenal
hPL. *See* human placental lactogen
human chorionic gonadotrophin (hCG), 52
human placental lactogen (hPL), 237
Humulus lupulus. *See* hops
hydatiform mole. *See* molar pregnancy
hydramnios, 131–132
Hydrastis canadensis. *See* golden seal
hydrosols. *See* flower waters
hyperemesis gravidarum, 146. *See also* pregnancy conditions
Hypericum perforatum. *See* St John's Wort
hypertension, 132, 171. *See also* pregnancy conditions
disorders, 132–133
herbs for, 133, 229
hypertonic state, 226
hypnobirthing, 190, 218. *See also* labour and birth
hypnotic, 311
hypoglycaemia, 133. *See also* pregnancy conditions
herbal treatment, 134–135
hypoglycaemic, 311
hypotensive, 311
hypothalamic-pituitary-adrenal (HPA), 243, 256
hypotonic state, 226
hyssop (*Hyssopus officinalis*), 87–88
Hyssopus officinalis. *See* hyssop

ice cream, 35. *See also* nutrition
Iceland moss (*Cetraria islandica*), 80
ICP. *See* intrahepatic cholestasis of pregnancy
IDA. *See* iron deficiency anaemia
immune
modulator, 311
system in pregnancy, 135–136
immunostimulant, 311
implantationbleeding, 52. *See also* pregnancy stages
implantation symptoms, 52
incontinence, 252. *See also* postpartum care
anal, 253

treatment, 252
urinary, 252
induction herbs, 202–203
infant fever, 293. *See also* fevers; newborn care
infantile diarrhea, 290–291. *See also* newborn care
infections, in infants 293. *See also* conditions of pregnancy
infusions, standard, 59–60. *See also* herbal pharmacy
inhalation analgesia, 217. *See also* labour and birth
inner sacred mother/mother goddess, 26–27
insomnia, 162. *See also* sleep disorders
instrumental delivery. *See* assisted birth
International Union for Conservation of Nature's Red List of Threatened Species. *See* IUCN
intolerances, 298. *See also* newborn allergies
intrahepatic cholestasis of pregnancy (ICP), 156, 161. *See also* skin disorders
intravenous (IV), 126
Inula helenium. See elecampane
in-vitro fertilisation (IVF), 25, 52, 137, 144
iodine, 38. *See also* nutrition
iron, 34. *See also* anaemia; nutrition
-rich foods, 108
-rich herbs, 109
tonic, 109–110
iron deficiency anaemia (IDA), 106
IUCN (International Union for Conservation of Nature's Red List of Threatened Species), 171
IV. *See* intravenous
IVF. *See* in-vitro fertilisation

jaundice, 294
Juglans cinerea. See butternut bark

kegels. *See* pelvic—floor exercises
kidney herbs, 140

LA. *See* linoleic acid
labour, 105. *See also* birthing pack
drops, 197–198
labour and birth, 189, 207
adjuncts to herbal treatment, 203
assisted birth, 220
birthing balls, 218
birthing options, 189–190
birthing pack, 197–201
breech presentation, 192–193
caesarean section, 221–222
Celtic tradition, 207–208
childbirth mystery, 207–208
conscious childbirth, 190
crowning, 215
epidural analgesia, 217–218
episiotomy, 220–221
essences for labour induction, 203
fear of childbirth, 190–191
first stage of labour, 211–214
"flowing fountain, the", 208
foetal monitoring, 219
herbal essences for, 203
herbal induction mix, 202–203
herbs to prepare for, 194–196
hormone changes in labour, 208–209
hypnobirthing, 190, 218
induction of, 201–203
induction of labour and post-term pregnancy, 201
inhalation analgesia, 217
medical induction, 219–220
medical pain relief in labour, 217
meditation, 208
monitoring, 219
music therapy, 218
pain in labour, 191
pain relief, 217–218
partus preparators, 194–196
perineal massage, 196
"place of treasure", 217
positive affirmation, 214–215
posterior presentation, 220
preparation for, 193–194
preparation for after birth, 196
ripening of cervix, 209
rupture of membranes, 210–211
second stage of labour, 214
signs of approaching labour, 209–210
stages of labour, 209
TENS machine, 218
third stage of labour, 215–217
vaginal birth after caesarean, 192
vaginal delivery and self-doubt, 191–192
water births, 218–219
labyrinths, 263
lactation, 267. *See also* pregnancy
benefits of breastfeeding, 267–268
blocked ducts, 277

candidiasis, 279–280
caution in, 10–11
contaminants in breastmilk, 272–273
engorgement, 273–274
essential oils, 12–15
establishing breastfeeding, 270–271
herbs contraindicated in, 8–10
herbs to breastfeeding mothers, 273
hormone changes involved in, 268–269
hormones involved in maintenance stage, 269
insufficient milk supply, 274–275
and lactogenesis, 268
laxative herbs with anthraquinones, 10
mastitis, 277–279
nipples, sore or cracked, 276–277
nutrition for breastfeeding, 271–272
oversupply of milk, 275–276
oxytocin, 268–269
stages, 269–270
steps of, 268
thrush, 279–280
weaning, 280
lactogenesis, 268
lady's mantle (*Alchemilla vulgaris*), 75
La Leche League, 271, 281
Lamium album. *See* white deadnettle
lanolin, 65
laryngotracheobronchitis, 296. *See also* respiratory illness
Lavandula angustifolia. *See* lavender
lavender (*Lavandula angustifolia*), 88, 121–122
laxative, 311
leg cramps, 145–146. *See also* pregnancy conditions
  herbs for, 229
lemon balm (*Melissa officinalis*), 89, 121–122
Leonurus cardiaca. *See* Motherwort
lesser celandine (*Ranunculus ficaria*), 92
LFTs. *See* liver function tests
light spotting, 104
limeflowers, 121
linden tree (*Tilia europaea*), 97
liniments, 64. *See also* herbal pharmacy
linoleic acid (LA), 38
liquorice (*Glycyrrhiza glabra*), 86
liver, 35. *See also* nutrition
liver function tests (LFTs), 161
lobelia (*Lobelia inflata*), 89
Lobelia inflata. *See* lobelia

lochia, 247. *See also* bleeding
loss, healing after. *See* healing after loss
lotions, 68. *See also* herbal pharmacy
low mood. *See* depression
low serum progesterone, 136
lying-in period, 239–240. *See also* postpartum care
lymphatic, 311

magnesium, 37. *See also* nutrition
ma huang (*Ephedra sinica*), 83
manganese, 36. *See also* nutrition
marc, 61
marigold (*Calendula officinalis*), 78
marshmallow (*Althaea officinalis*), 75
massage oil, 47–48, 177–178, 198–199, 229–230. *See also* birthing pack; exercise and lifestyle; conditions of pregnancy; healing after loss; postpartum care; newborn care
mastitis, 277. *See also* lactation
  herbal treatment, 279
  management of, 278–279
  signs of, 278
Materia Medica, 73
  agrimony (*Agrimonia eupatoria*), 74
  alfalfa (*Medicago sativa*), 89
  aniseed (*Pimpinella anisum*), 91
  apothecary's rose (*Rosa gallica*), 92
  arnica (*Arnica montana*), 76
  ashwagandha, winter cherry (*Withania somnifera*), 100
  beth root (*Trillium erectum*), 97–98
  bilberry (*Vaccinium myrtillus*), 98
  blackberry, bramble (*Rubus fructicosus*), 93
  Black Cohosh (*Cimicifuga racemosa*), 81–82
  black elder (*Sambucus nigra*), 94
  Black Haw (*Viburnum prunifolium*), 99–100
  Black Horehound (*Ballota nigra*), 77
  bladder wrack (*Fucus vesiculosis*), 84
  Blue Cohosh (*Caulophyllum thalictroides*), 79–80
  buchu (*Barosma betulina*), 78
  burdock (*Arctium Lappa*), 76
  butternut bark (*Juglans cinerea*), 88
  caraway (*Carum carvi*), 79
  castor oil plant (*Ricinus communis*), 92
  catnip, catnep, catmint (*Nepeta cataria*), 90
  cayenne pepper (*Capsicum minimum*), 79
  chaste tree (*Vitex agnus castus*), 100

chickweed (*Stellaria media*), 95
Chinese angelica (*Angelica sinensis*), 76
cinnamon (*Cinnamonum zeylandicum/verum*), 82
cleavers (*Galium aperine*), 85
common Comfrey (*Symphytum officinale*), 95–96
common lime/linden tree (*Tilia europaea*), 97
cornsilk (*Zea mays*), 100–101
couchgrass (*Agropyron repens*), 74–75
curled dock, yellow dock (*Rumex crispus*), 93
daisy (*Bellis perennis*), 78
damask rose (*Rosa damascene*), 92
damiana (*Turnera diffusa*), 98
dandelion (*Taraxacum officinale*), 96–97
dill (*Anethum graveolens*), 76
dog rose (*Rosa canina*), 92
Dong Quai (*Angelica sinensis*), 76
dosages for infants, 73
elecampane (*Inula helenium*), 88
eyebright (*Euphrasia officinalis*), 84
False Unicorn (*Chamaelirium luteum* (cultivated)), 80–81
fennel (*Foeniculum vulgare*), 84
fenugreek (*Trigonella foenum graecum*), 97
feverfew (*Tanacetum parthenium*), 96
garden angelica (*Angelica archangelica*), 76
garlic (*Allium sativum*), 75
German chamomile (*Chamomilla recutita, Matricaria chamomilla/recutita*), 81
ginger (*Zingiber officinalis*), 101
ginseng (*Panax Ginseng*), 90
Goat's Rue (*Galega officinalis*), 85
goldenrod (*Solidago virgaurea*), 95
golden seal (*Hydrastis canadensis*), 86–87
gotu cola (*Centella/Hydrocotyle asiatica*), 80
ground ivy (*Glechoma hederacea*), 86
guelder rose, cramp bark (*Viburnum opulus*), 99
hawthorn (*Crataegus monogyna/oxacanthoides*), 82
heartsease, pansy (*Viola tricolor*), 100
herb Robert (*Geranium robertianum*), 85–86
herbs especially suitable for babies, 73–101
herbs for pregnancy, lactation, and newborn, 73
hops (*Humulus lupulus*), 86
horsechestnut (*Aesculus hippocastanum*), 74
horsetail (*Equisetum arvense*), 83–84

hyssop (*Hyssopus officinalis*), 87–88
Iceland moss (*Cetraria islandica*), 80
lady's mantle (*Alchemilla vulgaris*), 75
lavender (*Lavandula angustifolia*), 88
lemon balm (*Melissa officinalis*), 89
lesser celandine (*Ranunculus ficaria*), 92
liquorice (*Glycyrrhiza glabra*), 86
lobelia (*Lobelia inflata*), 89
ma huang (*Ephedra sinica*), 83
marigold (*Calendula officinalis*), 78
marshmallow (*Althaea officinalis*), 75
meadowsweet (*Filipendula ulmaria*), 84
milk thistle (*Carduus marianus, Silybum marianum*), 79
milk vetch (*Astragalus membranaceus*), 77
Motherwort (*Leonurus cardiaca*), 89
mugwort (*Artemisia vulgaris*), 77
mullein (*Verbascum thapsus*), 99
myrrh (*Commiphora molmol, Commiphora myrrha*), 82
nettle (*Urtica dioica*), 98
oak (*Quercus robur/petraea*), 91–92
oats (*Avena sativa*), 77
partridge berry (*Mitchella repens*), 90
pasque flower (*Anemone pulsatilla*), 75
passionflower (*Passiflora incarnata*), 91
pellitory-of-the-wall (*Parietaria judaica*), 91
peppermint (*Mentha piperita*), 89–90
plantain (*Plantago lanceolata/major*), 91
purple cone flower (*Echinacea angustifolia, pallida,* and *purpurea*), 83
raspberry leaf, red raspberry leaf (*Rubus idaeus*), 93
red clover (*Trifolium pratense*), 97
Rosa species, 92
rose hips (*Rosa canina fructus*), 92–93
rosemary (*Rosemarinus officinalis*), 93
roseroot (*Rhodiola rosea*), 92
sage, red sage (*Salvia officinalis*), 94
saw palmetto (*Serenoa repens*), 95
senna (*Cassia acutifolia/angustifolia* spp.), 79
shepherd's purse (*Capsella bursa pastoris*), 78–79
Siberian ginseng (*Eleutherococcus senticosus*), 83
skullcap (*Scutellaria lateriflora*), 94–95
slippery elm (*Ulmus rubra*), 98
St John's Wort (*Hypericum perforatum*), 87
thyme (*Thymus vulgaris*), 97

tulsi/holy basil/sacred basil (*Ocimum tenuiflorum/sanctum*), 90
turmeric (*Curcuma longa*), 82
valerian (*Valeriana officinalis*), 98–99
vervain (*Verbena officinalis*), 99
white deadnettle (*Lamium album*), 88
wild indigo (*Baptisia tinctoria*), 77–78
wild yam (*Dioscorea villosa*), 82–83
witch hazel (*Hamamelis virginiana*), 86
wood betony (*Stachys betonica*), 95
yarrow (*Achillea millefolium*), 74
yellow gentian (*Gentiana lutea*), 85
yellow jasmine (*Gelsemium sempervirens*), 85
Matricaria chamomilla/recutita. See German chamomile
MCHC. *See* mean corpuscular haemoglobin concentration
MCV. *See* mean corpuscular volume
Meadowsweet (*Filipendula ulmaria*), 84, 165
meals, 34. *See also* nutrition
mean corpuscular haemoglobin concentration (MCHC), 107
mean corpuscular volume (MCV), 107
meats, 34. *See also* nutrition
Medicago sativa. *See* alfalfa
medical induction, 219–220. *See also* labour and birth
medicine bundle, 180. *See also* healing after loss
meditation for labour and birth, 208. *See also* labour and birth
melasma, 160. *See also* skin disorders
Melissa officinalis. *See* lemon balm
memory, 264
memory transfer, 264
menstruum, 61
Mentha piperita. *See* peppermint
meticillin-resistant *Staphylococcus aureus* (MRSA), 278
milk and dairy, 29–30. *See also* nutrition
milk, insufficient supply, 274. *See also* lactation
  herbal treatments, 275
  signs of, 274–275
milk oversupply, 275–276. *See also* lactation
milk thistle (*Carduus marianus*, *Silybum marianum*), 79
milk vetch (*Astragalus membranaceus*), 77
miscarriage, 136. *See also* healing after loss; pregnancy conditions
  acute threatened, 137–139
  alternative prescribing, 139–140

antiphospholipid syndrome, 143–144
  case study, 138–139
  completing, 140–141
  early, 175
  herbal approach to recurrent, 144
  low progesterone as cause of early, 136–137
  recurrent, 143
  tonics and balancers, 142–143
  uterine restorative formula, 143
  uterine restorative tonics, 142
Mitchella repens. *See* Partridge Berry
molar pregnancy, 125
mood swings, 122–123. *See also* emotional and stress-related conditions
morning sickness, 146
mother child bonding, 231. *See also* herbs for labour and delivery
Mother Goddess, 26–27, 305. *See also* sprays
motherhood, 25–27
Motherwort (*Leonurus cardiaca*), 89, 104–105, 121
MRSA. *See* meticillin-resistant *Staphylococcus aureus*
mucilaginous herbs, 63
mugwort (*Artemisia vulgaris*), 77, 141
mullein (*Verbascum thapsus*), 99
multiple pregnancy, 145. *See also* pregnancy conditions
muscle cramps, 145–146. *See also* pregnancy conditions
music therapy, 218. *See also* labour and birth
myrrh (*Commiphora molmol*, *Commiphora myrrha*), 82

nappy rash, 294. *See also* newborn care
  herbal treatments, 294–295
  management, 294
nasal inhaler tubes, 234
nausea & vomiting in pregnancy (NVP), 146. *See also* pregnancy conditions
  essential oils, 149
  herbal treatment, 147–149
nausea, 229. *See also* herbs for labour and delivery
NEC. *See* necrotising enterocolitis
necrotising enterocolitis (NEC), 268
neonatal jaundice, 294. *See also* newborn care
Nepeta cataria. *See* catmint; catnep; catnip
nervines, 140, 311
nettle (*Urtica dioica*), 98
neuralgesic, 311

neural tube defects, 24, 35
newborn allergies, 284. *See also* newborn care
    bottle fed babies, 285
    care of breastfeeding mothers, 287
    cow's milk allergy, 284–285
    elimination diets, 286
    environmental allergies, 287
    herbal treatment for food allergy and intolerance, 286
    suspect foods for breastfeeding mothers, 285
newborn care, 283. *See also* newborn allergies
    adapting to life, 283–284
    atopic dermatitis, 291–292
    baby blessing herbs, 297–298
    candida infection, 287–288
    colic, 288–289
    common conditions, 284
    constipation, 289–290
    cradle cap, 290
    diarrhea, 290–291
    ear infections, 291
    eczema, 291–292
    eye conditions, 292
    herbs to bless new baby, 297
    infections and fevers, 293
    intolerances, 284–287
    jaundice, 294
    nappy rash, 294–295
    otitis media, 291
    reflux, 295
    respiratory illness, 295–296
    seborrhoeic dermatitis, 290
    signs of serious illness, 284
    sleep problems, 296
    thrush, 287–288
    umbilical care, 296
    vomiting, 297
NHS. *See* UK National Health Service
nipple sore or crack, 276. *See also* lactation
    herbal treatments, 276–277
non-native herbs, 1–2. *See also* herbal prescribing and safety
nose bleeds, 149. *See also* pregnancy conditions
nourishing oils, 196
nutrition, 29
    antioxidants, 38
    caffeine, 33
    calcium, 37
    carbohydrates and fibre, 38
    chromium, 37
    cravings, 32
    essential fatty acids, 38
    essential nutrients in pregnancy, 35–39
    folic acid, 35
    food allergy, 30
    food hygiene, 33
    foods and substances to avoid, 33–35
    healthy eating in pregnancy, 29–31
    healthy vegan diet, 30
    herb tea, 3
    ice cream, 35
    iodine, 38
    iron, 34
    liver, 35
    magnesium, 37
    manganese, 36
    milk and dairy, 29–30
    pâté, 34
    peanuts, 35
    poultry, 34
    pre-and probiotics, 38–39
    protein, 38
    raw or partially cooked eggs, 34
    raw or under-cooked meats, 34
    salt, 33
    selenium, 36
    shellfish and raw fish, 34
    soft and blue cheeses, 34
    supplements, 31
    tobacco, 33
    unpasteurised milks, 34
    vegetarians and vegans, 30–31
    vitamin A, 36
    vitamin C, 36
    vitamin D, 35–36
    vitamin E, 36
    water, 32–33
    weight gain, 32
    zinc, 36
nutritional anaemia, 108. *See also* anaemia
NVP. *See* nausea & vomiting in pregnancy

oak (*Quercus robur/petraea*), 91–92
oats (*Avena sativa*), 77
oatstraw, 121–122
obstetric care, 2–3
obstetric cholestasis. *See* intrahepatic cholestasis of pregnancy
occiput-posterior position (OP), 220
Ocimum tenuiflorum/sanctum. *See* holy basil; sacred basil; tulsi

oedema, 150. *See also* pregnancy conditions
    herbal treatment, 150–151
oestrogen, 55–56. *See also* second trimester; third trimester
oestrogenic, 311
oligohydramnios, 130. *See also* pregnancy conditions
    herbal treatment, 131
OP. *See* occiput-posterior position
ophthalmic, 311
opioid pain relief, 217. *See also* labour and birth
os, 101
otitis media, 291
overactive bladder, 252
oxymel, 62
oxytocic, 311
oxytocin, 208–209, 237–238, 268–269

pain, 229–230. *See also* pregnancy conditions; herbs for labour and delivery; postpartum care
    in labour, 191
    -relieving endorphins, 209
palpitations, 151. *See also* pregnancy conditions
pampering massage oil, 241
Panax Ginseng. See ginseng
pancreatic, 311
panic, 230. *See also* herbs for labour and delivery
pansy (*Viola tricolor*), 100
Parietaria judaica. See pellitory-of-the-wall
Partridge Berry (*Mitchella repens*), 90, 139–140, 195
parturient, 311
partus preparators, 194–196, 312. *See also* labour and birth
pasque flower (*Anemone pulsatilla*), 75, 261
Passiflora incarnata. See passionflower
passionflower (*Passiflora incarnata*), 91, 121, 123
pâté, 34. *See also* nutrition
peanuts, 35. *See also* nutrition
pellitory-of-the-wall (*Parietaria judaica*), 91
pelvic. *See also* exercise and lifestyle; postpartum care; pregnancy conditions
    floor exercises, 42, 253
    instability, 151
    pain. *See* back/pelvic pain
pelvic girdle pain (PGP), 151. *See also* pregnancy conditions

pelvic organ prolapse (POP), 257. *See also* postpartum care
    herbal treatment, 258
pemphigoid gestationis (PG), 161. *See also* skin disorders
PEP. *See* polymorphic eruption of pregnancy
PEP, 160–161. *See also* skin disorders
peppermint (*Mentha piperita*), 89–90
perfluorinated chemicals (PFCs), 272
perineal. *See also* herbs for labour and delivery; labour and birth; postpartum care
    care, 230
    healing, 253
    herbal treatment, 254
    massage, 196
    trauma, 261
pessaries, 66. *See also* herbal pharmacy
PFCs. *See* perfluorinated chemicals
PG. *See* pemphigoid gestationis
PGP. *See* pelvic girdle pain
physiomedicalism, 1–2. *See also* herbal prescribing and safety
pilewort, 170
Pimpinella anisum. See aniseed
placenta, 54. *See also* first trimester; pregnancy conditions capsules, 222
    praevia, 151–152
placental abruption, 152. *See also* pregnancy conditions
placental site trophoblastic tumour (PSTT), 125
"place of treasure", 217
Plantago lanceolata/major. See plantain
plantain (*Plantago lanceolata/major*), 91
polyhydramnios, 131. *See also* pregnancy conditions
    herbal treatment, 132
polymorphic eruption of pregnancy (PEP), 160
polyvinyl chloride (PVC), 272
POP. *See* pelvic organ prolapse
posterior presentation, 220. *See also* labour and birth
postnatal depression. *See* postpartum depression
postnatal tonic, 200. *See also* birthing pack
postpartum. *See also* postpartum care
    conditions, 244
    depression, 255–257
    endometritis, 249
    hair loss. *See* postpartum telogen effluvium
    prolapse, 257–258

thyroiditis, 262–263
tonics, 242–243, 261
wraps, 241–242
postpartum care, 237
    afterpains, 244–245
    anaemia, 245
    back pain, 245
    birth trauma, 245–247
    bleeding, 247
    blessing ceremony for new mother, 241
    caesarean section, 247–248
    caring in fourth trimester, 237–244
    constipation, 248
    diet and exercise, 242
    emotional and stress-related conditions, 248–249
    endocrine balance, 243–244
    endometritis, 249–250
    fatigue, 250–251
    hair loss, 251–252
    herbal treatment, 242
    hormonal changes after birth, 237–238
    hormonal imbalance, 243
    incontinence, 252–253
    lying-in period, 239–240
    pelvic floor exercises, 253
    pelvic organ prolapse, 257–258
    perineal healing, 253–254
    postpartum conditions, 244
    postpartum depression, 255–257
    postpartum tonics, 242–243
    postpartum wraps, 241–242
    scar tissue, 259–260
    seven-circuit labyrinth, 240
    sexual dysfunction, 260–262
    sitz baths and vaginal steaming, 244
    supporting new mother, 238–239
    thyroiditis, postpartum, 262–263
postpartum depression, 255. *See also* postpartum care
    additional supports, 257
    essential oils, 257
    flower essences, 257
    herbal treatment, 256
postpartum haemorrhage (PPH), 107, 216, 231. *See also* herbs for labour and delivery
postpartum telogen effluvium (PPTE), 251
post-term pregnancy, 201
post-traumatic stress disorder (PTSD), 175, 245
poultices, 68. *See also* herbal pharmacy

PPA. *See* prevalence of postpartum anaemia
PPH. *See* postpartum haemorrhage
PPROM. *See* preterm prelabour rupture of membranes
PPTE. *See* postpartum telogen effluvium
practitioner self care, 184–185. *See also* healing after loss
prebiotics, 38–39, 126. *See also* nutrition
pre-eclampsia/eclampsia, 152. *See also* pregnancy conditions
    treatment, 154
pregnancies, assisted, 25, 137, 144
pregnancy, 25. *See also* lactation
    atopic eruption of, 160
    caution in, 10–11
    ectopic, 119–120, 175
    essential nutrients in, 35–39
    essential oils contraindicated in, 15
    essential oils safe in, 12–13
    healthy diet for, 29
    healthy eating in, 29–31
    heightened sensitivity of, 4
    herbal care in uncomplicated, 21–22
    herbs contraindicated in, 8–10
    infections, 135
    laxative herbs with anthraquinones, 10
    molar, 125
    -related pelvic girdle pain, 151
    screening, 23–25
pregnancy conditions, 103
    abdominal pain and cramps, 104–106
    allergy, 106
    anaemia, 106–110
    back pain, 111–113
    bacterial vaginosis, 167
    bleeding, 113–114
    breast changes, 114–115
    Candida albicans, 115–116
    candidiasis, 115–116
    carpal tunnel syndrome, 116
    cervix, conditions of, 117–118
    constipation, 118–119
    dizziness and fainting, 119
    eclampsia, 152–154
    ectopic pregnancy, 119–120
    emotional and stress-related conditions, 120–123
    epistaxis, 149
    fatigue and exhaustion, 123–124
    gestational diabetes, 124–125

gestational trophoblastic disease, 125
group B streptococcus, 126–127
gums, 127
haemorrhoids, 168–170
headaches, 127–128
heartburn, 128
herbal treatment, 103
herpes, genital, 129
hydramnios, 130–132
hyperemesis gravidarum, 146–149
hypertension and hypertensive disorders, 132–133
hypoglycaemia, 133–135
immune system in pregnancy, 135–136
miscarriage, 136–144
multiple pregnancy, 145
muscle cramps, leg cramps, 145–146
nausea & vomiting in pregnancy, 146
nose bleeds, 149
oedema, 150–151
oligohydramnios, 130–132
palpitations, 151
pelvic girdle pain, 151
pelvic instability, 151
pelvic pain, 111–113
placental abruption, 152
placenta praevia, 151–152
polyhydramnios, 130–132
pre-eclampsia, 152–154
pregnancy infections, 135
preterm labour, 154
preterm membrane rupture, 154–155
pruritis, 155–157
restless legs syndrome, 157–158
rhinitis, 158–159
ruptured ectopic, 120
sciatica, 111–113
skin disorders, 159–161
sleep disorders, 161–162
stillbirth, 162–163
stress incontinence, 167
stretch marks, 163–164
urgent medical attention, 103
urinary tract conditions, 164–166
vaginal infections, 167
vaginitis, 167
varicose veins, 168–170
vulvovaginal, 115–116
pregnancy stages, 51
    conception, 51–52
    first trimester, 53–55
    gestational age, 52–53
    implantation bleeding, 52
    implantation symptoms, 52
    second trimester, 55–56
    third trimester, 56–57
    trimesters, 53
premature rupture of membranes (PROM), 130, 155
    risk of, 210
prescribing herbs. *See* herbal prescribing and safety
preterm, 154. *See also* pregnancy conditions
    labour, 105–106, 154
preterm prelabour rupture of membranes (PPROM), 127, 154–155. *See also* pregnancy conditions
prevalence of postpartum anaemia (PPA), 245
primigravidae, 56. *See also* second trimester
probiotics, 38–39. *See also* nutrition
    foods, 126
progesterogenic, 312
progesterone, 53, 56. *See also* first trimester; third trimester
progesterone insufficiency. *See* low serum progesterone
progressive muscle relaxation, 45. *See also* exercise and lifestyle
prolactin, 209. *See also* third trimester
    levels, 56
PROM. *See* premature rupture of membranes
protein, 38. *See also* nutrition
pruritic urticarial papules and plaques of pregnancy (PUPPP), 160, 172
pruritis, 155. *See also* pregnancy conditions; skin disorders
    herbal treatment, 156–157
PSTT. *See* placental site trophoblastic tumour
psychotropic, 312
PTSD. *See* post-traumatic stress disorder
PUPPP. *See* pruritic urticarial papules and plaques of pregnancy
purgative, 312
purple cone flower (*Echinacea angustifolia, pallida,* and *purpurea*), 83
PVC. *See* polyvinyl chloride

Quercus robur/petraea. *See* oak
quickening, 56. *See also* second trimester

RAADP. *See* routine antenatal anti-D prophylaxis

Ranunculus ficaria. See lesser celandine
raspberry leaf (*Rubus idaeus*), 93, 139, 194–195. *See also* birthing pack
    tea, 198
RDAs. *See* recommended daily allowances
rebozos. *See* postpartum—wraps
recommended daily allowances (RDAs), 31, 39
recurrent abortion. *See* recurrent pregnancy loss
recurrent miscarriage, 143. *See also* miscarriage
    herbal approach to, 144
recurrent pregnancy loss (RPL), 143
red clover (*Trifolium pratense*), 97
Red Ginseng, 198
red raspberry leaf (*Rubus idaeus*), 93
red sage (*Salvia officinalis*), 94
reduced decoction, 60. *See also* herbal pharmacy
Reference Nutrient Intake (RNI), 35, 39
reflux, 295
refrigerant, 312
relaxant herbal tea, 104
relaxation, 43–47. *See also* exercise and lifestyle
relaxin, 53–54, 167, 209, 269. *See also* first trimester
reproduction, assisted, 25, 137, 144
rescue. *See also* healing after loss
    essence, 185
    spray, 178, 200
respiratory illness, 295. *See also* newborn care
    bronchiolitis, 296
    chest infections, 295
    laryngotracheobronchitis, 296
respiratory syncytial virus (RSV), 296
rest, 43. *See also* exercise and lifestyle
restless legs syndrome (RLS), 157. *See also* pregnancy conditions
    treatments, 158
restlessness, 296
retained placenta, 231–232. *See also* herbs for labour and delivery
retroplacental haemorrhage. *See* placental abruption
rhinitis, 158–159. *See also* pregnancy conditions
Rhodiola rosea. See roseroot
rhubarb leaves, 274
rhythmic breathing, 44. *See also* exercise and lifestyle
Ricinus communis. See castor oil plant
rigid os, 230. *See also* herbs for labour and delivery
ritual and ceremony for bereaved parents, 178. *See also* healing after loss

RLS. *See* restless legs syndrome
RNI. *See* Reference Nutrient Intake
room spray with vibrational essences, 199–200. *See also* birthing pack
Rosa canina. See dog rose
Rosa canina fructus. See rose hips
Rosa damascene. See damask rose
Rosa gallica. See apothecary's rose
Rosa spp. *See* Rose
Rose (*Rosa* spp.), 92 123, 176. *See also* healing after loss
rose hips (*Rosa canina fructus*), 92–93
Rosemarinus officinalis. See rosemary
rosemary (*Rosemarinus officinalis*), 93, 178. *See also* healing after loss
roseroot (*Rhodiola rosea*), 92
routine antenatal anti-D prophylaxis (RAADP), 24
RPL. *See* recurrent pregnancy loss
RSV. *See* respiratory syncytial virus
rubefacient, 312
Rubus fructicosus. See blackberry; bramble
Rubus idaeus. See raspberry leaf; red raspberry leaf
Rumex crispus. See curled dock; yellow dock
ruptured ectopic pregnancy, 120. *See also* pregnancy conditions
rupture of membranes, 210–211. *See also* labour and birth

SACN. *See* Scientific Advisory Committee on Nutrition
sacred basil (*Ocimum tenuiflorum/sanctum*), 90
Sacred Birthing, 200, 304. *See also* sprays
sacred rose bath, 181. *See also* healing after loss
Sacred Space, 200, 305. *See also* sprays
sage (*Salvia officinalis*), 94
salt, 33. *See also* nutrition
Salvia officinalis. See red sage; sage
Sambucus nigra. See black elder
saw palmetto (*Serenoa repens*), 95
SBP. *See* systolic blood pressure
scar tissue, 259. *See also* postpartum care
    castor oil packs, 260
    herbal treatment, 259–260
    scar breakdown oil, 260
sciatica, 111–113. *See also* pregnancy conditions
Scientific Advisory Committee on Nutrition (SACN), 39
Scutellaria lateriflora. See skullcap
seborrhoeic dermatitis, 290

seborrhoeic eczema, 209
second trimester, 55. *See also* pregnancy stages
    Braxton Hicks contractions, 56
    foetus growth, 55
    oestrogen, 55–56
    primigravidae, 56
    quickening, 56
sedative, 312
    nerviness, 121
selenium, 36. *See also* nutrition
semen, human, 202
senna (*Cassia acutifolia/angustifolia* spp.), 79
Serenoa repens. See saw palmetto
seven-circuit labyrinth, 240. *See also* postpartum care
sex, 43. *See also* exercise and lifestyle
sexual dysfunction, 260. *See also* postpartum care
    herbal treatment for pain, 261
    herbs for low libido, 261–262
SG. *See* striae gravidarum
shepherd's purse (*Capsella bursa pastoris*), 78–79
shock, clinical, 232. *See also* herbs for labour and delivery
sialagogue, 312
Siberian ginseng (*Eleutherococcus senticosus*), 83
sitz baths, 67, 141, 244. *See also* herbal pharmacy; postpartum care
skin disorders, 159–161 *See also* pregnancy conditions; pruritis
    atopic eczema, 160
    intrahepatic cholestasis of pregnancy, 161
    melasma or chloasma, 160
    pemphigoid gestationis, 161
    PEP, 160–161
    topical applications, 161
skin disorders, infants, *See* newborn care
skullcap (*Scutellaria lateriflora*), 94–95, 122–123
sleep disorders, 161. *See also* emotional and stress-related conditions; pregnancy conditions
    herbal treatment, 162, 296
slippery elm (*Ulmus rubra*), 98, 128
smudge, 185. *See also* healing after loss
Solidago virgaurea. See goldenrod
soul. *See also* healing after loss; vibrational essences
    loss, 185
    medicine, 301–302
spasmolytic, 312
SPD. *See* symphysis pubis dysfunction
sphincter damage, anal, 253

spiritual perspectives on pregnancy loss, 184. *See also* healing after loss
splenic, 312
spontaneous abortion. *See* miscarriage
sprays, 304. *See also* vibrational essences
    happy healthy baby, 305
    Mother Goddess, 305
    sacred birthing, 304
    sacred space, 305
Stachys betonica. See wood betony
standard decoctions, 60. *See also* herbal pharmacy
standard infusions, 59–60. *See also* herbal pharmacy
steam inhalations, 66. *See also* herbal pharmacy
Stellaria media. See chickweed
stillbirth, 162–163, 176. *See also* pregnancy conditions; healing after loss
stimulant, 312
St John's Wort (*Hypericum perforatum*), 87, 112, 116, 122
stomachic, 312
stress incontinence, 167. *See also* incontinence; pregnancy conditions
stretch marks, 163. *See also* pregnancy conditions; striae gravidarum
    herbal treatment, 163–164
    preventative massage oil, 163–164
striae gravidarum (SG), 163–164
styptic/haemostatic, 312
succus, 62
supplements, 31. *See also* nutrition
suppositories, 66. *See also* herbal pharmacy
suspect foods for breastfeeding mothers, 285. *See also* newborn allergies
swimming or floating, 41. *See also* exercise and lifestyle
sympathomimetic, 312
symphysis pubis dysfunction (SPD), 151
Symphytum officinale. See common Comfrey
synergy in herbal prescription, 5. *See also* herbal prescribing and safety
synthetic oxytocin, 223
syrups, 63. *See also* herbal pharmacy
systolic blood pressure (SBP), 171

Tanacetum parthenium. See feverfew
Taraxacum officinale. See dandelion
tears, 232. *See also* herbs for labour and delivery
tea, warming herb, 148, 242
TENS machine. *See* transcutaneous electrical neurostimulation machine

termination, 175. *See also* healing after loss
third trimester, 56. *See also* pregnancy stages
    approaching delivery, 57
    Braxton Hicks contractions, 57
    corticotrophin-releasing hormone, 56
    oestrogen and progesterone, 56
    prolactin levels, 56
thrush, 279–280, 287–288
thyme (*Thymus vulgaris*), 97
Thymus vulgaris. *See* thyme
thyroiditis, postpartum, 262–263. *See also* postpartum care
thyroid stimulating hormone (TSH), 89
Tilia europaea. *See* common lime; linden tree
tinctures, 60–62. *See also* herbal pharmacy; herbal prescribing and safety
    alcohol in, 4, 62
    dosages, 61
    dried herb, 61
    from fresh herbs, 60–61
    home-made, 61
    and powders, 4
    for relaxation and pain relief, 198
    strength and quality, 5
    for vaginal candidiasis, 116
    vinegar, 62
tobacco, 33. *See also* nutrition
tonic, 312
toxaemia. *See* pre-eclampsia/eclampsia
transcutaneous electrical neurostimulation machine (TENS machine), 218. *See also* labour and birth
transvaginal cervical 'stitch' (TVC), 117
trauma, birth, 245–247. *See also* postpartum care
Trifolium pratense. *See* red clover
Trigonella foenum graecum. *See* fenugreek
Trillium erectum. *See* beth root
trimester, 53. *See also* postpartum care; pregnancy stages
    abdominal pain, 104
    blessing ceremony for new mother, 241
    diet and exercise, 242
    endocrine balance, 243–244
    first, 53–55
    herbal treatment, 242
    hormonal changes after birth, 237–238
    hormonal imbalance, 243
    lying-in period, 239–240
    postpartum tonics, 242–243
    postpartum wraps, 241–242
    second, 55–56

    seven-circuit labyrinth, 240
    sitz baths and vaginal steaming, 244
    supporting new mother, 238–239
    third, 56–57
    women care in fourth, 237–244
trophorestorative, 312
TSH. *See* thyroid stimulating hormone
tulsi (*Ocimum tenuiflorum/sanctum*), 90
turmeric (*Curcuma longa*), 82
Turnera diffusa. *See* damiana
TVC. *See* transvaginal cervical 'stitch'
two-way communication, 55. *See also* first trimester

UHT (ultra-heat treated), 34
UK National Health Service (NHS), 264
Ulmus rubra. *See* slippery elm
ultra-heat treated. *See* UHT
ultrasound, 24
umbilical care, 296. *See also* newborn care
uncomplicated pregnancy, herbal care, 21–22. *See also* herbal care of pregnant woman
United Plant Savers, 2, 16
unpasteurised milks, 34. *See also* nutrition
urge incontinence, 252
urinary frequency, 164
urinary tract conditions, 164. *See also* pregnancy conditions
    herbal treatment, 165–166
    measures for cystitis, 165
    urinary frequency, 164
urinary tract infection (UTI), 105, 164–165
Urtica dioica. *See* nettle
uterine
    antiseptic tonics, 250
    restorative formula, 143
    restorative tonics, 142
uterine infection, 249. *See also* postpartum care
    herbal treatment, 249–250
uterine restorative formula, 143
UTI. *See* urinary tract infection

Vaccinium myrtillus. *See* bilberry
vaginal. *See also* herbal pharmacy; labour and birth; postpartum care; pregnancy conditions
    delivery and self-doubt, 191–192
    infections, 167
    self-examination, 204
    steaming, 67–68, 141, 244

vaginal birth after caesarean (VBAC), 192.
    See also labour and birth
vaginal fumigation. *See* vaginal—steaming
vaginitis, 167. *See also* pregnancy conditions
valerian (*Valeriana officinalis*), 98–99, 112, 122
Valeriana officinalis. *See* valerian
varicose veins, 168. *See also* pregnancy
        conditions
    herbal treatments, 169
    internal medicine, 170
    local applications, 169–170
    measures for, 168–169
varicosities, 168
vasoconstrictor, 312
vasodilator, 312
vasomotor rhinitis of pregnancy. *See* rhinitis
vasoprotective, 312
VBAC. *See* vaginal birth after caesarean
vegan diet, 30. *See also* nutrition
vegetarians, 30–31. *See also* nutrition
Ventouse, 192
Verbascum thapsus. *See* mullein
Verbena officinalis. *See* vervain
vervain (*Verbena officinalis*), 99, 122–123, 140
vibrational essences, 121, 140, 178, 246, 301.
        See also flower essences; healing
        after loss
    choosing for patient, 303
    happy healthy baby, 305
    in herbal practice, 303
    internal use of, 303–304
    key qualities of, 305–306
    medicine for soul, 301–302
    for mind, body, emotions, and spirit, 302
    Mother Goddess, 305
    in pregnancy and lactation, 302
    room spray with, 199–200
    sacred birthing, 304
    sacred space, 305
    sprays, 185, 304
    suggested essences, 306–307
    topical application, 304
    working mechanism, 302
vibrational medicine, 301–302
Viburnum opulus. *See* cramp bark; guelder rose
Viburnum prunifolium. *See* Black Haw
vinegars, 62. *See also* herbal pharmacy
vinyl. *See* polyvinyl chloride
Viola tricolor. *See* heartsease; pansy

vitamin. *See also* nutrition
    A, 36
    C, 36
    D, 35–36
    E, 36
Vitex, 242–243
Vitex agnus castus. *See* Chaste Tree
vomiting, 297. *See also* newborn care
vulnerary, 312
vulvar varicosities, 168, 170, 231–233, 253.
        See also herbs for labour and delivery
vulvovaginal candidiasis, 115–116. *See also*
        pregnancy conditions

wakefulness, 296
warming teas, 148, 242
warm sitz baths, 258
water, 32–33. *See also* labour and birth; nutrition
    births, 218–219
weaning, 280. *See also* lactation
WED. *See* Willis-Ekbom disease
weight gain, 32. *See also* nutrition
Western herbal medicine, 2
white deadnettle (*Lamium album*), 88
WHO. *See* World Health Organisation
whole plant, 5
wild indigo (*Baptisia tinctoria*), 77–78
wild yam (*Dioscorea villosa*), 82–83, 106
Willis-Ekbom disease (WED), 157
winter cherry (*Withania somnifera*), 100
witch hazel (*Hamamelis virginiana*), 86, 169
Withania somnifera. *See* ashwagandha;
        winter cherry
wood betony (*Stachys betonica*), 95
World Health Organisation (WHO), 106, 216

yarrow (*Achillea millefolium*), 74
yellow dock (*Rumex crispus*), 93
yellow gentian (*Gentiana lutea*), 85
yellow jasmine (*Gelsemium sempervirens*), 85
yew, 179. *See also* healing after loss
Ylang-Ylang essential oil, 262
yoga, 41. *See also* exercise and lifestyle
yoni steaming. *See* vaginal—steaming

Zea mays. *See* cornsilk
zinc, 36. *See also* nutrition
Zingiber officinalis. *See* ginger
zona pellucida, 52

www.ingramcontent.com/pod-product-compliance
Lightning Source LLC
Chambersburg PA
CBHW080354030426
42334CB00024B/2875